Emergency Chest Radiology

Tae Jung Kim • Kyung Hee Lee
Yeon Hyeon Choe • Kyung Soo Lee

Emergency Chest Radiology

Springer

Tae Jung Kim
Department of Radiology
Samsung Medical Center
Sungkyunkwan University School of Medicine
Seoul
Korea (Republic of)

Kyung Hee Lee
Department of Radiology
Seoul National University
Bundang Hospital
Seongnam-si
Kyonggi-do
Korea (Republic of)

Yeon Hyeon Choe
Department of Radiology
Samsung Medical Center
Sungkyunkwan University School of Medicine
Seoul
Korea (Republic of)

Kyung Soo Lee
Department of Radiology
Samsung Medical Center
Sungkyunkwan University School of Medicine
Seoul
Korea (Republic of)

ISBN 978-981-33-4398-6 ISBN 978-981-33-4396-2 (eBook)
https://doi.org/10.1007/978-981-33-4396-2

This Springer imprint is published by the registered company Springer Nature Singapore Pte Ltd.
The registered company address is: 152 Beach Road, #21-01/04 Gateway East, Singapore 189721, Singapore

To my beloved parents who taught me faithfulness and dedication, and to my wife, Jeong Soo, and son, Minjune, for their unconditional support and patience.

—T.J.K

To my parents for their endless love, support, and encouragement.

—K.H.L

To my wife, Mi Kyung, and my children, Joo Young and Jooae, for their love and encouragement.

—Y.H.C

To my sons Joo Hwang Lee and Joo Young Lee who are currently shoulder to shoulder with me in medicine, and my beloved wife Kyung Sook Yi. They have always stood by me throughout my medical life.

—K.S.L

Preface

The reliance on imaging for diagnosis and management decisions in various medical disciplines has been continuously evolving, and this is typically reflected in the emergency setting where an accurate and rapid diagnosis is critical for the patients' life. The capability of identifying key imaging features that are crucial for a timely and accurate diagnosis is difficult to achieve and requires a thorough understanding of the pathophysiology and imaging features of the specific diseases.

This book will provide an up-to-date review of every aspect of emergency chest radiology for inpatients as well as for patients admitted to emergency departments with chest trauma, infection, postoperative complications, and cardiovascular emergencies. This comprehensive book is unsurpassed as a valuable source of practical information on the imaging diagnosis of acutely ill and injured patients. To this end, the wide spectrum of chest and cardiovascular emergencies is systematically categorized and typical imaging manifestations of these emergent conditions in the current state-of-the-art imaging modalities are illustrated in detail. In addition, this book contains detailed information on the pathophysiology of diseases and the mechanisms of trauma that are the very basics for imaging diagnosis. This book is ideal for all members of the emergency team, general, thoracic and emergency radiologists, radiology residents, and medical students.

I am immensely grateful to the other three authors, Dr. Kyung Hee Lee, Dr. Yeon Hyeon Choe, and Dr. Kyung Soo Lee, for their motivation, everlasting enthusiasm, wisdom, and dedication throughout the writing and editing of this book. Moreover, I would like to thank the Springer team for their great efforts in the process of planning and producing this book.

Seoul, Korea

Tae Jung Kim

Contents

1 Traumatic Lung Injuries

1.1 Introduction

Blunt thoracic trauma is associated with a high risk of morbidity and mortality. The first description of thoracic trauma appears in the Edwin Smith Papyrus from ancient Egypt, written circa 1600 BC [1]. Hippocrates recognized that hemoptysis after rib fracture was a more severe injury than a simple rib fracture [2]. After head trauma, blunt chest trauma is the second leading cause of morbidity and mortality in patients with trauma [3]. Motor vehicle accidents are the predominant cause of blunt thoracic injury, followed by motorcycle crashes, pedestrian versus auto injuries, and falls from great heights [3, 4]. Thoracic injuries are frequently accompanied by multiple other injuries, including those of the abdomen, head, and extremities. Diagnostic imaging has become a critical component in the diagnosis and treatment of patients with chest trauma. A portable chest radiograph is usually used for initial screening of obvious chest traumas. CT is more sensitive than chest radiography in detecting various thoracic injuries. With the advent of multi-detector CT technologies, routine use of thin-section axial images and multiplanar reformations became possible, and the widespread use of whole-body CT in multi-trauma patients minimizes the rate of missed injuries and decreases the mortality rate.

1.2 Pulmonary Contusion

1.2.1 Mechanism of Injury

Pulmonary contusion is the most common lung injury after blunt thoracic trauma, occurring in approximately 30–70% of patients [5, 6]. Pulmonary contusion is defined as focal parenchymal injury with hemorrhage and edema formation in the alveoli and interstitium, resulting in disruption of alveolar–capillary integrity without accompanying major parenchymal disruption. There are three basic mechanisms of pulmonary contusion [7]: (1) bursting effects at the gas/liquid interfaces of the alveoli, (2) inertial effects that occur when low-density alveolar tissue is stripped from heavier hilar structures as they accelerate at different rates, and (3) implosion effects due to rebound or overexpansion of gas bubbles after passage of a pressure wave. The lung is similar to other air-containing organs such as intestines and eardrums in its vulnerability to blast effects. Contusions can occur when the chest wall is compressed against the lung parenchyma, by shearing of the lung tissue across bony structures, from rib fractures, or by previously formed pleural adhesions tearing the lung tissue. Contusion in the opposite site of the lung may be seen (contrecoup contusion).

Pulmonary contusion leads to pathophysiologic changes depending on the extent and sever-

T. J. Kim et al., *Emergency Chest Radiology*, https://doi.org/10.1007/978-981-33-4396-2_1

ity of injury, such as ventilation/perfusion mismatch, intrapulmonary shunt, increased lung water, and loss of pulmonary compliance, which result clinically in hypoxemia, hypercapia, and increased work of breathing [8]. Patients with pulmonary contusion may present with respiratory symptoms such as dyspnea, tachypnea, and hemoptysis.

Pulmonary hemorrhage is the typical histologic finding in lung contusion. Animal studies have demonstrated that pulmonary contusion shows progressive changes [9, 10]. Interstitial hemorrhage is followed by interstitial edema in 1–2 h. At 24 h, massive edema develops due to extravascular leakage of proteins, red blood cells, and inflammatory cells in the air spaces along with fibrin deposition. At 48 h, more fibrin, cell debris, and many inflammatory cells have accumulated, and the lymphatics are dilated and filled with protein. It has been suggested that the healing process is almost complete 7–10 days after traumatic lung injury, with little residual fibrosis [11].

1.2.2 Imaging Diagnosis

The complex pathophysiology of pulmonary contusion is reflected on chest radiograph and CT as ill-defined, patchy ground-glass opacity in mild contusion, to widespread areas of consolidation in more severe injury. Pulmonary contusion typically presents as a localized increased opacity adjacent to the area of direct trauma with a non-anatomical distribution, which is different from the areas of opacity seen in pneumonia in that they are not confined within the anatomic limits of the various segments and lobes [6] (Figs. 1.1 and 1.2). Contusion frequently accompanies fractures of the adjacent bony thorax (Fig. 1.1c), which are often absent in the pediatric population owing to greater musculoskeletal elasticity [12, 13]. It is important to note that the evidence of contusion may not be radiologically evident within 6 h after trauma. CT is more sensitive in detecting pulmonary contusion compared with chest radiographs. An animal study using a canine model found that 100% of pulmonary contusions were demonstrated on CT, compared with 38% on chest radiograph [14]. On CT, sparing of 1–2 mm of subpleural lung may be seen, especially in children [15]. Contusion develops within 6 h and usually resolves in 7 days (Fig. 1.1c), but severe contusion may persist for up to 14 days [16, 17]. Pulmonary opacities that do not resolve or progress beyond this period more likely indicate pulmonary laceration or complications such as aspiration, pneumonia, or fat embolism, rather than pulmonary contusion [18].

CT may be helpful in predicting clinical course and outcome in patients with pulmonary contusion. Wagner and Jamieson suggested that the percentage of airspace consolidation on CT may predict the need for ventilator support in patients with pulmonary contusion [19]. In that study, all patients required mechanical ventilation when more than 28% of the airspace was involved. Miller et al. measured the volume of contusion on CT and suggested that contusion volume was an independent predictor of development of subsequent acute respiratory distress syndrome (ARDS). They found that 82% of patients with greater than 20% contusion developed ARDS, while only 22% of patients with less than 20% contusion developed ARDS [20].

1.3 Pulmonary Laceration

1.3.1 Mechanism of Injury

Pulmonary laceration is defined as a traumatic disruption of the lung parenchyma that results in the formation of a cavity that is filled with blood or air [19]. A traumatic, blood-filled lung cyst is also called a pulmonary hematoma. Four types of pulmonary laceration have been defined according to the mechanisms of injury. Type I lacerations are the most common; these are caused by rupture or shearing of the lung parenchyma due to sudden compression of the chest wall, are often centrally located, and maybe up to 8 cm in diameter (Fig. 1.3). Type II lacerations are located in a paraspinal area secondary to a traumatic shift of the lower lobes across the spine, and are often

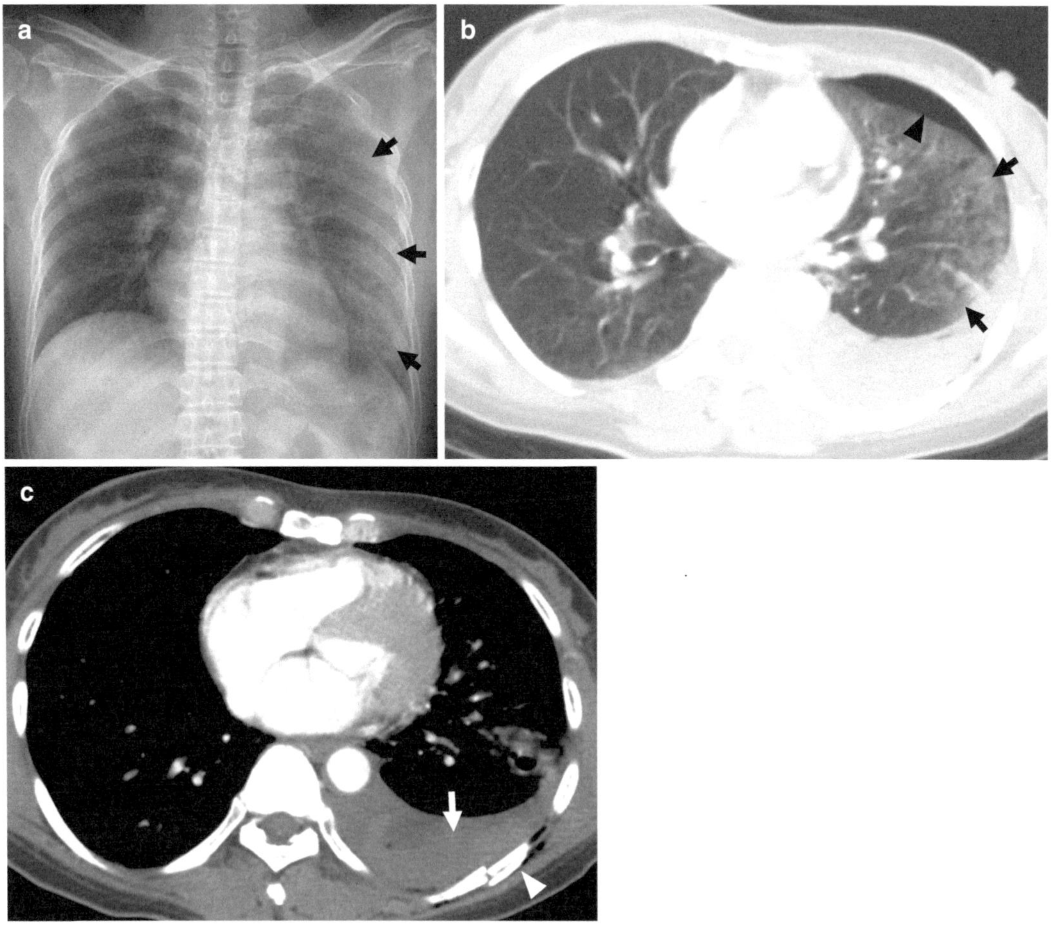

Fig. 1.1 Pulmonary contusion in a 52-year-old woman who suffered a motor vehicle accident. (**a**) Chest radiograph shows diffuse and ill-defined increased opacity in the left lung (arrows). (**b**) Lung window image of a CT scan obtained at the level of the left atrium shows diffuse ill-defined ground-glass opacity in the left upper and lower lobes (arrows). Also note the small pneumothorax (arrowhead). (**c**) Mediastinal window image of an enhanced CT scan depicts hyperdense pleural effusion, suggesting hemothorax (arrow). Also, note the rib fracture (arrowhead) in the left posterior thorax

elongated in shape (Fig. 1.4). Type III lacerations are caused by a direct puncture of the lungs by a fractured rib; these are the second most common type of laceration and usually occur in older patients (Fig. 1.5). Finally, type IV lacerations are tears of the lung adjacent to previously formed dense pleural adhesions [5, 6, 16]. Immediately after trauma, pulmonary laceration is often obscured on CT as well as chest radiograph by an accompanying pulmonary contusion, and becomes apparent over the next 2–3 days as the contusion gradually resolves [21].

1.3.2 Imaging Diagnosis

Pulmonary lacerations are often round or ovoid in shape owing to elastic recoil of the lung parenchyma, and may have a thin rim of hyperdense pseudomembrane, representing adjacent compressed lung parenchyma. Pulmonary laceration may demonstrate an air–fluid level or air meniscus, depending on the time course of blood coagulation and lysis in the cavity. Pulmonary hematoma presents as a well-circumscribed, round area of increased attenuation

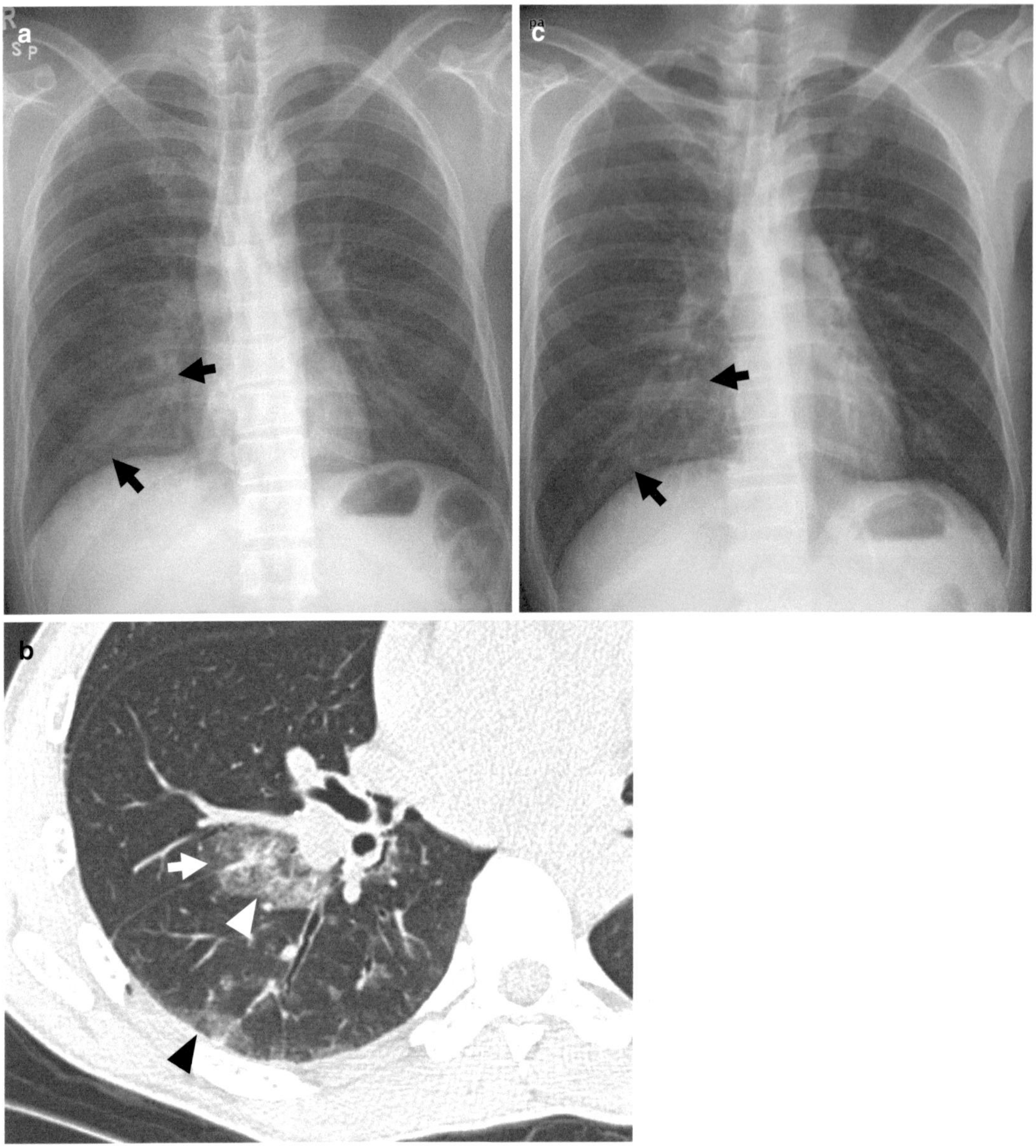

Fig. 1.2 Pulmonary contusion in a 38-year-old man after a fall from a rooftop. (**a**) Chest radiograph shows ground-glass opacities in the right lower lung zone (arrows). (**b**) Lung window image of a CT scan obtained at the level of the right middle lobar bronchus demonstrates ill-defined ground-glass opacities in the right middle (arrow) and lower (arrowheads) lobes showing nonanatomical distribution, which is a means of distinguishing injury from infectious pneumonia. (**c**) Follow-up chest radiograph taken 5 days after the initial event demonstrates resorption of pulmonary contusion in the right lower lung zone (arrows)

on CT (Fig. 1.3c). Typically, pulmonary laceration takes weeks to months to resolve completely. During the resorption process, some lacerations may appear as thin-walled lung cysts, referred to as posttraumatic pneumatoceles, or solid pulmonary nodules. Correlation with the previous radiological studies as well as trauma history aids in accurate diagnosis. Potential complications of pulmonary laceration include lung abscess formation due to secondary infection, enlargement of the cavity due to the ball-valve effect, and formation of a bronchopleural fistula in cases of peripheral laceration [22].

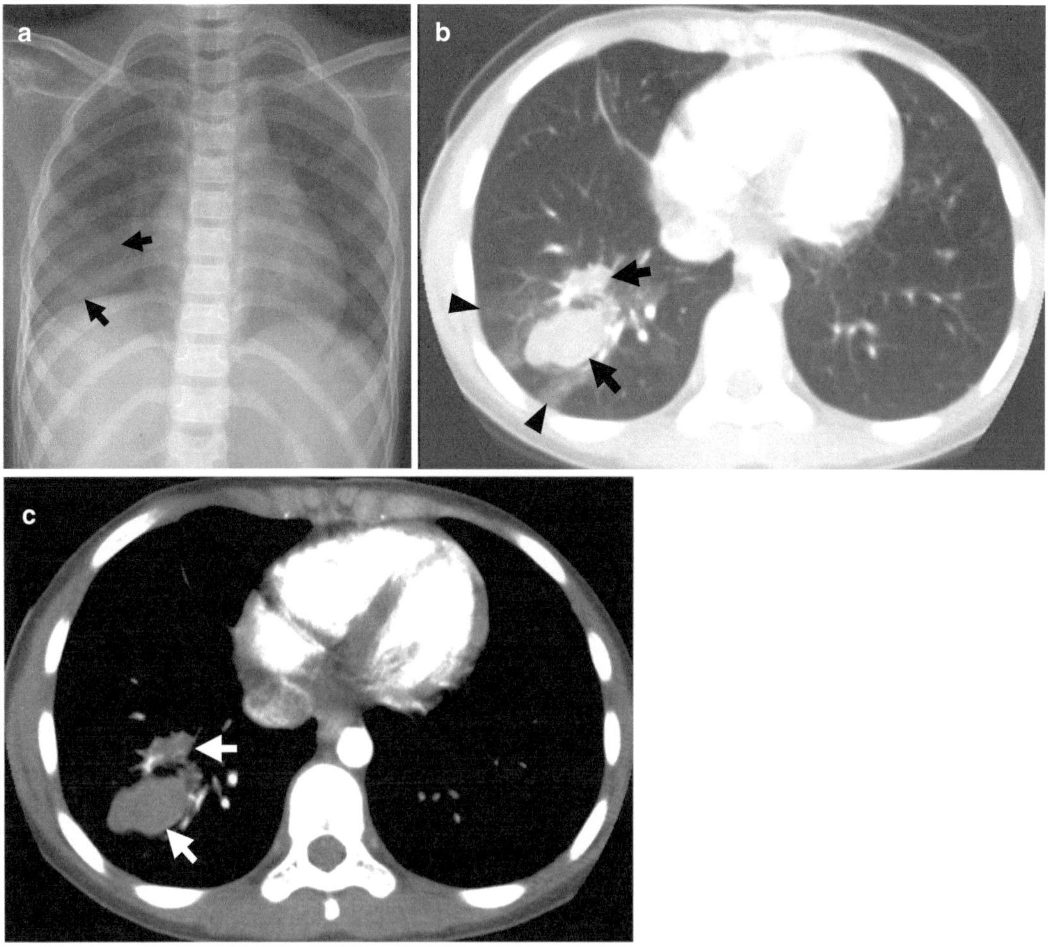

Fig. 1.3 Type I pulmonary laceration in a 9-year-old boy with a history of a fall from a great height. (**a**) Chest radiograph shows a localized area of increased opacity in the right lower lung zone (arrows). (**b**) Lung window image of a CT scan obtained at the level of the left ventricle demonstrates type I pulmonary lacerations in an ovoid shape in the right lower lobe (arrows). Also, note surrounding ground-glass opacities representing either pulmonary contusion or hemorrhage (arrowhead). (**c**) Mediastinal window image of an enhanced CT scan depicts the hyperdense nature of the lesion, representing a hematoma in the lacerated parenchyma (arrows)

1.4 Traumatic Lung Herniation

Herniation of the lung through a traumatically induced thoracic wall defect is a rare occurrence. The anterior thorax is the site of predilection for lung herniation because it lacks muscular support compared to the posterior thorax, which is supported by the trapezius, latissimus dorsi, and rhomboid muscles [23]. Lung herniation is most often asymptomatic. However, surgical correction is necessary if lung herniation is accompanied by incarceration or worsened by positive pressure ventilation. CT can be used to clearly define the extent of lung herniation as well as associated traumatic injuries in the chest wall and pleural space (Fig. 1.6).

1.5 The Roles of Imaging Studies and Recommended Protocols in Traumatic Lung Injury

Imaging studies are critical for establishing a diagnosis and treatment plan for patients with traumatic lung injury. Chest radiography is the initial imaging modality for standard workup of

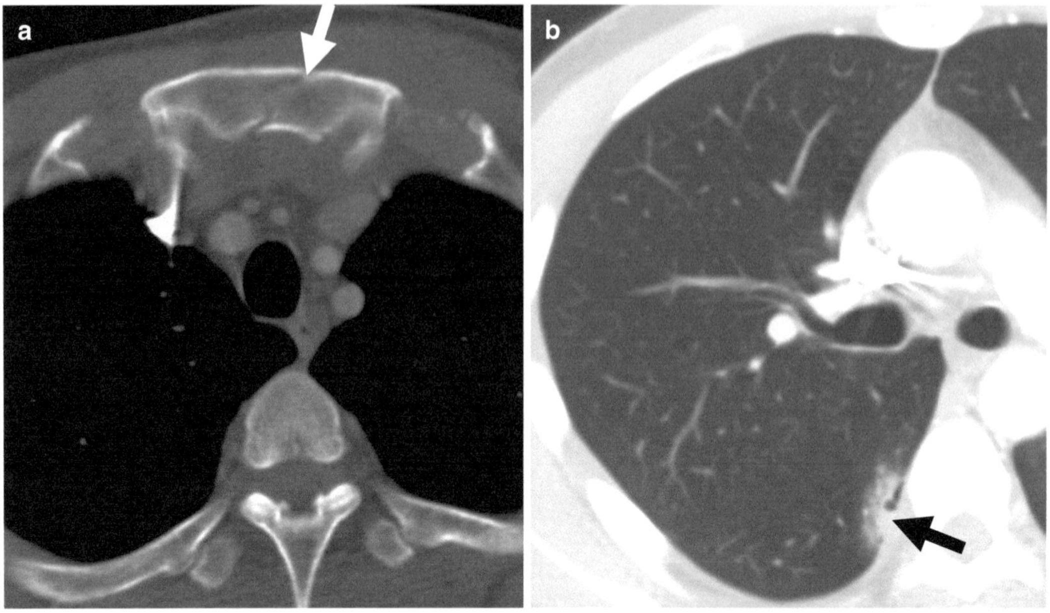

Fig. 1.4 Type II pulmonary laceration in a 30-year-old man with a dashboard injury from a motor vehicle accident. (**a**) Bone window image of a CT scan obtained at the level of the arch vessels shows sternal fracture (arrow), suggesting high-energy trauma. (**b**) Lung window image of a CT scan obtained at the level of the right main stem bronchus demonstrates a type II pulmonary laceration in an elongated shape in the paravertebral area of the right lower lobe (arrow), which occurred due to compression of alveoli against the vertebrae

acute thoracic trauma, and is typically performed as a portable anteroposterior radiograph with the patient in a supine position. Obvious chest injuries such as rib fracture, large pneumothorax, or hemothorax can easily be detected during this initial workup. CT of the chest, either alone or as part of a whole-body scan, is generally the next imaging study if additional workup is required. Small pneumothorax, hemothorax, pulmonary contusion or laceration, and tracheobronchial injuries can be successfully visualized by CT. Scans should be acquired at thin detector configurations so that multiplanar reformations can be reconstructed from the thin axial images. MRI is not commonly used in the acute trauma setting, but can be used in stabilized patients for subsequent detailed evaluation of vascular, cardiac, spinal, and bone and joint injuries. Ultrasound can be used as a complementary tool for detecting pneumothorax, hemothorax, and pericardial effusion.

1.6 Summary

Pulmonary contusion and laceration are the most common lung parenchymal injuries that result from blunt thoracic trauma. Pulmonary contusion represents focal hemorrhage and edema in the lung parenchyma without major parenchymal disruption. Pulmonary contusion typically shows a nonanatomical distribution, not confined within the anatomic limits of the lungs, which differs from pneumonia. Pulmonary laceration is a traumatic disruption of the lung parenchyma, resulting in cavity formation. Four types of pulmonary lacerations have been described according to the mechanism of injury. Imaging plays a vital role in demonstrating pulmonary parenchymal injury and any associated injuries and also provides information that is essential to establishing a treatment plan, as it grants a better understanding of the extent and mechanism of injuries.

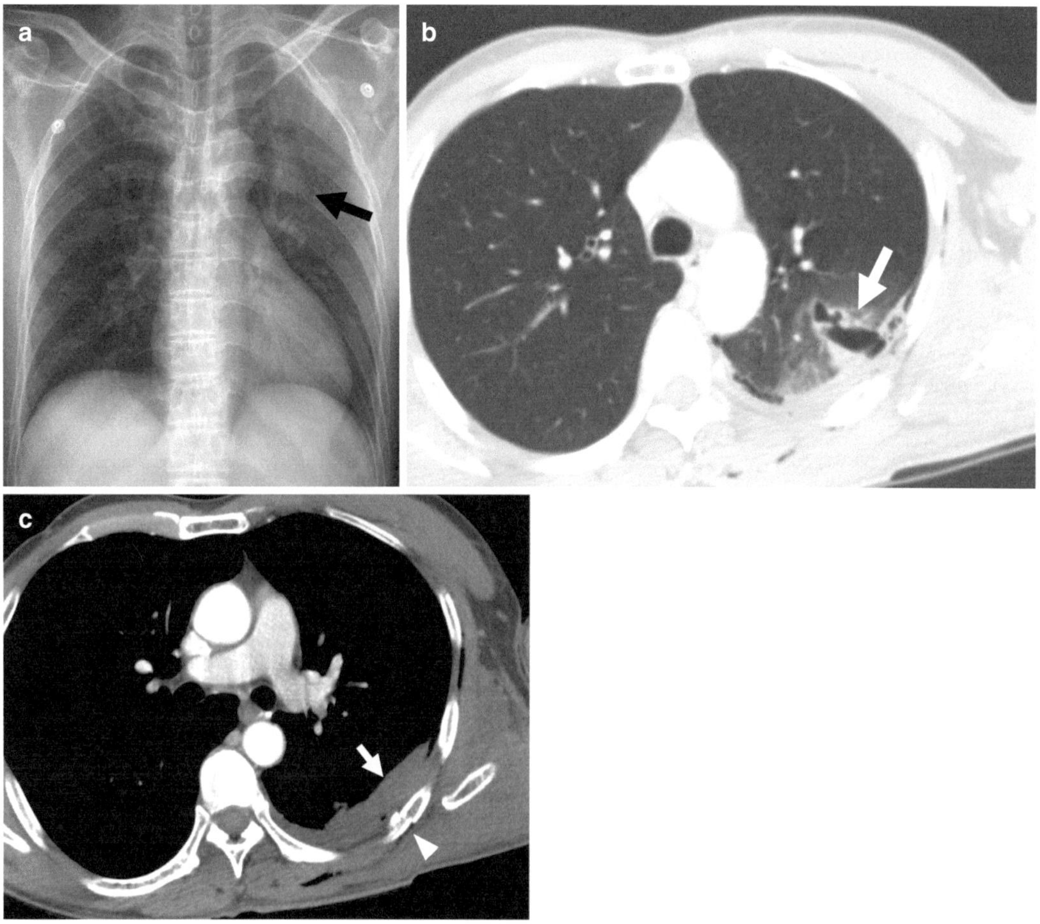

Fig. 1.5 Type III pulmonary laceration in a 38-year-old man who suffered a motor vehicle accident. (**a**) Portable chest radiograph taken with the patient in a supine position shows a localized area of increased opacity in the left upper lung zone (arrow). (**b**) Lung window image of a CT scan obtained at the level of the aortic arch demonstrates a type II pulmonary laceration in a tubular shape (arrow), which was caused by direct puncture of the lung by a fractured rib. (**c**) Mediastinal window image of an enhanced CT scan depicts a hemothorax (arrow) and rib fracture (arrowhead) in the left thorax

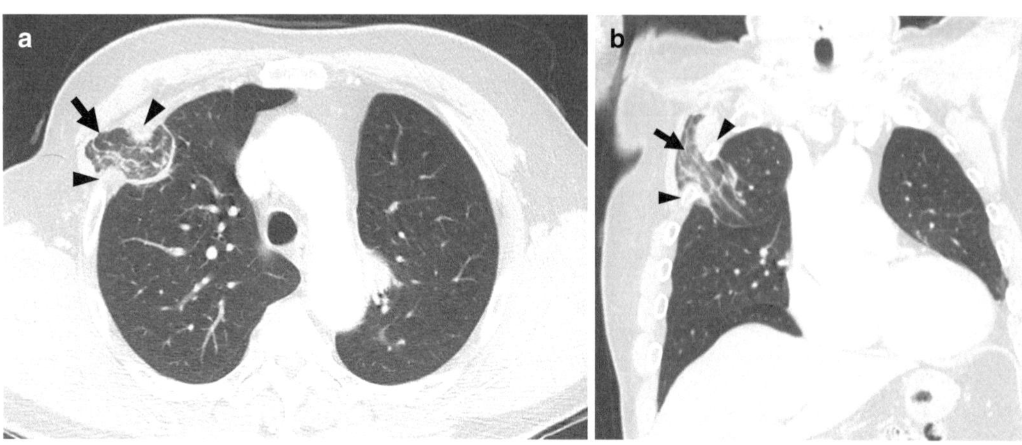

Fig. 1.6 Traumatic lung herniation in a 65-year-old man with a history of rib fracture. (**a**, **b**). Axial (**a**) and coronal (**b**) lung window images of a CT scan obtained at the level of the aortic arch demonstrate a focal herniation of the right upper lobe (arrow) through the chest wall defect (arrowheads) due to a previous rib fracture

Key Points

- On CT, pulmonary contusion manifests as a poorly defined area of consolidation and ground-glass opacity, usually in the lung periphery adjacent to the area of direct trauma with a nonanatomical distribution.
- On CT, pulmonary laceration is characterized by the presence of localized air collection in an area of consolidation.
- Traumatic lung injury typically shows a nonanatomical distribution, not confined within the anatomic limits of the lungs, which differs from pneumonia.

References

1. Breasted JH. The Edwin Smith Surgical Papyrus: published in facsimile and hieroglyphic transliteration with translation and commentary in two volumes. JAMA. 1931;96(18):1534. https://doi.org/10.1001/jama.1931.02720440082042.
2. Withington ET. Hippocrates, vol. 3. Cambridge, MA: Harvard University Press; 1959. p. 307–13.
3. Karmy-Jones R, Jurkovich GJ. Blunt chest trauma. Curr Probl Surg. 2004;41(3):211–380. https://doi.org/10.1016/j.cpsurg.2003.12.004.
4. Peterson RJ, Tepas JJ III, Edwards FH, Kissoon N, Pieper P, Ceithaml EL. Pediatric and adult thoracic trauma: age-related impact on presentation and outcome. Ann Thorac Surg. 1994;58(1):14–8. https://doi.org/10.1016/0003-4975(94)91063-4.
5. Cohn SM. Pulmonary contusion: review of the clinical entity. J Trauma. 1997;42(5):973–9. https://doi.org/10.1097/00005373-199705000-00033.
6. Wagner RB, Crawford WO Jr, Schimpf PP. Classification of parenchymal injuries of the lung. Radiology. 1988;167(1):77–82. https://doi.org/10.1148/radiology.167.1.3347751.
7. Clemedson CJ. Blast injury. Physiol Rev. 1956;36(3):336–54. https://doi.org/10.1152/physrev.1956.36.3.336.
8. Garzon AA, Seltzer B, Karlson KE. Physiopathology of crushed chest injuries. Ann Surg. 1968;168(1):128–36. https://doi.org/10.1097/00000658-196807000-00015.
9. Casley-Smith JR, Eckert P, Foldi-Borcsok E. The fine structure of pulmonary contusion and the effect of various drugs. Br J Exp Pathol. 1976;57(5):487–96.
10. Fulton RL, Peter ET. The progressive nature of pulmonary contusion. Surgery. 1970;67(3):499–506.
11. Moseley RV, Vernick JJ, Doty DB. Response to blunt chest injury: a new experimental model. J Trauma. 1970;10(8):673–83. https://doi.org/10.1097/00005373-197008000-00008.
12. Nakayama DK, Ramenofsky ML, Rowe MI. Chest injuries in childhood. Ann Surg. 1989;210(6):770–5. https://doi.org/10.1097/00000658-198912000-00013.
13. Roux P, Fisher RM. Chest injuries in children: an analysis of 100 cases of blunt chest trauma from motor vehicle accidents. J Pediatr Surg. 1992;27(5):551–5. https://doi.org/10.1016/0022-3468(92)90443-b.
14. Schild HH, Strunk H, Weber W, et al. Pulmonary contusion: CT vs plain radiograms. J Comput Assist Tomogr. 1989;13(3):417–20.
15. Donnelly LF, Klosterman LA. Subpleural sparing: a CT finding of lung contusion in children. Radiology. 1997;204(2):385–7. https://doi.org/10.1148/radiology.204.2.9240524.
16. Goodman LR, Putman CE. The S.I.C.U. chest radiograph after massive blunt trauma. Radiol Clin North Am. 1981;19(1):111–23.
17. Wiot JF. The radiologic manifestations of blunt chest trauma. JAMA. 1975;231(5):500–3. https://doi.org/10.1001/jama.1975.03240170042020%JJAMA.
18. Kaewlai R, Avery LL, Asrani AV, Novelline RA. Multidetector CT of blunt thoracic trauma. Radiographics. 2008;28(6):1555–70. https://doi.org/10.1148/rg.286085510.
19. Wagner RB, Jamieson PM. Pulmonary contusion. Evaluation and classification by computed tomography. Surg Clin North Am. 1989;69(1):31–40. https://doi.org/10.1016/s0039-6109(16)44732-8.
20. Miller PR, Croce MA, Bee TK, et al. ARDS after pulmonary contusion: accurate measurement of contusion volume identifies high-risk patients. J Trauma. 2001;51(2):223–8.; discussion 229–230. https://doi.org/10.1097/00005373-200108000-00003.
21. Miller LA. Chest wall, lung, and pleural space trauma. Radiol Clin North Am. 2006;44(2):213–24., viii. https://doi.org/10.1016/j.rcl.2005.10.006.
22. Shanmuganathan K, Mirvis SE. Imaging diagnosis of nonaortic thoracic injury. Radiol Clin North Am. 1999;37(3):533–51., vi. https://doi.org/10.1016/s0033-8389(05)70110-x.
23. Maurer E, Blades B. Hernia of the lung. J Thorac Surg. 1946;15:77–98.

Traumatic Airway Injuries

2

2.1 Introduction

Tracheobronchial injuries are relatively uncommon, occurring in only 0.5% of all patients with multiple injuries managed in major trauma centers [1]. Tracheobronchial injuries are life threatening, with more than 75% of patients with blunt tracheobronchial trauma dying before they reach the emergency department [2]. There are two types of tracheobronchial injuries. Penetrating injuries can be caused by laceration or from projectile injuries to the neck or chest. Blunt injuries can occur from motor vehicle accidents or fall from great heights. Pneumomediastinum and pulmonary interstitial emphysema are defined as abnormal gas collection in the mediastinum and pulmonary interstitium, respectively, and mainly occur because of alveolar rupture due to increased alveolar pressure. This chapter concentrates on blunt tracheobronchial injuries that occur between the intrathoracic trachea and the main stem bronchi, pneumomediastinum, and pulmonary interstitial emphysema.

2.2 Tracheobronchial Injury

2.2.1 Mechanism of Injury

Three potential mechanisms of blunt tracheobronchial injuries have been proposed [3]. First, sudden compression of the thoracic cage is the most common pattern of injury associated with tracheobronchial disruption. It is postulated that this produces a decrease in the anteroposterior diameter and a widening of the transverse diameter. Then, lateral expansion of the lungs causes traction on the trachea at the carina. Airway injury occurs if this lateral force exceeds the limits of tracheobronchial elasticity. Second, airway rupture may occur as a consequence of high intraluminal airway pressure. Pressure in the trachea suddenly increases due to compression of the lungs, trachea, and main bronchi between the sternum and the spine. If the glottis is closed at the time of impact, rupture may occur if the intraluminal airway pressure exceeds the elasticity of the main airway. These types of airway injuries most commonly occur at the junction between the membranous and the cartilaginous airway or between cartilaginous rings. The third potential mechanism is a rapid deceleration injury that generates shearing forces at the cricoid cartilage and carina, which are relatively well-fixed to surrounding structures [4].

Fractures of the bronchi are more common than those of the trachea, constituting approximately 80% of all airway injuries. The main bronchi 1–2 cm distal to the carina is the most frequently involved location, and the right side is more frequently involved than the left [5, 6].

Symptoms and signs of tracheobronchial injuries include cough, dyspnea, hemoptysis, and shock. Tracheobronchial injuries are most often accompanied by pneumothorax, pneumomediastinum, and subcutaneous emphysema.

T. J. Kim et al., *Emergency Chest Radiology*, https://doi.org/10.1007/978-981-33-4396-2_2

Subcutaneous emphysema in the cervical or thoracic region is the most common finding, seen in 65–87% of patients [7].

Early diagnosis of tracheobronchial injuries is very important because unrecognized injuries may eventually lead to airway stenosis and stricture, for which resection rather than reparative surgery is usually warranted [2].

2.2.2 Imaging Diagnosis

The most common radiographic findings of tracheobronchial injuries are the presence of pneumothorax, pneumomediastinum, and subcutaneous emphysema [8] (Fig. 2.1). Subcutaneous emphysema initially involves the neck and upper thorax and later becomes generalized [9]. Tracheobronchial laceration or fracture may cause bronchial obstruction and atelectasis of the ipsilateral lung. In case of complete bronchial transection, the ipsilateral lung may fall posterolaterally away from the hilum ("fallen lung sign"), which is a pathognomonic but uncommon finding [10–12] (Fig. 2.1). The presence of a persistent pneumothorax, even with chest tube placement and suction, pneumothorax, and pneumomediastinum in the absence of pleural effusion, or mediastinal or cervical subcutaneous emphysema in a patient who is not receiving positive pressure ventilation should raise the concern of possible tracheobronchial injury. Overdistention or herniation of an endotracheal cuff may be seen in tracheal laceration. CT can be used to identify the tear site in tracheobronchial injuries. Disruption of the bronchial wall can be visualized on CT. An endotracheal cuff that has herniated through the tracheal defect may show a "Mickey Mouse head" appearance on CT [13]. An acute change in the caliber or acute angulation of the airways can also suggest tracheobronchial injury (Figs. 2.1b and 2.2). The presence of mediastinal air adjacent to the airways is an indirect sign of tracheobronchial tear [13, 14]. Free air detected at the level of the carina is consistent with main bronchial injury [14, 15]. In case of suspected tracheobronchial injury on CT, immediate bronchoscopy should be attempted to confirm the diagnosis and evaluate the extent of injury.

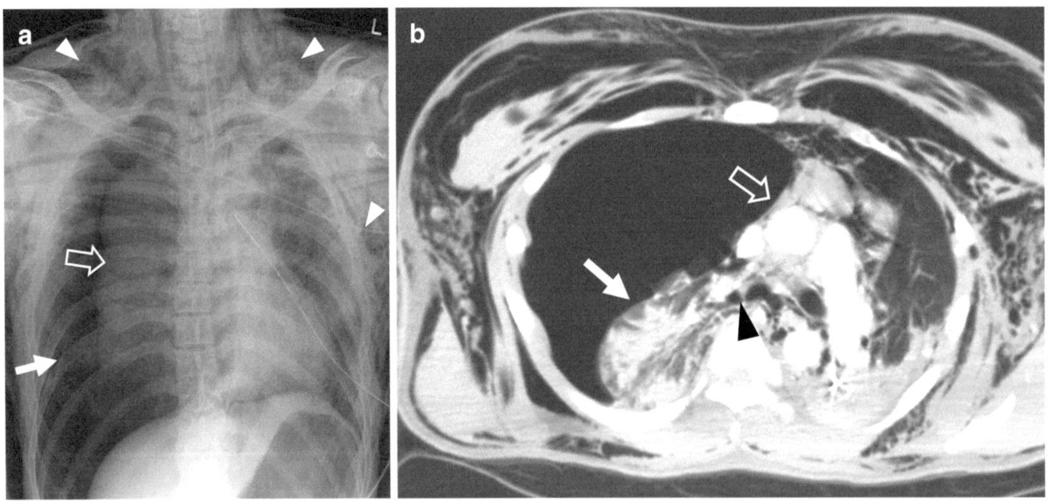

Fig. 2.1 Bronchial laceration in a 50-year-old woman who suffered a motor vehicle accident. (**a**) Portable chest radiograph shows a large pneumothorax (arrow) and extensive subcutaneous emphysema (arrowheads). Note right lung collapse (open arrow). (**b**) Lung window image of a CT scan obtained at the level of the aortic arch shows a large pneumothorax and pneumomediastinum with extensive subcutaneous emphysema. Acute change in the caliber is noted in the right main bronchus, suggesting bronchial laceration (arrowhead). The right lung is collapsed and displaced inferior to the right hilum ("fallen-lung sign") (arrow). Also note mediastinal shifting (open arrow), suggesting tension pneumothorax. Laceration of the right main bronchus was identified during surgery

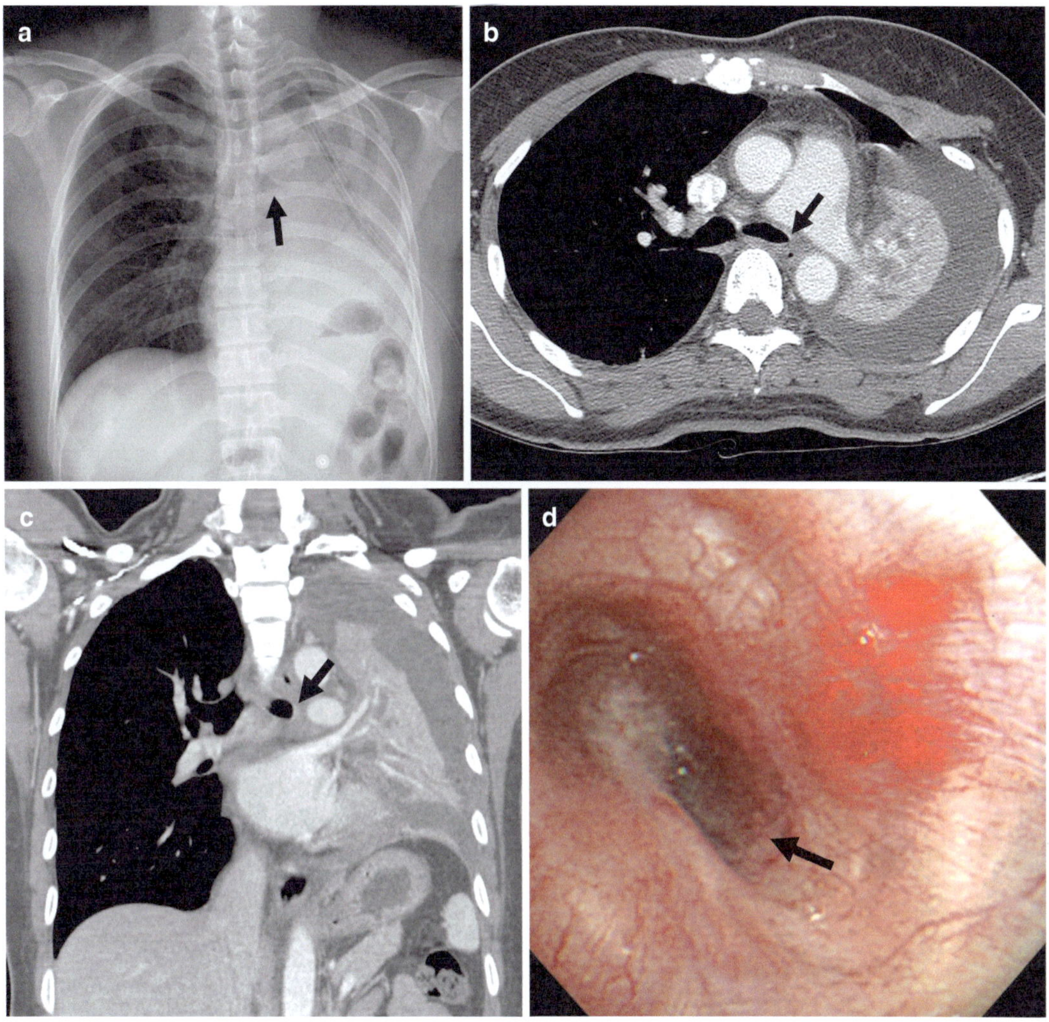

Fig. 2.2 Bronchial laceration in a 45-year-old woman who suffered a motor vehicle accident. (**a**) Chest radiograph shows abrupt cut-off of the left main bronchus (arrow). Total atelectasis of the left lung is persistent although a chest tube is placed in the left hemothorax due to pneumothorax, which strongly suggests bronchial injury. (**b**, **c**) Axial and coronal CT scans demonstrate abrupt cut-off of the left main bronchus (arrow). Also note the total collapse of the left lung with hydropneumothorax. (**d**) Bronchoscopy reveals complete obstruction at the proximal left main bronchus (arrow) due to laceration. Surgery confirmed the bronchial laceration and resection and anastomosis of the left main bronchus was performed

2.3 Pneumomediastinum

2.3.1 Etiology and Pathogenesis

Pneumomediastinum is defined as the presence of gas in the mediastinal space. Gas within the mediastinum may originate from the following sites: the lungs, airways, esophagus, neck, and abdominal cavity [16]. The most common mechanism of pneumomediastinum is the extension of gas from airspaces in the lung parenchyma into the interstitium and thence into the mediastinum. A sudden increase in alveolar pressure with airway closure results in rupture of alveoli adjacent to bronchovascular bundles. Gas moves to the hilum and mediastinum along the peribronchovascular interstitium [16, 17]. Development of pneumomediastinum is closely related to certain conditions that result in a sudden increase in

Table 2.1 Causes of pneumomediastinum

Lungs
Alveolar rupture associated with elevated alveolar pressure
Deep respiratory maneuvers: strenuous exercise, forced vital capacity breaths
Valsalva maneuvers
Weight lifting
Smoking marihuana or cocaine
Asthma
Vomiting
Artificial ventilation
Closed chest trauma
Sudden drop in atmospheric pressure: rapid ascent of a scuba diver or pilot
Infection: tuberculosis, histoplasmosis, dental or retropharyngeal infection
Blunt, or penetrating chest trauma
Airways
Tracheobronchial laceration
Bronchial stump dehiscence
Bronchoscopy
Tracheostomy
Esophagus
Esophageal perforation: Boerhaave syndrome
Esophagoscopy
Esophageal carcinoma
Neck
Surgical procedure in the neck
Dental extraction
Abdominal cavity
Perforation of the hollow viscus
Surgical procedure in the abdomen
Idiopathic

alveolar pressure. Such conditions and diseases are summarized in Table 2.1. Tracheobronchial laceration and esophageal perforation, which can be traumatic, iatrogenic, or spontaneous, can progress to pneumomediastinum. Gas can also enter the mediastinum from the head and neck (e.g., from tracheostomy, laryngeal injury, or facial fracture), the retroperitoneum (e.g., from a perforated duodenal ulcer or perforated diverticulitis), or the chest wall (e.g., from a thoracostomy site). Pneumopericardium can occur by the same mechanism as that which causes pneumomediastinum. Gas probably enters the pericardium along the venous sheath of the pericardial reflections, in which the level of support from the overlying soft tissue is weak. Pneumomediastinum usually has a benign clinical course, and conservative management is indicated. Complications include pneumothorax due to stretching of the mediastinal pleura and hypotension due to impaired venous return to the heart [18].

2.3.2 Imaging Diagnosis

Pneumomediastinum is manifested by lucent streaks or focal bubble-like or larger collections of gas outlining the mediastinal structures on radiographs (Fig. 2.3). The gas shadow is typically more evident on the left side. On posteroanterior projection, the laterally displaced mediastinal pleura produces a thin longitudinal line parallel to the border of the heart (Figs. 2.3 and 2.4). This line is created by both the parietal pleura and the visceral pleura of the lung, in contrast to the visceral pleural line in cases of pneumothorax. There are several radiographic signs related to pneumomediastinum: continuous diaphragm sign, Naclerio's V sign, ring-around-the-artery sign, thymic spinnaker-sail sign, and extrapleural air sign.

2.3.2.1 Continuous Diaphragm Sign [19] (Fig. 2.3)

This is a radiographic sign of pneumomediastinum or pneumopericardium if lucency is seen above the diaphragm, or of pneumoperitoneum if lucency is seen below the diaphragm. Normally, the central portion of the diaphragm cannot be discretely visualized on chest radiographs as it merges with the cardiac silhouette. If the diaphragm can be seen continuously across the midline, this is highly suggestive of free gas within the mediastinum or pericardium. Compared to pneumomediastinum, pneumopericardium is almost always associated with pericardial fluid, leading to obliteration of the central portion of the diaphragm on radiographs taken with the patient in an erect position. Also, air in the pericardial space demonstrates a change in position on follow-up radiographs taken in different body positions [20].

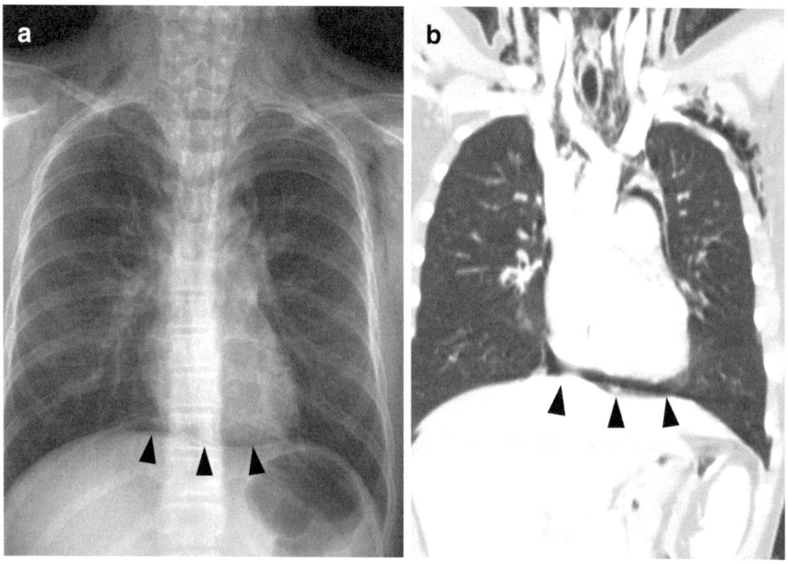

Fig. 2.3 Pneumomediastinum in a 28-year-old woman with abrupt onset of retrosternal pain. (**a**) Chest radiograph shows pneumomediastinum outlining the central portion of the diaphragm (arrowheads), a finding known as the "continuous diaphragm sign." Also note pneumomediastinum outlining the mediastinal structures and extensive subcutaneous emphysema in the neck and axillary area. (**b**) Coronal lung window image of a CT scan demonstrates free gas within the central portion of the lower mediastinum just above the diaphragm (arrow heads)

2.3.2.2 Naclerio's V Sign (Fig. 2.5)

This sign is named after Emil A. Naclerio, an American thoracic surgeon, who first described it in 1957 [21]. It is a V-shaped air collection in the left lower thorax. One limb of the V is produced by mediastinal gas outlining the left lower lateral mediastinal border. The other limb is produced by gas between the parietal pleura and medial left hemidiaphragm. This sign was originally described in patients with esophageal perforation but is not specific to that condition.

2.3.2.3 Ring-Around-the-Artery Sign [22] (Fig. 2.6)

This is seen on lateral chest radiographs; it appears as a well-defined lucency along or surrounding the right pulmonary artery.

2.3.2.4 Extrapleural Air Sign [23]

This is defined as the presence of gas between the parietal pleura and the diaphragm. On a lateral projection, the gas forms a radiolucent pocket of gas posterior to the dome of the hemidiaphragm.

2.3.2.5 Thymic Spinnaker-Sail Sign [24] (Figs. 2.7 and 2.8)

This is a sign of pneumomediastinum present on neonatal chest radiograph. It refers to the thymus being outlined by air with each lobe displaced laterally and appearing like spinnaker sails due to mediastinum. It is distinct from the sail sign of the normal thymus seen in neonates.

2.4 Pulmonary Interstitial Emphysema

2.4.1 Pathophysiology

Pulmonary interstitial emphysema (PIE) refers to collection of gases within the peribronchovascular sheaths, interlobular septa, and visceral pleura [25]. PIE essentially, if not exclusively, occurs in preterm neonates with immature lungs, usually after mechanical ventilation therapy, but it may also occur in adults associated with virtually any phenomenon that increases intrapulmonary pressure or lung volume [26]. One autopsy study demonstrated that PIE is most commonly associated

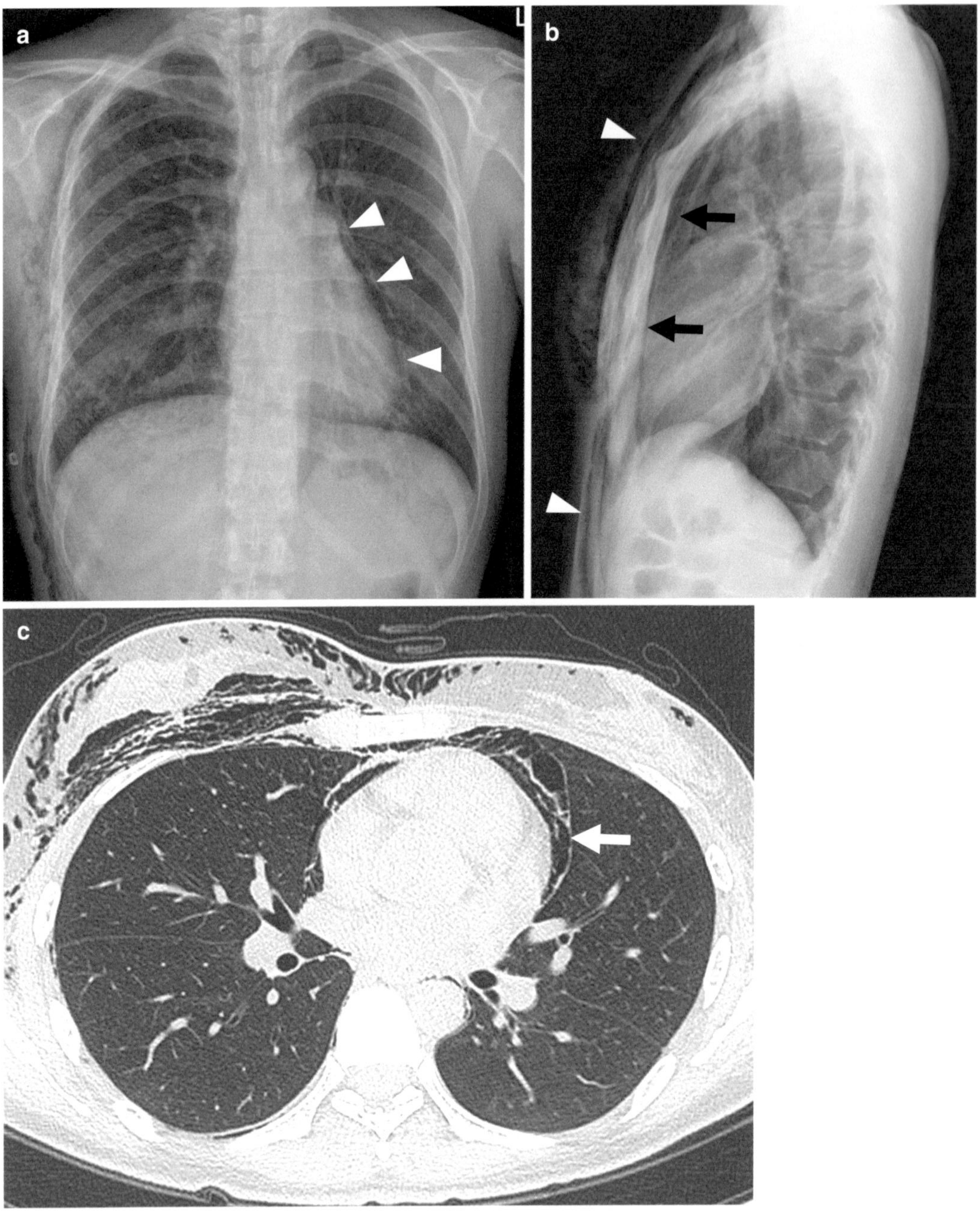

Fig. 2.4 Spontaneous pneumomediastinum in a 23-year-old woman. (**a**) Chest radiograph demonstrates a long linear opacity parallel to the left heart border (arrowheads), representing the laterally displaced mediastinal pleura. Note the mottled lucencies in the right lower thorax, suggesting extensive subcutaneous emphysema. (**b**) Lateral radiograph demonstrates retrosternal pneumomediastinum (arrows) and subcutaneous emphysema in the chest and abdominal walls (arrowheads). (**c**) Lung window image of a CT scan at the level of the aortic root shows pneumomediastinum and subcutaneous emphysema with lateral displacement of the mediastinal pleura (arrow)

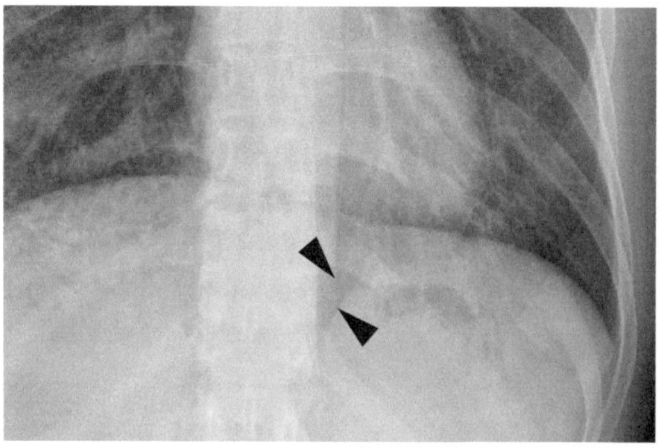

Fig. 2.5 Naclerio's V sign in a 23-year-old woman with pneumomediastinum. Magnified view of a chest radiograph demonstrates an air lucency outlining the medial portion of the left hemidiaphragm and the lower lateral mediastinal border (arrowheads)

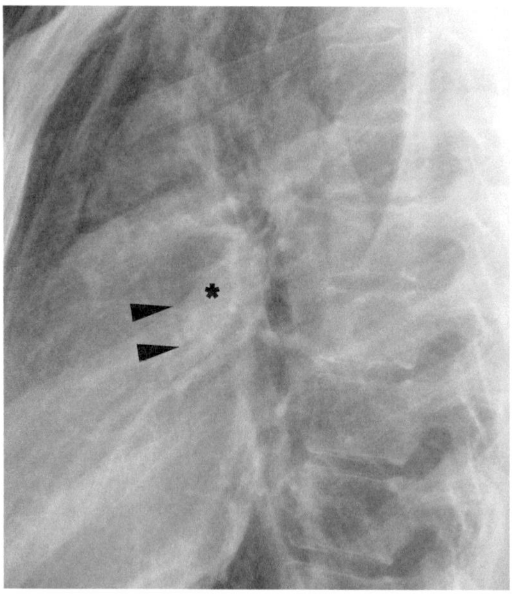

Fig. 2.6 Ring-around-the artery sign in a 32-year-old woman with pneumomediastinum. Magnified view of a lateral radiograph demonstrates a curvilinear air lucency (arrowheads) along the anterior surface of the right pulmonary artery (asterisk)

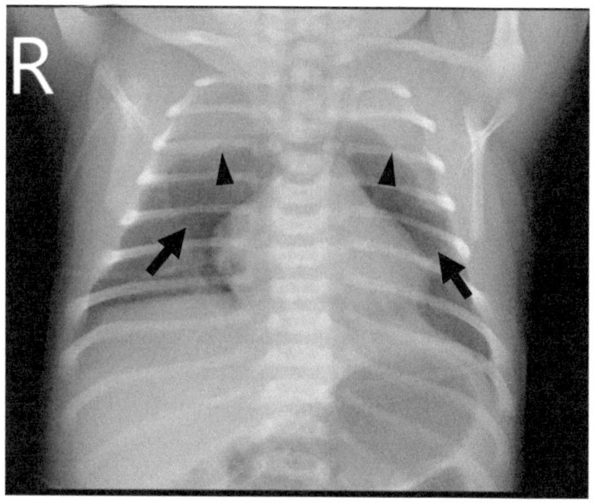

Fig. 2.7 Pneumomediastinum in an infant with chest wall retraction. Supine chest radiograph demonstrates pneumomediastinum outlining the cardiac border (arrows). Both lobes of the thymus (arrowheads) are lifted due to the air in the mediastinum

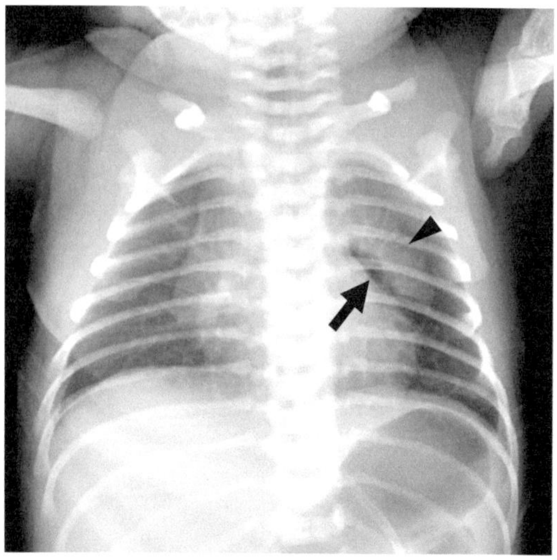

Fig. 2.8 Thymic spinnaker-sail sign in an infant with pneumomediastinum. Supine chest radiograph demonstrates elevation and lateral displacement of the left lobe of the thymus (arrow head) due to air in the mediastinum (arrow), creating a thymic spinnaker-sail sign

with usual interstitial pneumonia and a history of prior mechanical ventilation [27]. In neonate placed on mechanical ventilator support or continuous positive airway pressure, increased alveolar pressure, and poor compliance of the lungs may result in rupture of the alveoli. Air then escapes into the adjacent pulmonary interstitium and lymphatics. Pulmonary interstitial emphysema may resolve spontaneously, but may persist or progress with prolonged air leakage, causing pneumomediastinum, pneumothorax, pneumopericardium, or subcutaneous emphysema.

2.4.2 Imaging Diagnosis

PIE appears as linear or cystic radiolucencies in the interstitium radiating from the hilum [28] (Fig. 2.9a). The affected segment is often hyperexpanded, and pneumomediastinum or pneumothorax may be seen as well. PIE is rarely recognized radiographically in adults, likely because of other superimposed radiographic abnormalities such as subcutaneous emphysema and parenchymal opacities [29]. PIE appears as perivascular lucent or low-attenuating halos and small cysts on CT [28] (Fig. 2.10). CT allows for better visualization of associated barotrauma such as pneumothorax or pneumomediastinum, and helps differentiate persistent PIE from other hyperlucent lesions such as congenital lobar emphysema and congenital pulmonary airway malformation [30] (Figs. 2.9 and 2.10).

2.5 Summary

Tracheobronchial injury is a rare but potentially life-threatening condition with a high mortality rate. In patients with suspected tracheobronchial injuries, imaging plays a key role in demonstrating the airway injury, its complications, and any associated injuries, including pulmonary, vascular, and musculoskeletal injuries. Chest radiography and CT are the mainstays of imaging in these patients. The presence of pneumomediastinum and pulmonary interstitial emphysema are suggestive of tracheobronchial injuries and baro-

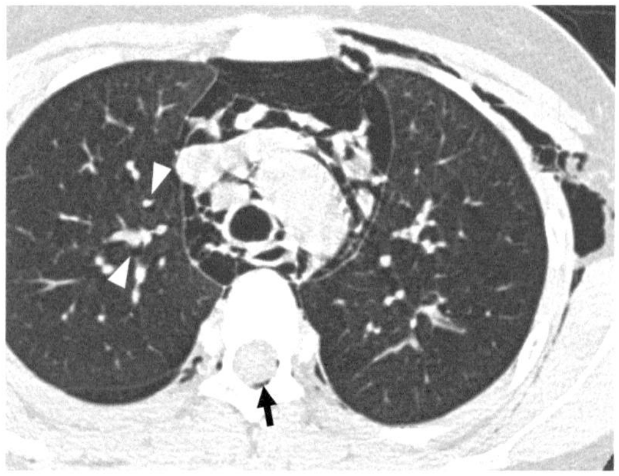

Fig. 2.10 Pulmonary interstitial emphysema in a 28-year-old woman with pneumomediastinum. Lung window images of a CT scan obtained at the level of the aortic arch demonstrate perivascular lucent halos (arrowhead) in the right upper lobe, suggesting pulmonary interstitial emphysema. Also note pneumomediastinum and pneumorrhachis (i.e., gas within the spinal canal) (arrow)

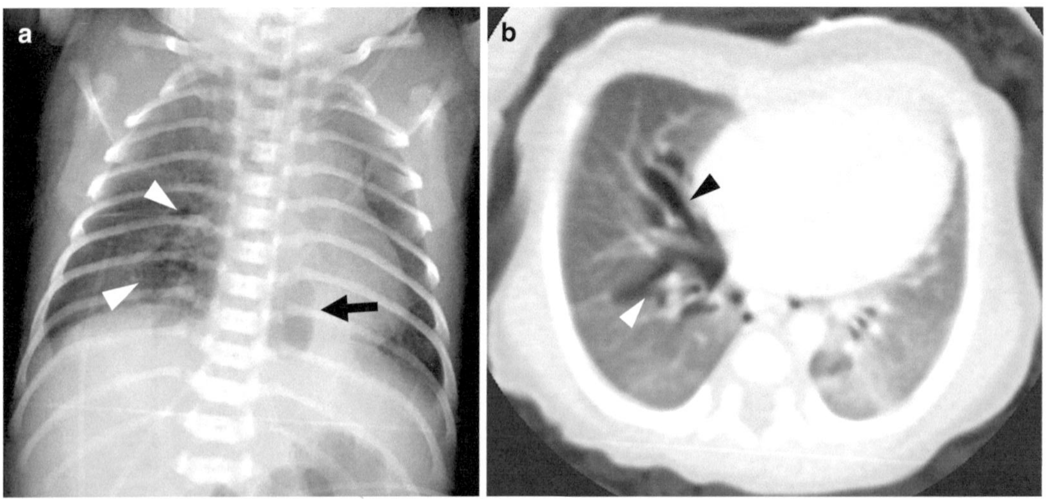

Fig. 2.9 Spontaneous pulmonary interstitial emphysema in an infant with respiratory distress syndrome. (**a**) Chest radiograph demonstrates multiple linear and cystic areas of lucency in the right infrahilar area (arrowheads), indicating pulmonary interstitial emphysema. Also note pneumomediastinum in the retrocardiac area (arrow). (**b**) Lung window image of a CT scan at the level of the left ventricle shows multiple cystic or tubular lucencies along the bronchovascular bundles in the right middle and lower lobes (arrowheads). Also note the diffuse ground-glass opacities in both lungs due to respiratory distress syndrome

trauma, respectively, and may manifest as characteristic imaging findings. Emergency radiologists and physicians should be familiar with the typical imaging findings of tracheobronchial injuries according to mechanism of injury, which ultimately influence treatment decisions.

Key Points

- Common CT findings of tracheobronchial injuries include disruption of the trachea or bronchial cartilage rings, acute change in the caliber or acute angulation of the airways, airway wall irregularity, bronchial obstruction and atelectasis of the ipsilateral lung, and overdistension of an endotracheal cuff.
- Radiographic signs related with pneumomediastinum include continuous diaphragm sign, Naclerio's V sign, ring-around-the-artery sign, thymic spinnaker-sail sign, and extrapleural air sign.
- Pulmonary interstitial emphysema represents air leakage into the pulmonary interstitium due to barotrauma and manifests as perivascular lucent or low-attenuating halos and small cysts on CT.

References

1. Gussack GS, Jurkovich GJ, Luterman A. Laryngotracheal trauma: a protocol approach to a rare injury. Laryngoscope. 1986;96(6):660–5. https://doi.org/10.1288/00005537-198606000-00013.
2. Bertelsen S, Howitz P. Injuries of the trachea and bronchi. Thorax. 1972;27(2):188–94. https://doi.org/10.1136/thx.27.2.188.
3. Kirsh MM, Orringer MB, Behrendt DM, Sloan H. Management of tracheobronchial disruption secondary to nonpenetrating trauma. Ann Thorac Surg. 1976;22(1):93–101. https://doi.org/10.1016/s0003-4975(10)63961-6.
4. Huh J, Milliken JC, Chen JC. Management of tracheobronchial injuries following blunt and penetrating trauma. Am Surg. 1997;63(10):896–9.
5. Barmada H, Gibbons JR. Tracheobronchial injury in blunt and penetrating chest trauma. Chest. 1994;106(1):74–8. https://doi.org/10.1378/chest.106.1.74.
6. Wiot JF. The radiologic manifestations of blunt chest trauma. JAMA. 1975;231(5):500–3.
7. Paraschiv M. Iatrogenic tracheobronchial rupture. J Med Life. 2014;7(3):343–8.
8. Unger JM, Schuchmann GG, Grossman JE, Pellett JR. Tears of the trachea and main bronchi caused by blunt trauma: radiologic findings. AJR Am J Roentgenol. 1989;153(6):1175–80. https://doi.org/10.2214/ajr.153.6.1175.
9. Larizadeh R. Rupture of the bronchus. Thorax. 1966;21(1):28–31. https://doi.org/10.1136/thx.21.1.28.
10. Oh KS, Fleischner FG, Wyman SM. Characteristic pulmonary finding in traumatic complete transection of a main-stem bronchus. Radiology. 1969;92(2):371–2. passim. https://doi.org/10.1148/92.2.371.
11. Kumpe DA, Oh KS, Wyman SM. A characteristic pulmonary finding in unilateral complete bronchial transection. Am J Roentgenol Radium Ther Nucl Med. 1970;110(4):704–6. https://doi.org/10.2214/ajr.110.4.704.
12. Petterson C, Deslauriers J, McClish A. A classic image of complete right main bronchus avulsion. Chest. 1989;96(6):1415–7. https://doi.org/10.1378/chest.96.6.1415.
13. Chen JD, Shanmuganathan K, Mirvis SE, Kileen KL, Dutton RP. Using CT to diagnose tracheal rupture. Am J Roentgenol. 2001;176(5):1273–80. https://doi.org/10.2214/ajr.176.5.1761273.
14. Scaglione M, Romano S, Pinto A, Sparano A, Scialpi M, Rotondo A. Acute tracheobronchial injuries: impact of imaging on diagnosis and management implications. Eur J Radiol. 2006;59(3):336–43. https://doi.org/10.1016/j.ejrad.2006.04.026.
15. Savas R, Alper H. Fallen lung sign: radiographic findings. Diagn Interv Radiol. 2008;14(3):120–1.
16. Cyrlak D, Milne EN, Imray TJ. Pneumomediastinum: a diagnostic problem. Crit Rev Diagn Imaging. 1984;23(1):75–117.
17. Macklin MT, Macklin CC. Malignant interstitial emphysema of the lungs and mediastinum as an important occult complication in many respiratory diseases and other conditions an interpretation of the clinical literature in the light of laboratory experiment. Medicine. 1944;23(4):281–358. https://doi.org/10.1097/00005792-194412000-00001.
18. Bejvan SM, Godwin JD. Pneumomediastinum: old signs and new signs. AJR Am J Roentgenol. 1996;166(5):1041–8. https://doi.org/10.2214/ajr.166.5.8615238.
19. Levin B. The continuous diaphragm sign. A newly-recognized sign of pneumomediastinum. Clin Radiol. 1973;24(3):337–8. https://doi.org/10.1016/s0009-9260(73)80050-9.
20. Felson B. The mediastinum. Semin Roentgenol. 1969;4(1):41–58.
21. Naclerio EA. The V sign in the diagnosis of spontaneous rupture of the esophagus (an early roentgen clue). Am J Surg. 1957;93(2):291–8. https://doi.org/10.1016/0002-9610(57)90781-x.
22. Hammond DI. The "ring-around-the-artery" sign in pneumomediastinum. J Can Assoc Radiol. 1984;35(1):88–9.

23. Lillard RL, Allen RP. The extrapleural air sign in pneumomediastinum. Radiology. 1965;85(6):1093–8. https://doi.org/10.1148/85.6.1093.
24. Moseley JE. Loculated pneumomediastinum in the newborn – a thymic spinnaker sail sign. Radiology. 1960;75(5):788–90. https://doi.org/10.1148/75.5.788.
25. Plenat F, Vert P, Didier F, Andre M. Pulmonary interstitial emphysema. Clin Perinatol. 1978;5(2):351–75.
26. Woodring JH. Pulmonary interstitial emphysema in the adult respiratory distress syndrome. Crit Care Med. 1985;13(10):786–91. https://doi.org/10.1097/00003246-198510000-00003.
27. Barcia SM, Kukreja J, Jones KD. Pulmonary interstitial emphysema in adults: a clinicopathologic study of 53 lung explants. Am J Surg Pathol. 2014;38(3):339–45. https://doi.org/10.1097/PAS.0000000000000130.
28. Hansell DM, Bankier AA, MacMahon H, McLoud TC, Muller NL, Remy J. Fleischner Society: glossary of terms for thoracic imaging. Radiology. 2008;246(3):697–722. https://doi.org/10.1148/radiol.2462070712.
29. Kemper AC, Steinberg KP, Stern EJ. Pulmonary interstitial emphysema: CT findings. AJR Am J Roentgenol. 1999;172(6):1642. https://doi.org/10.2214/ajr.172.6.10350307.
30. Donnelly LF, Frush DP. Localized radiolucent chest lesions in neonates: causes and differentiation. AJR Am J Roentgenol. 1999;172(6):1651–8. https://doi.org/10.2214/ajr.172.6.10350310.

3 Diaphragmatic Injuries

3.1 Introduction

Diaphragmatic injuries are rare and result from either blunt trauma or penetrating injuries. Traumatic diaphragmatic injuries frequently involve other serious injuries, such as rib fractures, pelvic fracture, splenic laceration or rupture, closed head injury, and liver laceration [1], which result in significant morbidity and mortality in the setting of trauma. Delayed diagnosis of diaphragmatic injuries is not uncommon because most diaphragmatic injuries are initially asymptomatic but may present with late symptoms of incarcerated viscera, or because associated injuries often obscure the findings of diaphragmatic rupture [2]. Given their tangential course, which evades delineation on routine axial cross-sectional imaging, identification of diaphragmatic abnormalities is often challenging. Several diagnostic signs are associated with diaphragmatic rupture, such as "dependent viscera sign," "collar sign," "hepatic collar sign," and "dangling diaphragm sign"; radiologists should be familiar with all of these signs to ensure early and accurate diagnosis of diaphragmatic injuries. Thoracic splenosis related with diaphragmatic rupture and the diagnostic pitfalls of diaphragmatic injuries will also be described in this chapter. Esophageal hiatal hernias (sliding and paraesophageal) are described in Chap. 5: Traumatic and nontraumatic esophageal emergency.

3.2 Diaphragmatic Rupture

3.2.1 Epidemiology and Mechanism of Injury

The frequency of penetrating and blunt diaphragmatic injuries varies across studies, but recently, several large studies reported a higher number of penetrating injuries than blunt diaphragmatic injuries [3–5]. Penetrating injuries are more common among young men: 91.4% of cases in the USA were male and the average age of US patients was 31 years [5]. Blunt diaphragmatic injuries are also more common in men: Men accounted for 67.9% of blunt diaphragmatic injuries, with an average age of 44 years. Compared with penetrating injury, blunt diaphragmatic injury is associated with a longer intensive care unit stay, longer duration of ventilator support, and higher mortality rate [5]. Blunt diaphragmatic injuries most often occur in a motor vehicle collision, a fall from a height, or a crushing blow. Several mechanisms have been suggested for the development of diaphragmatic rupture in blunt thoracic trauma. The most commonly accepted theory holds that, in a frontal impact such as a dashboard injury, a sudden increase in intra-abdominal pressure is transmitted to the fixed diaphragm, resulting in upward displacement of abdominal contents moving toward the low-pressure thorax. In a lateral thoracoabdominal impact, shearing stress on a stretched dia-

T. J. Kim et al., *Emergency Chest Radiology*, https://doi.org/10.1007/978-981-33-4396-2_3

phragm or avulsion of the diaphragm from its points of attachment result in diaphragmatic rupture [2, 6, 7]. Rupture may occur in any area, and the location and extent of tear varies and has no fixed pattern, but tears most frequently develop at the weakest portion of the diaphragm, which is the posterolateral surface along the embryonic fusion lines [8].

Diaphragmatic rupture occurs more often on the left side than on the right, with a ratio of approximately 3:1 [9]. This left-side predominance has been ascribed to multiple factors, including the buffer effect of the liver on the right side, greater weakness of the posterolateral aspect of the left hemidiaphragm, and underdiagnosis of right-sided injuries [2]. Indeed, a defect in the right hemidiaphragm may be sealed by the liver, and herniation may therefore be delayed or absent. In addition, it is easy to detect a diaphragmatic abnormality in the left upper abdomen, which has abundant fat deposits, while it may be difficult to detect a diaphragmatic defect due to higher attenuation of the hepatic parenchyma in the right upper abdomen [9].

Blunt diaphragmatic injuries are frequently associated with other injuries, such as pulmonary injury (48.7%), splenic injury (44.8%), liver injury (39.7%), pneumothorax (30%), and hemothorax (21.5%) [5]. These accompanying injuries have substantial clinical significance in the diagnosis of diaphragmatic injury because a diaphragmatic injury may be overlooked entirely or detection may be delayed due to accompanying injuries. Therefore, special attention should be given to the identification of diaphragmatic injuries, especially in polytrauma patients.

Following diaphragmatic rupture, intra-abdominal structures generally herniate into the thorax due to negative intrapleural pressure. The herniated contents depend on the location and size of the rupture. The most common herniated organs are the stomach, colon, spleen, and omentum in left-sided diaphragmatic rupture, and the liver and colon in right-sided rupture [10–12]. Delayed herniation of the intra-abdominal contents is common, which may make diagnosis at the time of initial chest radiography and CT more difficult. Such herniated contents frequently strangulate, particularly if the diagnosis is delayed beyond 24 h. Short-term mortality related with diaphragmatic rupture is low [13, 14], however, overall mortality resulting from other life-threatening injuries associated with diaphragmatic rupture varies from 10 to 40% [2, 3, 5, 7–15]. Unrecognized diaphragmatic injuries may result in delayed complications, such as strangulation of the hollow viscus, for which the reported mortality rate is as high as 66% [13, 15] (Fig. 3.1). Another unusual complication associated with diaphragmatic rupture is thoracic splenosis. Splenosis is defined as the autoimplantation of splenic tissue. Thoracic splenosis may occur after combined splenic and diaphragmatic injury from blunt trauma or gunshot wounds. Splenic implantation typically involves the left pleural space but, rarely, can be bilateral. Thoracic splenosis is usually asymptomatic and is typically an incidental finding on imaging performed for other reasons. It may mimic malignant pleural tumors (Fig. 3.2).

3.2.2 Imaging Diagnosis

Chest radiography, despite its inherent limitations, can provide useful information on diaphragmatic injury and serves as a baseline imaging modality in trauma settings. The reported sensitivity of initial radiography varies widely, from 17 to 65% [16, 17]. The reported sensitivity for left-sided diaphragmatic injuries (27–60%) is higher than that for right-sided injuries (approximately 17%) [17]. The most valuable signs of diaphragmatic rupture on chest radiograph are visualization of the herniated viscera above the diaphragm with constriction at the diaphragmatic defect (i.e., collar sign) (Fig. 3.3) and visualization of the tip of the nasogastric tube above the diaphragm [9, 18]. Other suggestive findings include unexplained elevation of the hemidiaphragm (4–6 cm from the contralateral diaphragm) (Fig. 3.3), irregularity of the diaphragmatic contour, and inability to visualize the diaphragm [2, 18, 19] (Fig. 3.1a).

CT is the mainstay for evaluation of suspected diaphragmatic injuries. Rapid scanning and rou-

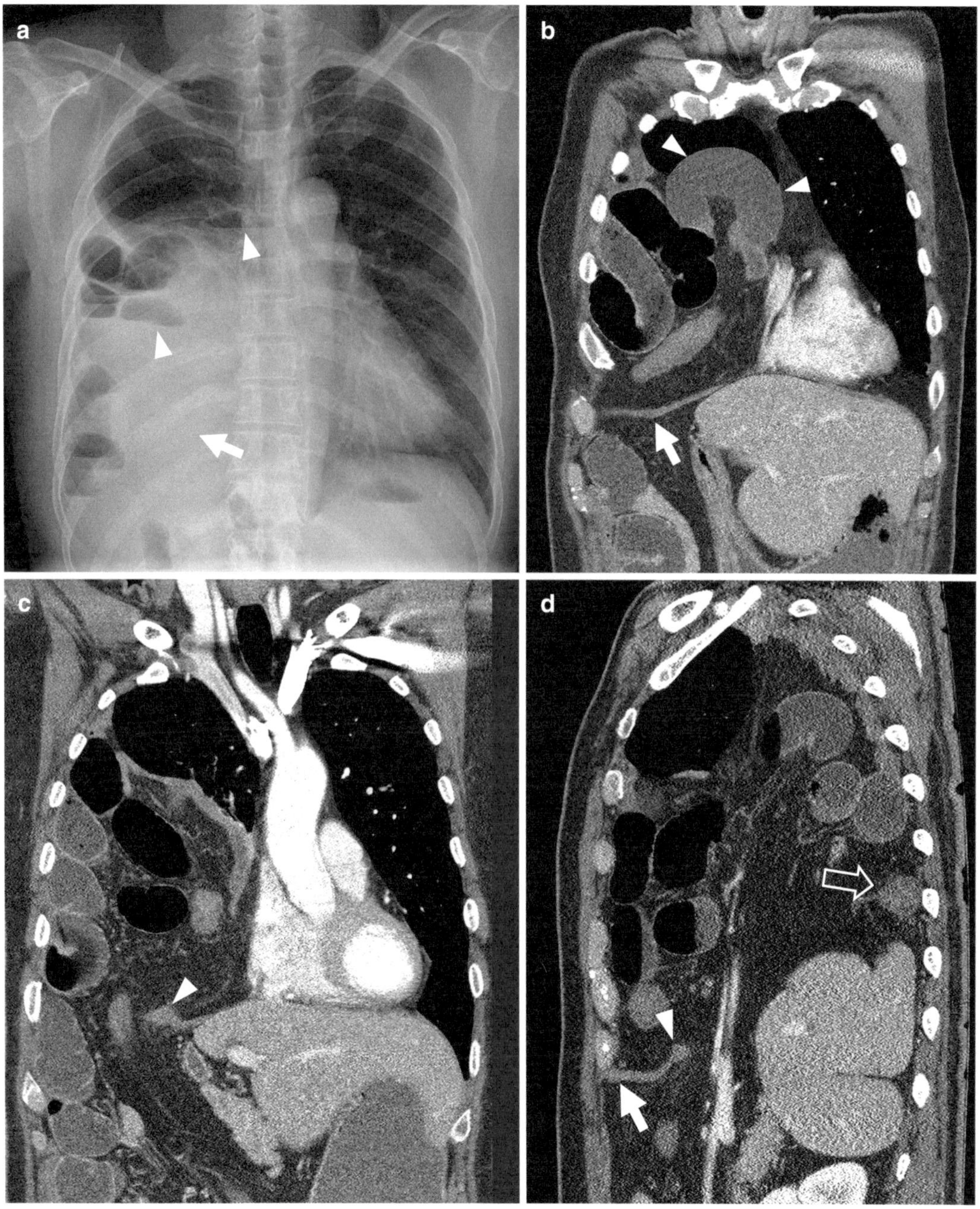

Fig. 3.1 Small bowel strangulation in a 68-year-old man with severe abdominal pain 30 years after sustaining a stab wound. (**a**) Chest radiograph shows multiple air-filled bowel loops within the lower portion of the right hemithorax (arrowheads). The right hemidiaphragm could not be clearly identified along any of its surface (arrow). (**b**) Coronal reformatted CT image shows a distended bowel loop with hypoenhancement of the bowel wall, suggesting strangulation. Note that the anterior part of the diaphragm is thickened (abnormally thick diaphragm sign) (arrow). (**c**) Coronal reformatted CT image shows a comma-shaped structure with soft-tissue attenuation (arrowhead), representing the torn-free edge of the right hemidiaphragm (dangling diaphragm sign). Also note herniated bowel loops and mesentery protruding through the large defect. (**d**) Sagittal reformatted CT image shows a triangular-shaped free edge of the torn diaphragm (dangling diaphragm sign) (arrowhead), the distal part of which appears thickened (abnormally thick diaphragm sign) (arrow). Also note the direct contact between the herniated bowel and mesentery and posterior chest wall (dependent viscera sign) (open arrow)

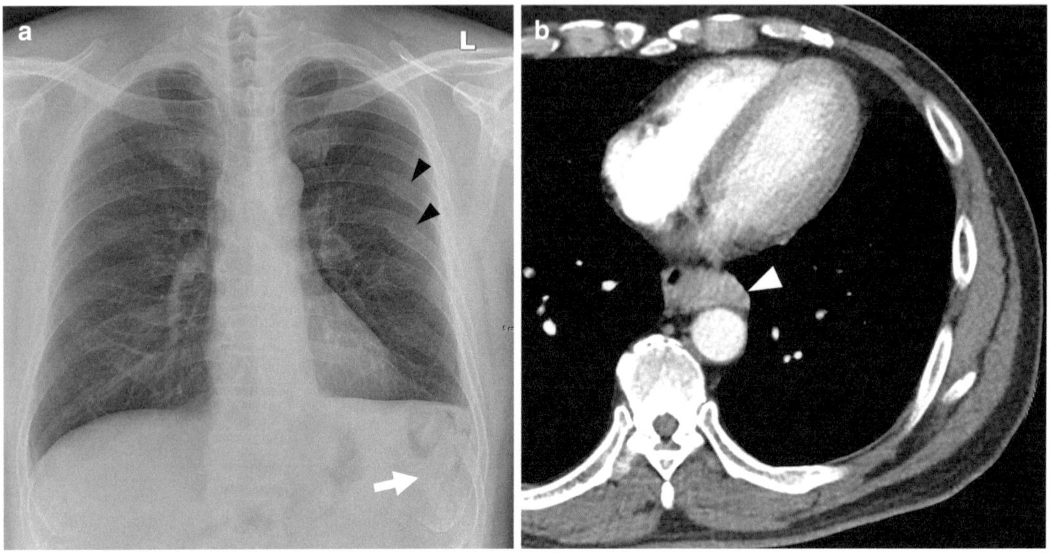

Fig. 3.2 Thoracic splenosis in an asymptomatic 56-year-old man who underwent repair of diaphragmatic rupture due to a motor vehicle accident 25 years prior. (**a**) Chest radiograph shows multiple old rib fractures (arrowheads), suggesting a previous trauma history. Also note a colonic loop in the left subdiaphragmatic area, replacing the splenic shadow (arrow). (**b**) Mediastinal window image of a CT scan obtained at the level of the interventricular septum shows a well-enhancing paraesophageal ovoid soft tissue mass (arrowhead). The diagnosis was confirmed by endoscopic ultrasound-guided fine-needle aspiration

tine multiplanar image reformation of up-to-date multi-detector CT (MDCT) have greatly improved the diagnostic performance of CT for diaphragmatic injuries. Its sensitivity currently ranges from 73 to 100%, with a specificity of 93–98% [20, 21]. CT signs of blunt diaphragmatic injuries can be classified into three groups: direct, indirect, and signs of uncertain or controversial origin (Table 3.1) [9].

3.2.2.1 Direct CT Signs

1. Visualized diaphragmatic defect: The visualized diaphragmatic defect sign represents a focal and abrupt loss of continuity in the diaphragm [9, 22]. The reported sensitivity and specificity range from approximately 17 to 90% and 90 to 100%, respectively [3, 9]. A defect is most easily visualized when aerated lung or abdominal fat abuts the diaphragm (Figs. 3.1, 3.2, 3.3, 3.4, 3.5, and 3.6). In contrast, parenchymal lesions at the base of the lungs or pleural or peritoneal fluid may obscure a focal diaphragmatic defect [23, 24]. Nontraumatic diaphragmatic defect, which is reported in 6% of asymptomatic adults, is part of the normal aging process and should be differentiated from traumatic defect [17].
2. Dangling diaphragm: The dangling diaphragm sign refers to visualization of the free edge of a torn diaphragm that curls inward, appearing as a comma-shaped soft tissue lesion [20] (Fig. 3.1c, d). This sign overlaps with the visualized diaphragmatic defect. The sensitivity and specificity of this sign have been reported as 54% and 98%, respectively [20].
3. Absent diaphragm: This sign refers to the absence of diaphragm in the area of a diaphragmatic injury. Absence of diaphragm represents a large defect, and, therefore, the abdominal contents are commonly found to have herniated through the defect (Fig. 3.4a). The sensitivity and specificity of this sign have been reported as 18–43% and 91%, respectively [25, 26]. Direct contact of the diaphragm with fluid or soft tissue lesions may be falsely interpreted as absence of diaphragm [27].

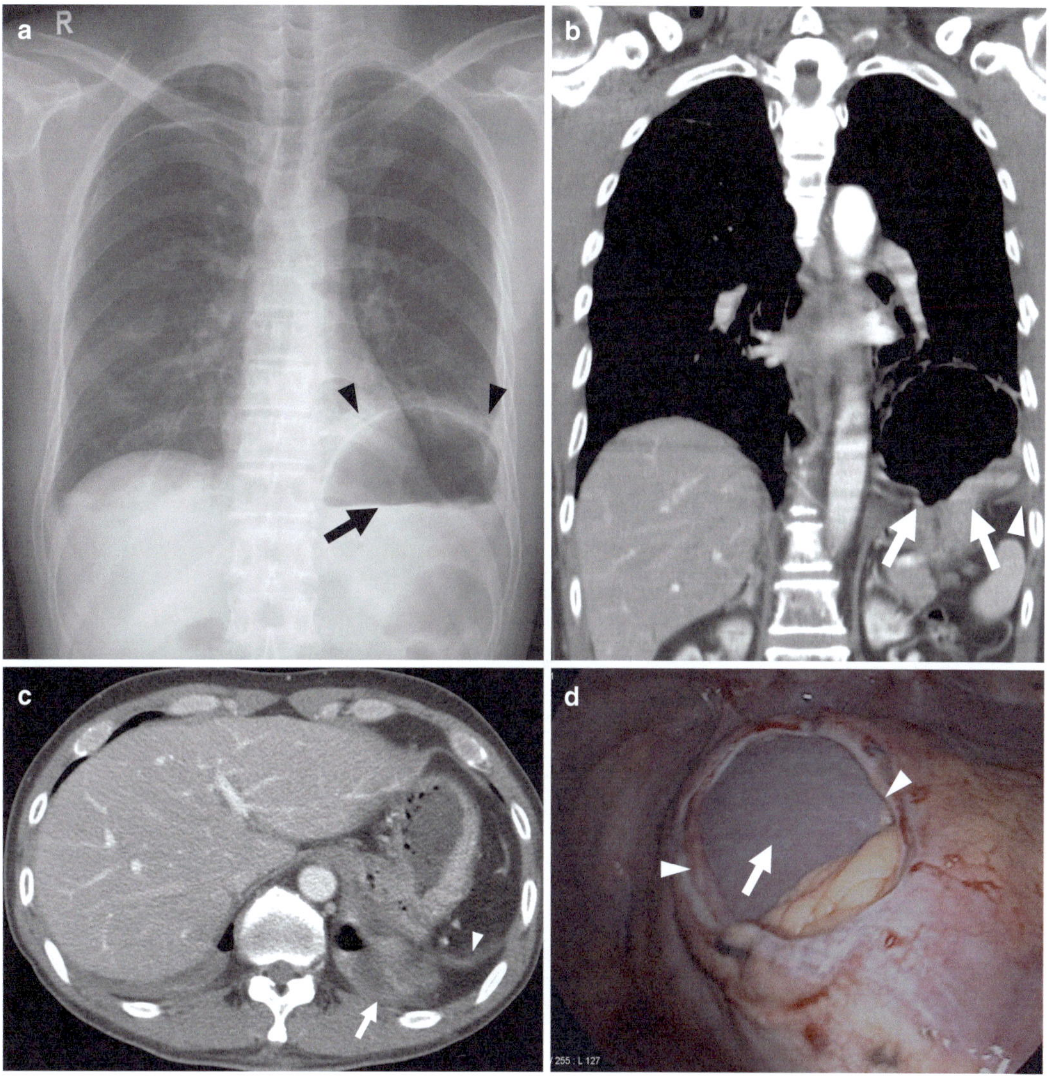

Fig. 3.3 Collar sign in a 49-year-old man after a motor vehicle accident. (**a**) Chest radiograph shows a distended stomach with an air-fluid level (arrow). Note the ill-defined increased opacity along the distended gastric fundus (arrowheads), suggesting adjacent atelectasis of the left lower lobe. (**b**) Coronal reformatted CT image clearly depicts herniation of the stomach through the diaphragmatic defect and waist-like constriction of the stomach (arrows). Note the thickened peripheral diaphragm (arrowhead). (**c**) Mediastinal window image of a CT scan obtained at the level of the left portal vein shows a herniated stomach (arrow) within the pleural cavity, peripheral to the diaphragm (abdominal contents peripheral to the diaphragm or lung sign) (arrowhead). (**d**) The diaphragmatic defect (arrowheads) was confirmed during surgery. Reduction of the herniated stomach (arrow) and diaphragmatic repair were performed

3.2.2.2 Indirect CT Signs Related to Herniation

1. Herniation through a defect: This sign refers to herniation of the peritoneal fat or abdominal organs into the thorax through a diaphragmatic defect [9] (Figs. 3.1, 3.3, 3.4, 3.5, 3.6, 3.7, and 3.8). The reported sensitivity and specificity of this sign are 50–95% and 98–100%, respectively [20, 23–26, 28]. The presence of intrathoracic space-occupying abnormalities, such

as a large hemothorax, or increased intrathoracic pressure due to positive pressure ventilation may hinder intrathoracic herniation of the abdominal contents into the thorax. Diaphragmatic hernias (e.g., Bochdalek or Morgagni hernias) are the most common diagnostic mimics of this sign (Figs. 3.9 and 3.10).

Table 3.1 Classification of CT signs of diaphragmatic rupture

Direct signs of diaphragmatic rupture
Visualized diaphragmatic defect
Dangling diaphragm
Absent diaphragm
Indirect signs related to herniation
Herniation through a defect
Collar sign
Hump and band sign
Dependent viscera sign
Abdominal contents peripheral to the diaphragm or lung
Elevated abdominal organs
CT signs of uncertain or controversial origin
Abnormally thick diaphragm
Diaphragmatic and peridiaphragmatic extravasation of contrast medium
Fractured rib

2. Collar sign: The collar sign refers to the waist-like constriction of the herniated organs at the site of a diaphragmatic defect. This sign is best appreciated on coronal or sagittal reformatted images (Fig. 3.3). The overall sensitivity and specificity of this sign have been reported as 44–64% and 98–100%, respectively [20, 23–26, 28]. Herniation of the liver through a right-side defect (i.e., hepatic collar sign) is relatively infrequent due to the size and consistency of the liver (Figs. 3.7 and 3.8). Diaphragmatic slips may result in indentations in abdominal structures (Figs. 3.7 and 3.8). A respiratory motion artifact may mimic the narrowed appearance of the abdominal organs.
3. Hump and band sign: The hump sign is a subset of the collar sign on the right side; the "hump" refers to the shape of the herniated liver through a right-sided diaphragmatic defect. The "band" corresponds to an area of hypoattenuation of the herniated liver at the level of the diaphragmatic defect on contrast-enhanced images [29] (Fig. 3.7). It has been hypothesized that compression from the ruptured diaphragm results in hypoperfusion of

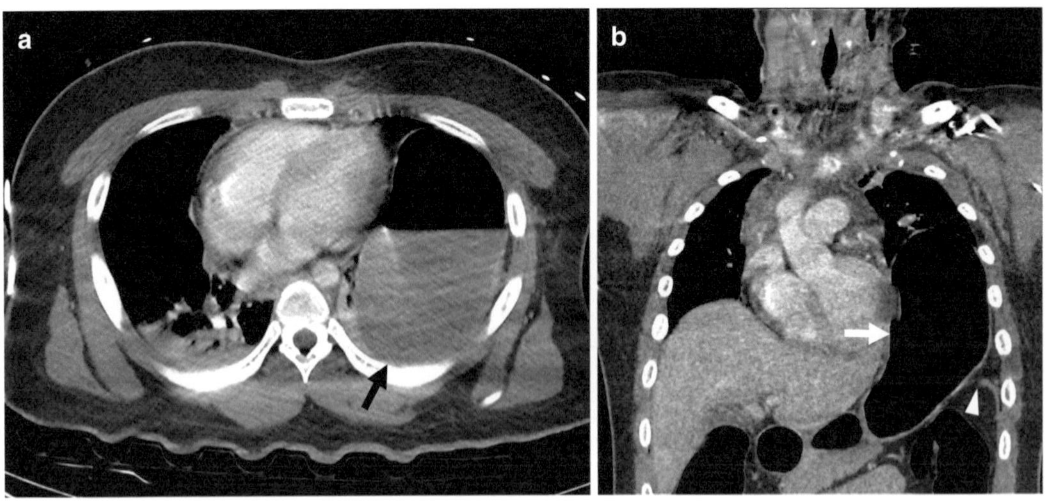

Fig. 3.4 Left-sided diaphragmatic rupture in a 20-year-old man after a motor vehicle accident. (**a**) Mediastinal window image of a CT scan obtained at the level of the left ventricle shows a complete absence of the left hemidiaphragm (absent diaphragm sign). The stomach is in a dependent position and contacts the posterior thoracic wall (dependent viscera sign) (arrow). (**b**) Coronal reformatted CT image shows herniation of the stomach into the left hemithorax (herniation through a defect sign) (arrow). A segment of the diaphragm not visible in (**a**) is depicted in its normal horizontal orientation (arrowhead)

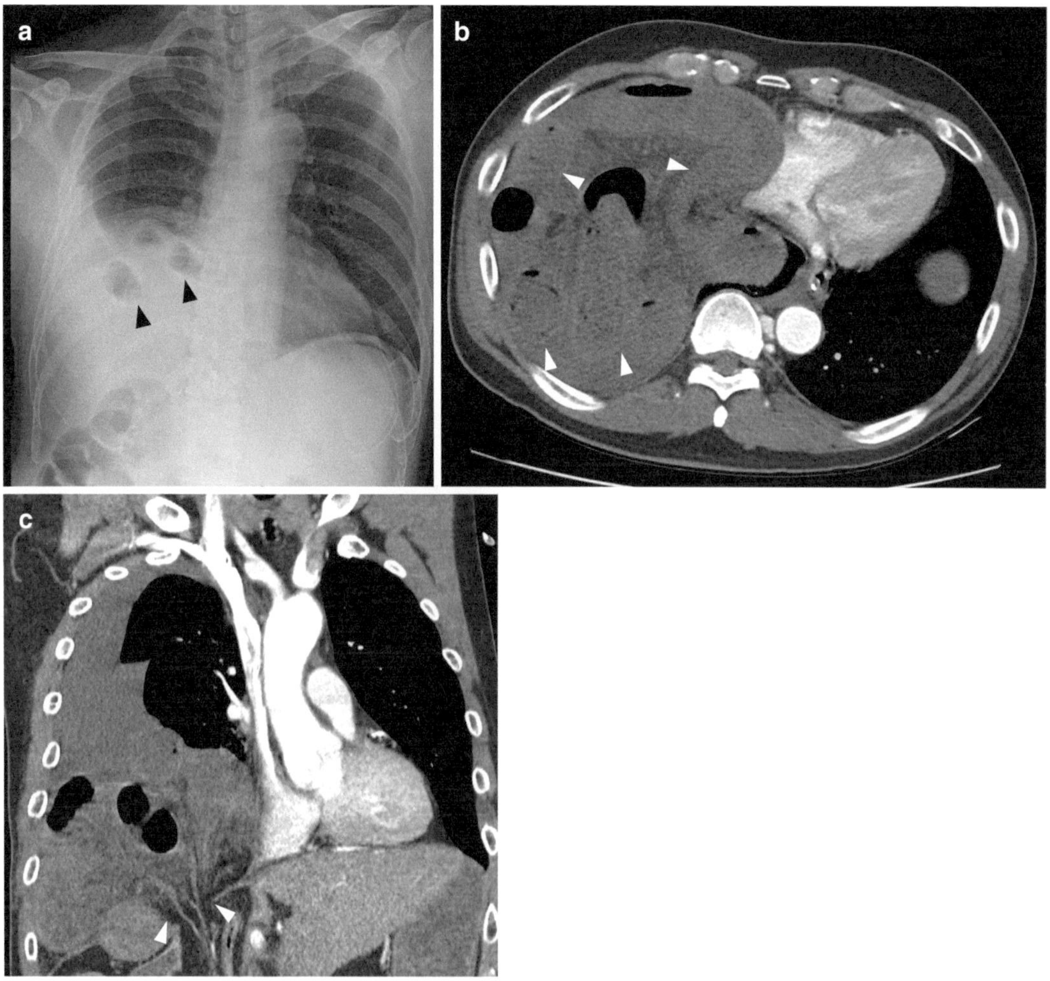

Fig. 3.5 Strangulation of the jejunum in a 45-year-old man who was in a motor vehicle accident 10 years prior. (**a**) Chest radiograph shows multiple air-filled small bowel loops in the right lower thorax (arrowheads). (**b**) Mediastinal window image of a CT scan obtained at the level of the left ventricle shows thickening and hypoenhancement of the herniated jejunal loops (arrowheads), suggestive of strangulation. The herniated abdominal contents contact the right posterior chest wall (dependent viscera sign). (**c**) Coronal reformatted CT image clearly depicts the diaphragmatic defect (arrowheads), through which jejunal loops and mesenteric vessels herniate into the thorax (herniation through a defect sign)

the liver parenchyma at the site of herniation. Similar to the collar sign, the hump and band signs are best appreciated on coronal and sagittal reformatted images. The reported sensitivities are 50–83% for the hump sign and 33–42% for the band sign [29, 30]. The specificity of these signs have not been reported in the literature. A high right hemidiaphragm and motion-related artifacts may mimic a hump sign.

4. Dependent viscera sign: The dependent viscera sign appears when herniated viscera (bowel or solid organs) are no longer supported posteriorly by an injured diaphragm and fall to a dependent position against the posterior ribs, without interposition of the lungs [31] (Figs. 3.1, 3.3–3.5, and 3.7). On the right side, the upper third of the liver or bowel will about the posterior right ribs, and on the left side, the stomach, bowel, or spleen will be

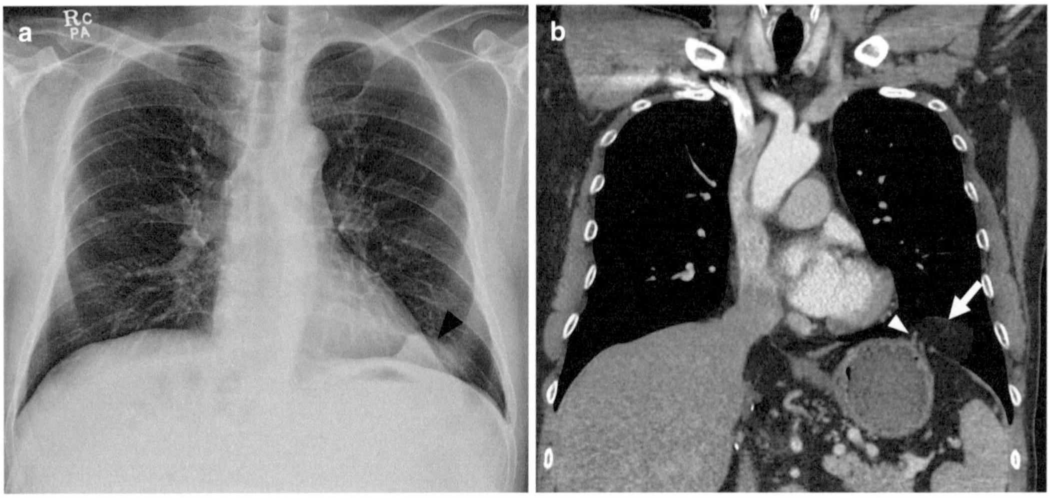

Fig. 3.6 Mesenteric herniation in a 48-year-old man with a focal diaphragmatic defect who had a history of blunt abdominal trauma 5 years prior. (**a**) Chest radiograph shows a sharply demarcated opacity above the left hemidiaphragm (arrowhead). (**b**) Coronal reformatted CT image shows herniated mesenteric fat (arrow) and mesenteric vessels (arrowhead) through a focal defect in the left hemidiaphragm

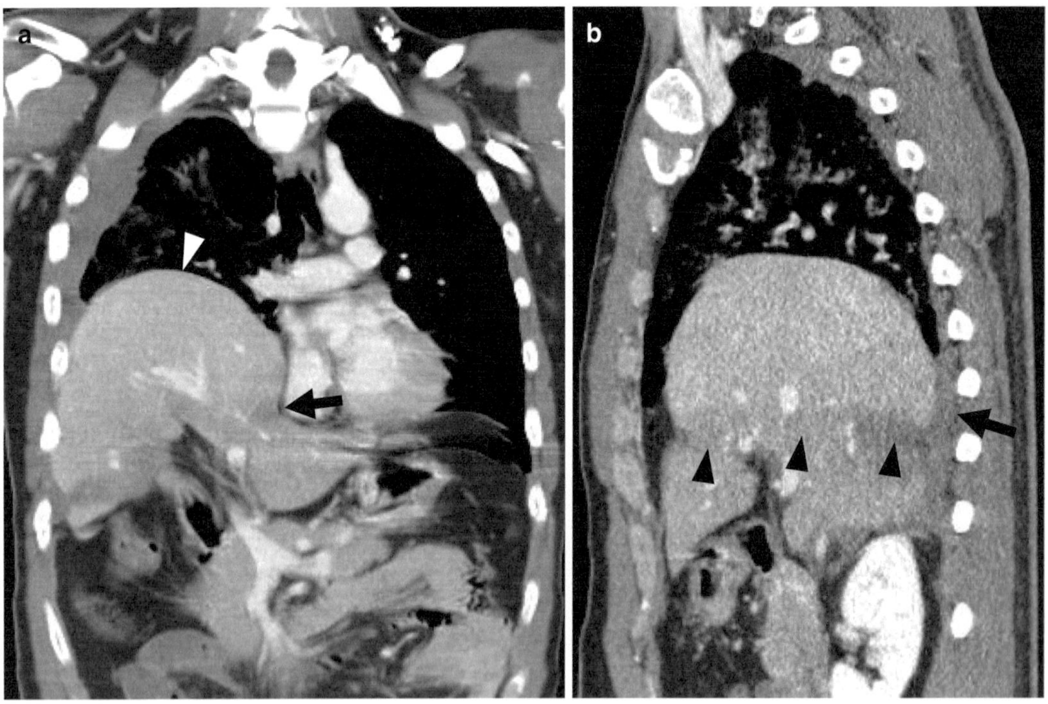

Fig. 3.7 Right-sided blunt diaphragmatic rupture in a 44-year-old man after a motor vehicle accident. (**a**) Coronal reformatted CT image shows herniation of the liver (arrowhead) through a diaphragmatic rupture (hump sign), with constriction at the defect (collar sign) (arrow). (**b**) Sagittal reformatted CT image depicts band-like hypoattenuation (band sign) (arrowheads) extending across the base of the defect. Also note the thickened diaphragm due to rupture with retraction (arrow), which was confirmed at surgery (abnormally thick diaphragm sign)

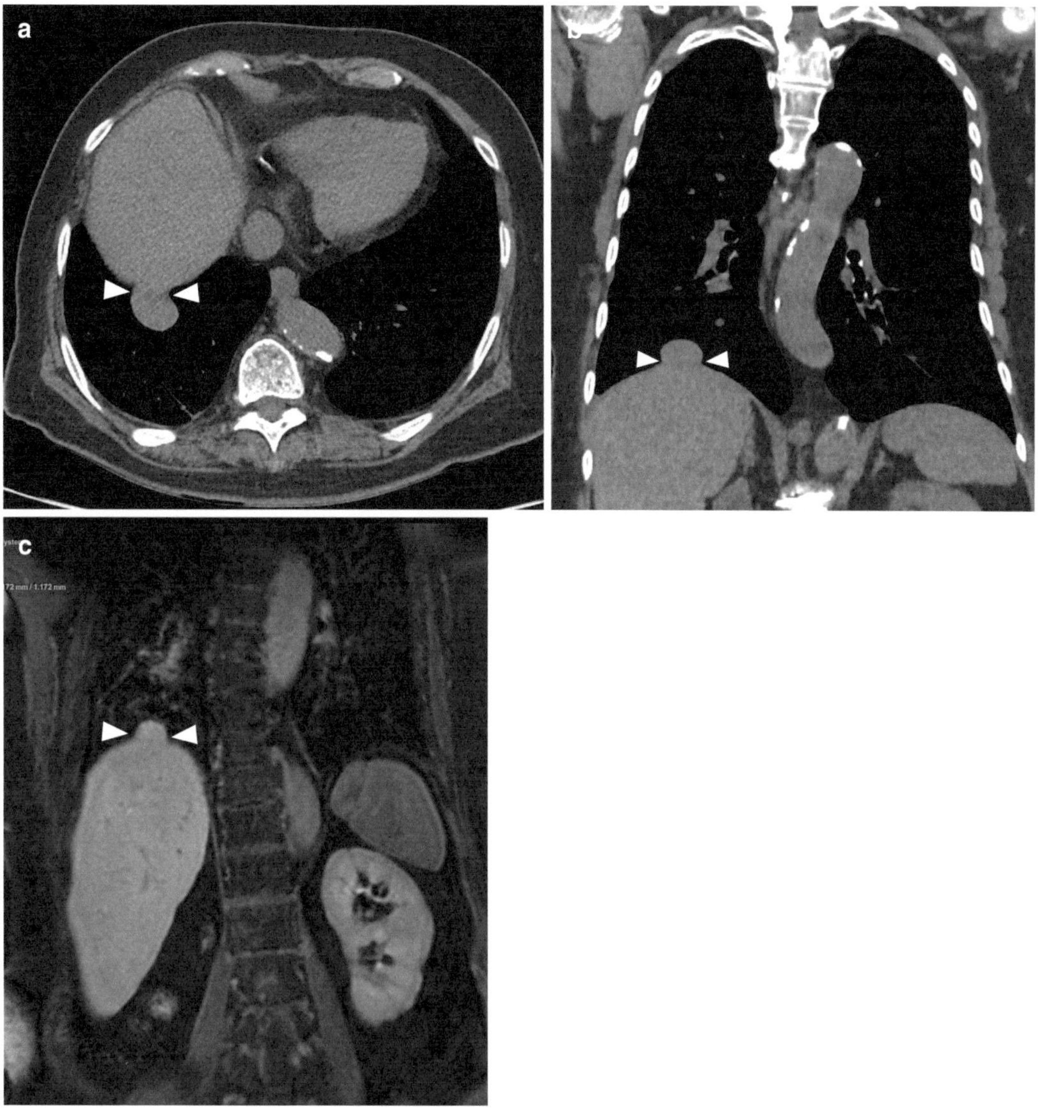

Fig. 3.8 Hepatic collar sign in a 72-year-old woman who underwent wedge resection of the right lower lobe due to metastatic colon cancer 3 years prior. (**a**) Mediastinal window image of a CT scan obtained at the level of the liver dome shows a well-defined mass in the right lower thorax, abutting the liver (arrowheads). (**b**) Coronal reformatted CT image demonstrates an ovoid mass in the right lower thorax abutting the diaphragm. Focal herniation of the liver was suspected rather than metastasis, considering the suspicious constriction at the diaphragm (arrowheads). (**c**) Coronal contrast-enhanced magnetic resonance image clearly demonstrates a focal herniation of the liver (arrowheads), presumably through a focal diaphragmatic defect due to a previous surgery

in contact with the posterior left ribs [31]. The reported sensitivity is 54–90%, with a specificity of 98–100% [20, 26, 29–31]. Cases of congenital hernia without a history of trauma may include this sign. This sign has low sensitivity for detection of a small defect, a rupture in an anterior location, and a rupture with a large pleural effusion [32].

5. Abdominal contents peripheral to the diaphragm or lungs: On an axial image of a normal diaphragm, all structures outside the domed upper contour are located in the thoracic cavity, while the structures inside the diaphragmatic contour are in the abdominal cavity. If abdominal organs or fat are seen outside of the normal upper contour of the

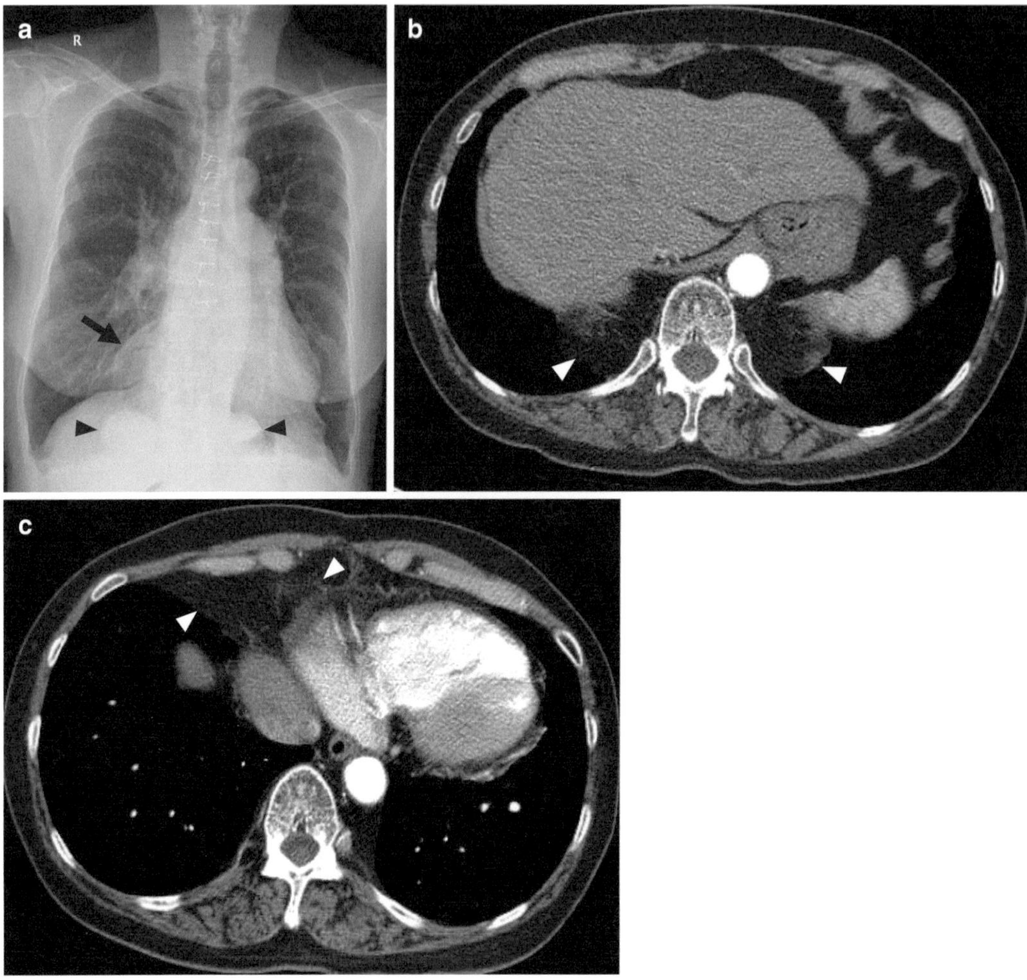

Fig. 3.9 Incidentally detected Bochdalek hernia and Morgagni hernia in an asymptomatic 75-year-old woman. (**a**) Chest radiograph shows bilateral paravertebral soft tissue masses (arrowheads) and a less dense opacity in the right cardiophrenic angle (arrow). (**b**) Mediastinal window image of a CT scan demonstrates bilateral herniation of abdominal fat (arrowheads) into the thorax (Bochdalek hernia). (**c**) Mediastinal window image of a CT scan demonstrates herniation of abdominal fat (arrowheads) into the thorax through a defect in the right anteromedial hemidiaphragm (Morgagni hernia)

diaphragm, they have herniated into the thoracic cavity [33] (Fig. 3.3c). The sensitivity and specificity of this sign have not been reported.

6. Elevated abdominal organs: Since the height of normal diaphragms varies, one cannot diagnose diaphragmatic rupture with only unilateral elevation of the abdominal organs, but this sign can increase the confidence of a diagnosis of diaphragmatic rupture when accompanied by other suggestive findings (Figs. 3.1, 3.3, and 3.5). Several studies have reported that elevation of the hemidiaphragm more than 5 cm (for right-sided rupture) and 4 cm (for left-sided rupture) above the contralateral hemidiaphragm is suggestive of diaphragmatic rupture. The reported sensitivity and specificity of the elevated abdominal organs sign are 50–83% and 89–99%, respectively [20, 26, 29, 30]. The pitfalls of this sign include diaphragmatic palsy, eventration (Fig. 3.11), atelectasis, and subpulmonic effusion.

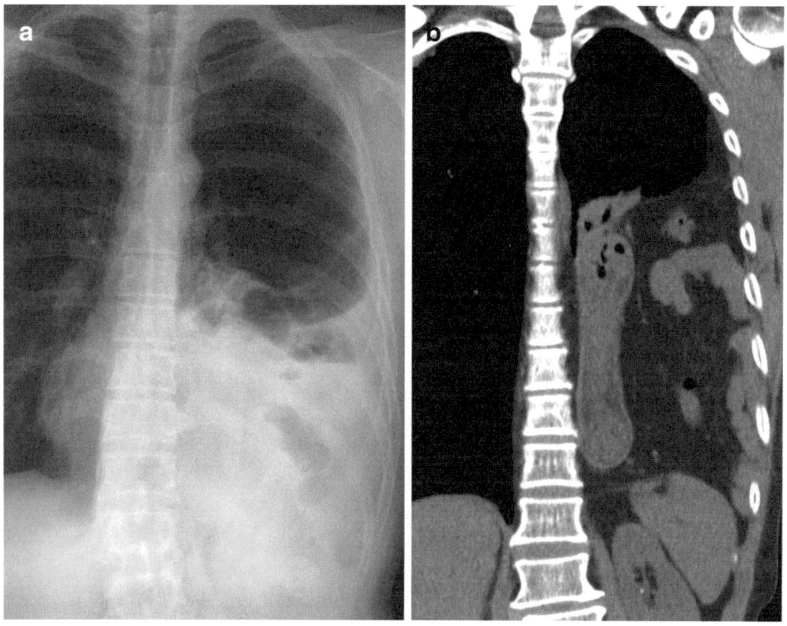

Fig. 3.10 Bochdalek hernia in a 58-year-old man with intermittent abdominal discomfort. (**a**) Chest radiograph shows multiple air-filled bowel loops in the left hemithorax. (**b**) Coronal reformatted CT image demonstrates herniation of the stomach, small bowel, and mesenteric fat into the left hemithorax through a defect in the posterior diaphragm (Bochdalek hernia)

3.2.2.3 CT Signs of Uncertain or Controversial Origin

1. Abnormally thick diaphragm: Thickening of the diaphragm is thought to be caused by retraction of the ruptured diaphragm (Figs. 3.1b, 3.3b, and 3.7b). There is no consensus on the optimal site for measurement of diaphragmatic thickness, but it is generally considered abnormally thickened by subjective comparison with the contralateral diaphragm at the same level [34]. Thickening may also be seen in cases of partial rupture with associated hematoma or edema. The reported sensitivity and specificity of this sign are 56–75% and 96%, respectively [26, 30, 34]. One of the limitations of this sign is that it does not allow radiologists to distinguish a full-thickness rupture requiring surgical repair from a partial-thickness tear, which usually does not require surgery. Moreover, hemorrhage or fluid accumulation near the diaphragm may mimic thickening of the diaphragm [26, 34].
2. Diaphragmatic and peridiaphragmatic extravasation of contrast medium: Extravasation of arterial contrast medium from the diaphragm is a rare but highly specific sign of diaphragmatic injury. It is predominantly seen in penetrating diaphragmatic injury. However, it is difficult to distinguish between intrinsic diaphragmatic bleeding and bleeding from adjacent organs. Therefore, this sign should be regarded as an auxiliary finding that is suggestive of a diaphragmatic injury. The reported sensitivity of this sign is low (0–12%), but the specificity is between 93 and 98% [20, 25, 26].
3. Fractured rib: The fractured rib sign is present when a juxtadiaphragmatic costal bone fragment faces the diaphragm and directly causes diaphragmatic perforation [22, 26]. The reported sensitivity of this sign is low, and no specificity has been reported [26].

3.3 Diagnostic Pitfalls in CT

The most common nontraumatic diaphragmatic hernias occur through the esophageal hiatus. These are described in detail in Chap. 5. Less common forms include Bochdalek hernia and Morgagni hernia. Diaphragmatic eventration is a common incidental finding, especially in individuals aged 60 years and above, which

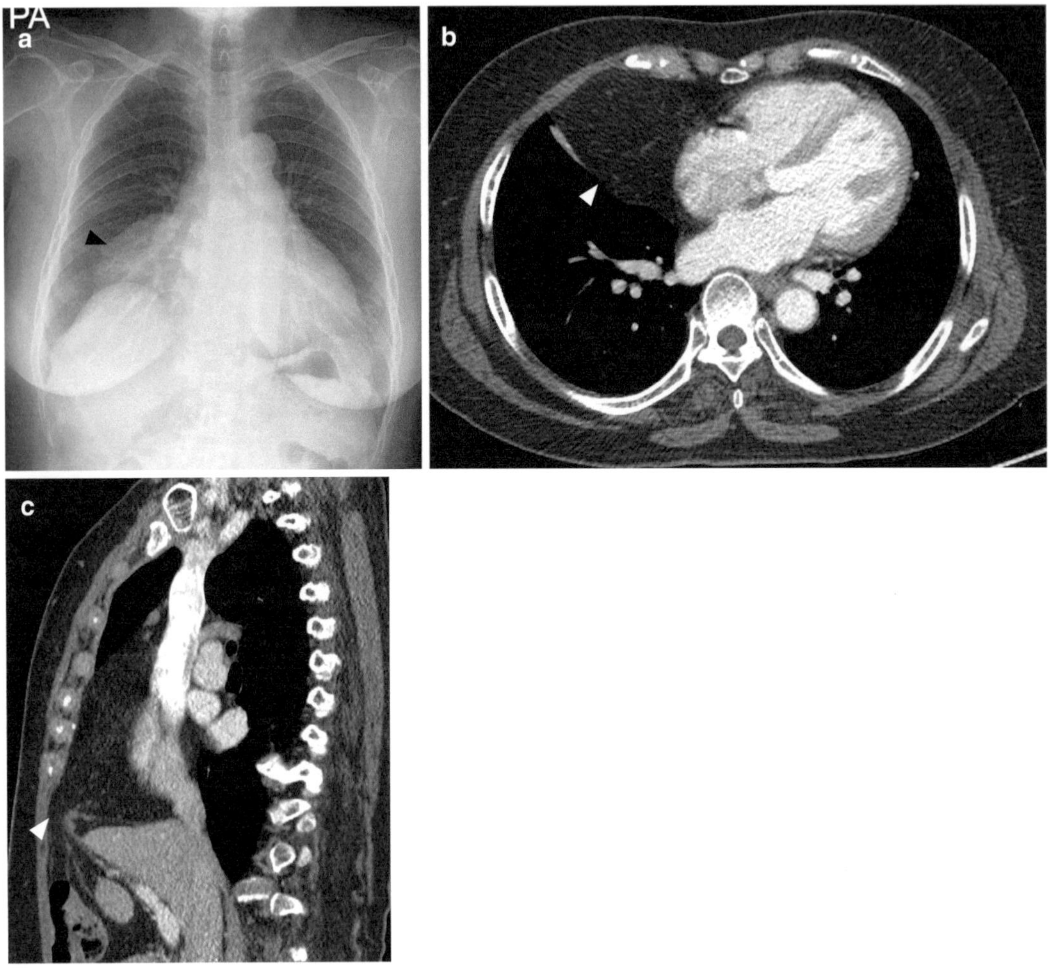

Fig. 3.11 Morgagni hernia in an asymptomatic 68-year-old woman. (**a**) Chest radiograph shows a large mass (arrowhead) bulging from the right cardiophrenic angle. Note the relatively less dense opacity of the mass, indicating fatty contents. (**b**) Mediastinal window image of a CT scan obtained at the level of the left atrium shows herniation of abdominal fat in the right cardiophrenic region (arrowhead). (**c**) Sagittal reformatted CT image clearly demonstrates herniation of abdominal fat (arrowhead) into the right thorax through a defect in the right anteromedial diaphragm

should be differentiated from other diaphragmatic abnormalities, as it is of no clinical significance [35].

3.3.1 Bochdalek Hernia

Bochdalek hernia in infants is a congenital diaphragmatic defect resulting from failure of the posterolateral diaphragmatic foramina to fuse in utero. On the contrary, Bochdalek hernia in adults occurs through a weak area, the pleuroperitoneal canal, and manifests as a person ages, in the presence of obesity and emphysema. The prevalence of such hernias increases with age, suggesting that they are acquired rather than congenital [36]. Bochdalek hernias are more common on the left than on the right, presumably due to the protective effect of the liver [36, 37]. On chest radiograph, Bochdalek hernia presents as a focal bulging contour in the hemidiaphragm or as a paravertebral mass adjacent to the posteromedial aspect of the hemidiaphragm (Fig. 3.9a). The typical location and the lower density of soft tissue than usual due to its high-fat content are suggestive of Bochdalek hernia [38, 39] (Figs. 3.9 and 3.10). Diagnostic confirmation and identification of herniated contents are easily done with CT. Coronal or sagittal reformatted images can be useful to demonstrate the defect (Figs. 3.9 and 3.10).

3.3.2 Morgagni Hernia

Morgagni hernia is uncommon, and maybe an incidental finding on imaging studies. Because the left side is protected by the heart, most herniations occur in the right cardiophrenic angle. The defects are developmental in origin, but hernias are more common in adults than in children, and are often associated with conditions that increase intra-abdominal pressure, including obesity, severe effort, or trauma [40, 41]. Morgagni hernia presents as a smooth, well-defined opacity in the right cardiophrenic angle on radiograph, and may resemble other cardiophrenic angle masses, including pericardial cysts, prominent pericardial fat pads, or other masses (Figs. 3.9 and 3.11). The diagnosis of Morgagni hernia is easily made with CT because of the presence of fat or abdominal contents between the costal and sternal attachments of the diaphragm in the right anteromedial location. The hernia may contain omentum, colon, stomach, liver, or small bowel [42, 43] (Figs. 3.9 and 3.11).

3.3.3 Diaphragmatic Eventration

Diaphragmatic eventration is a partial or complete diaphragmatic muscular defect comprising a thin structure that allows intra-abdominal contents to be elevated into the thoracic cavity. The diagnosis is often confused with a diaphragmatic hernia, which is a complete protrusion of the intra-abdominal contents through a diaphragmatic defect. A partial eventration typically affects only a segment of the hemidiaphragm; paralysis or palsy, by comparison, affects the entire hemidiaphragm. The typical location of eventration is the anteromedial portion of the right hemidiaphragm (Fig. 3.12). Total eventration of the diaphragm typically occurs in males on the left side [44] (Fig. 3.13). It is difficult to distinguish a total diaphragmatic eventration

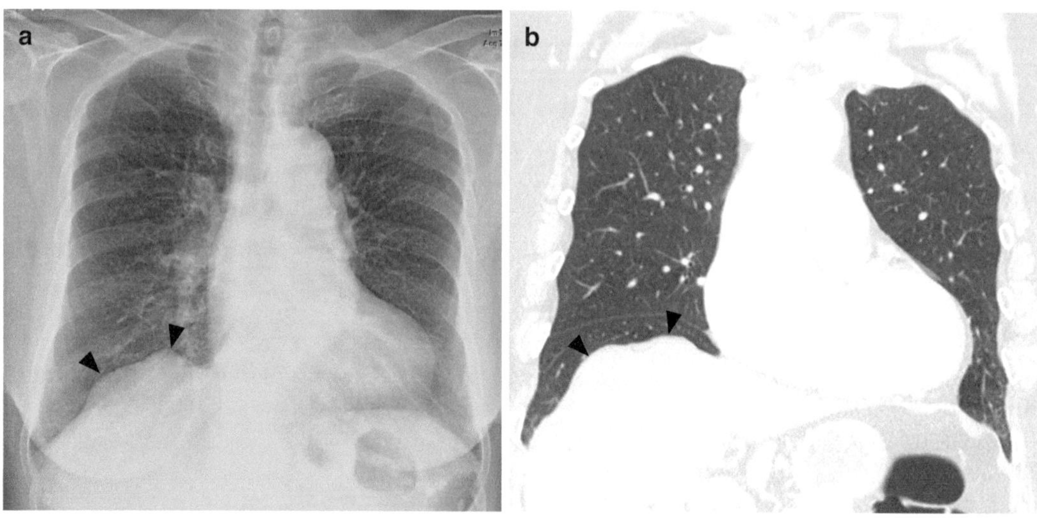

Fig. 3.12 Partial diaphragmatic eventration in an asymptomatic 71-year-old man. (**a**) Chest radiograph shows an elevation of the anteromedial portion of the right hemidiaphragm (arrowheads). (**b**) Coronal reformatted CT image demonstrates focal elevation of the anteromedial portion of the right hemidiaphragm (arrowheads) (partial eventration). Note the absence of atelectasis in the adjacent right lower lobe

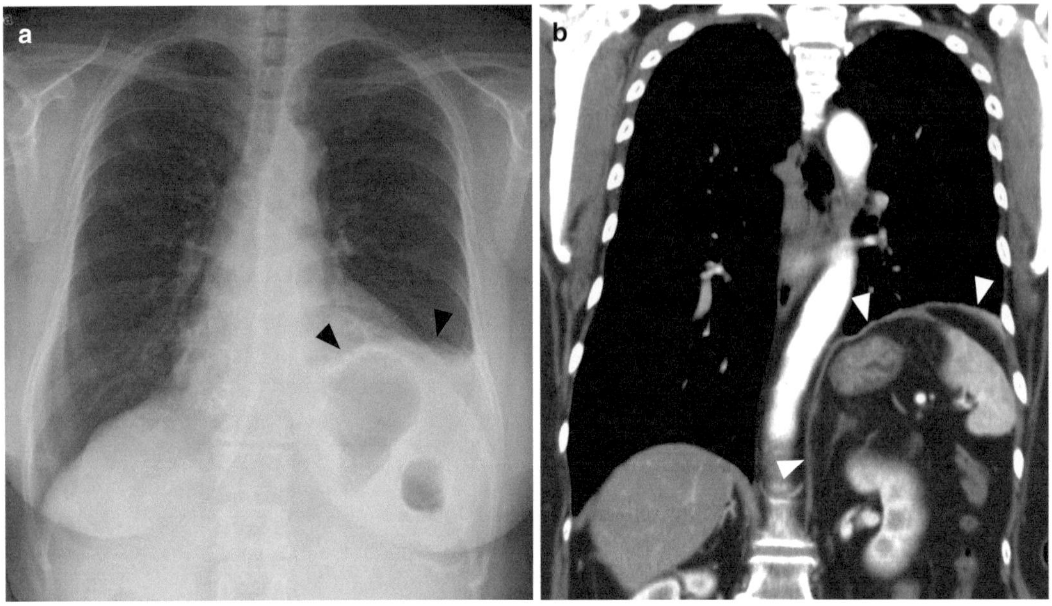

Fig. 3.13 Total diaphragmatic eventration in a 72-year-old woman. (**a**) Chest radiograph shows elevation of the left hemidiaphragm (arrowheads). (**b**) Coronal reformatted CT image demonstrates elevation of the entire left hemidiaphragm and abdominal organs without loss of continuity (total eventration) (arrowheads). Also note the absence of atelectasis in the adjacent left lower lobe

from diaphragmatic paralysis. A diaphragmatic eventration typically does not include atelectasis in the adjacent lung because the motion of the eventrated diaphragm is normal, whereas paralysis of the diaphragm often does include atelectasis (Figs. 3.12 and 3.13). Fluoroscopy and real-time ultrasonography typically reveal an inspiratory lag followed by delayed downward motion of the eventrated diaphragm [43].

3.4 Summary

In this chapter, we discussed diagnosis of diaphragmatic rupture, focusing on the epidemiology, mechanisms, and imaging features. Delayed diagnosis of diaphragmatic injuries is common because most injuries are initially asymptomatic and associated injuries often obscure the findings of diaphragmatic rupture. In order to accurately diagnose diaphragmatic injuries, it is important to understand the mechanisms of trauma and to suspect the possibility of diaphragmatic injuries. Diaphragmatic injuries are frequently accompanied by specific clues on imaging studies, such as the dependent viscera sign or collar sign, which are very helpful for diagnosis; emergency radiologists and physicians responsible for patients with suspected diaphragmatic injuries should be familiar with these imaging features. Thoracic splenosis is a rare condition that can occur in patients with a history of diaphragmatic rupture and may mimic neoplastic diseases in the thorax. Understanding diaphragmatic hernia, which can mimic diaphragmatic injury, will also aid in accurate diagnosis of diaphragmatic injuries.

Key Points

- Diaphragmatic rupture occurs more often on the left side than on the right, in a ratio of approximately 3:1, which is explained by the buffer effect of the liver, greater weakness of the left hemidiaphragm, and underdiagnosis of right-sided injuries.
- Direct signs of diaphragmatic injuries include the "visualized diaphragmatic defect," "dangling diaphragm sign," and "absent diaphragm sign." "Dangling diaphragm" refers to visual-

ization of the free edge of a torn diaphragm, which appears as a comma-shaped soft tissue lesion.

- Indirect CT signs of diaphragmatic injuries include "herniation through a defect," "collar sign," "hump and band sign," "dependent viscera sign," "abdominal contents peripheral to the diaphragm or lung," and "elevated abdominal organs."
- CT signs of uncertain or controversial origin include "abnormally thick diaphragm," "diaphragmatic and peridiaphragmatic extravasation of contrast medium," and "fractured rib."

References

1. Meyers BF, McCabe CJ. Traumatic diaphragmatic hernia. Occult marker of serious injury. Ann Surg. 1993;218(6):783–90. https://doi.org/10.1097/00000658-199312000-00013.
2. Shah R, Sabanathan S, Mearns AJ, Choudhury AK. Traumatic rupture of diaphragm. Ann Thorac Surg. 1995;60(5):1444–9. https://doi.org/10.1016/0003-4975(95)00629-Y.
3. Hammer MM, Flagg E, Mellnick VM, Cummings KW, Bhalla S, Raptis CA. Computed tomography of blunt and penetrating diaphragmatic injury: sensitivity and inter-observer agreement of CT Signs. Emerg Radiol. 2014;21(2):143–9. https://doi.org/10.1007/s10140-013-1166-0.
4. Gao JM, Du DY, Li H, et al. Traumatic diaphragmatic rupture with combined thoracoabdominal injuries: difference between penetrating and blunt injuries. Chin J Traumatol. 2015;18(1):21–6. https://doi.org/10.1016/j.cjtee.2014.07.001.
5. Fair KA, Gordon NT, Barbosa RR, Rowell SE, Watters JM, Schreiber MA. Traumatic diaphragmatic injury in the American College of Surgeons National Trauma Data Bank: a new examination of a rare diagnosis. Am J Surg. 2015;209(5):864–8.; discussion 868–869. https://doi.org/10.1016/j.amjsurg.2014.12.023.
6. Leaman PL. Rupture of the right hemidiaphragm due to blunt trauma. Ann Emerg Med. 1983;12(6):351–7. https://doi.org/10.1016/s0196-0644(83)80464-8.
7. de la Rocha AG, Creel RJ, Mulligan GW, Burns CM. Diaphragmatic rupture due to blunt abdominal trauma. Surg Gynecol Obstet. 1982;154(2):175–80.
8. Shorr RM, Crittenden M, Indeck M, Hartunian SL, Rodriguez A. Blunt thoracic trauma. Analysis of 515 patients. Ann Surg. 1987;206(2):200–5. https://doi.org/10.1097/00000658-198708000-00013.
9. Desir A, Ghaye B. CT of blunt diaphragmatic rupture. Radiographics. 2012;32(2):477–98. https://doi.org/10.1148/rg.322115082.
10. Sarna S, Kivioja A. Blunt rupture of the diaphragm. A retrospective analysis of 41 patients. Ann Chir Gynaecol. 1995;84(3):261–5.
11. Perlman SJ, Rogers LF, Mintzer RA, Mueller CF. Abnormal course of nasogastric tube in traumatic rupture of left hemidiaphragm. AJR Am J Roentgenol. 1984;142(1):85–8. https://doi.org/10.2214/ajr.142.1.85.
12. Estrera AS, Platt MR, Mills LJ. Traumatic injuries of the diaphragm. Chest. 1979;75(3):306–13. https://doi.org/10.1378/chest.75.3.306.
13. Chen JC, Wilson SE. Diaphragmatic injuries: recognition and management in sixty-two patients. Am Surg. 1991;57(12):810–5.
14. Boulanger BR, Milzman DP, Rosati C, Rodriguez A. A comparison of right and left blunt traumatic diaphragmatic rupture. J Trauma. 1993;35(2):255–60. https://doi.org/10.1097/00005373-199308000-00014.
15. Reber PU, Schmied B, Seiler CA, Baer HU, Patel AG, Buchler MW. Missed diaphragmatic injuries and their long-term sequelae. J Trauma. 1998;44(1):183–8. https://doi.org/10.1097/00005373-199801000-00026.
16. Patlas MN, Leung VA, Romano L, Gagliardi N, Ponticiello G, Scaglione M. Diaphragmatic injuries: why do we struggle to detect them? Radiol Med. 2015;120(1):12–20. https://doi.org/10.1007/s11547-014-0453-5.
17. Iochum S, Ludig T, Walter F, Sebbag H, Grosdidier G, Blum AG. Imaging of diaphragmatic injury: a diagnostic challenge? Radiographics 2002;22 Spec No(suppl_1):S103–16; discussion S116-108. https://doi.org/10.1148/radiographics.22.suppl_1.g02oc14s103.
18. Gelman R, Mirvis SE, Gens D. Diaphragmatic rupture due to blunt trauma: sensitivity of plain chest radiographs. AJR Am J Roentgenol. 1991;156(1):51–7. https://doi.org/10.2214/ajr.156.1.1898570.
19. Groskin SA. Selected topics in chest trauma. Radiology. 1992;183(3):605–17. https://doi.org/10.1148/radiology.183.3.1584904.
20. Desser TS, Edwards B, Hunt S, Rosenberg J, Purtill MA, Jeffrey RB. The dangling diaphragm sign: sensitivity and comparison with existing CT signs of blunt traumatic diaphragmatic rupture. Emerg Radiol. 2010;17(1):37–44. https://doi.org/10.1007/s10140-009-0819-5.
21. Magu S, Agarwal S, Singla S. Computed tomography in the evaluation of diaphragmatic hernia following blunt trauma. Indian J Surg. 2012;74(4):288–93. https://doi.org/10.1007/s12262-011-0390-7.
22. Holland DG, Quint LE. Traumatic rupture of the diaphragm without visceral herniation: CT diagnosis. AJR Am J Roentgenol. 1991;157(1):17–8. https://doi.org/10.2214/ajr.157.1.2048513.
23. Killeen KL, Mirvis SE, Shanmuganathan K. Helical CT of diaphragmatic rupture caused by blunt trauma. AJR Am J Roentgenol. 1999;173(6):1611–6. https://doi.org/10.2214/ajr.173.6.10584809.
24. Murray JG, Caoili E, Gruden JF, Evans SJ, Halvorsen RA Jr, Mackersie RC. Acute rupture of the diaphragm

due to blunt trauma: diagnostic sensitivity and specificity of CT. AJR Am J Roentgenol. 1996;166(5):1035–9. https://doi.org/10.2214/ajr.166.5.8615237.
25. Worthy SA, Kang EY, Hartman TE, Kwong JS, Mayo JR, Muller NL. Diaphragmatic rupture: CT findings in 11 patients. Radiology. 1995;194(3):885–8. https://doi.org/10.1148/radiology.194.3.7862996.
26. Nchimi A, Szapiro D, Ghaye B, et al. Helical CT of blunt diaphragmatic rupture. AJR Am J Roentgenol. 2005;184(1):24–30. https://doi.org/10.2214/ajr.184.1.01840024.
27. Sliker CW. Imaging of diaphragm injuries. Radiol Clin North Am. 2006;44(2):199–211., vii. https://doi.org/10.1016/j.rcl.2005.10.003.
28. Shanmuganathan K, Killeen K, Mirvis SE, White CS. Imaging of diaphragmatic injuries. J Thorac Imaging. 2000;15(2):104–11. https://doi.org/10.1097/00005382-200004000-00005.
29. Rees O, Mirvis SE, Shanmuganathan K. Multidetector-row CT of right hemidiaphragmatic rupture caused by blunt trauma: a review of 12 cases. Clin Radiol. 2005;60(12):1280–9. https://doi.org/10.1016/j.crad.2005.06.013.
30. Chen HW, Wong YC, Wang LJ, Fu CJ, Fang JF, Lin BC. Computed tomography in left-sided and right-sided blunt diaphragmatic rupture: experience with 43 patients. Clin Radiol. 2010;65(3):206–12. https://doi.org/10.1016/j.crad.2009.11.005.
31. Bergin D, Ennis R, Keogh C, Fenlon HM, Murray JG. The "dependent viscera" sign in CT diagnosis of blunt traumatic diaphragmatic rupture. AJR Am J Roentgenol. 2001;177(5):1137–40. https://doi.org/10.2214/ajr.177.5.1771137.
32. Larici AR, Gotway MB, Litt HI, et al. Helical CT with sagittal and coronal reconstructions: accuracy for detection of diaphragmatic injury. AJR Am J Roentgenol. 2002;179(2):451–7. https://doi.org/10.2214/ajr.179.2.1790451.
33. Heiberg E, Wolverson MK, Hurd RN, Jagannadharao B, Sundaram M. CT recognition of traumatic rupture of the diaphragm. AJR Am J Roentgenol. 1980;135(2):369–72. https://doi.org/10.2214/ajr.135.2.369.
34. Leung JC, Nance ML, Schwab CW, Miller WT Jr. Thickening of the diaphragm: a new computed tomography sign of diaphragm injury. J Thorac Imaging. 1999;14(2):126–9. https://doi.org/10.1097/00005382-199904000-00012.
35. Okuda K, Nomura F, Kawai M, Arimizu N, Okuda H. Age related gross changes of the liver and right diaphragm, with special reference to partial eventration. Br J Radiol. 1979;52(623):870–5. https://doi.org/10.1259/0007-1285-52-623-870.
36. Gale ME. Bochdalek hernia: prevalence and CT characteristics. Radiology. 1985;156(2):449–52. https://doi.org/10.1148/radiology.156.2.4011909.
37. Mullins ME, Stein J, Saini SS, Mueller PR. Prevalence of incidental Bochdalek's hernia in a large adult population. AJR Am J Roentgenol. 2001;177(2):363–6. https://doi.org/10.2214/ajr.177.2.1770363.
38. De Martini WJ, House AJ. Partial Bochdalek's herniation; computerized tomographic evaluation. Chest. 1980;77(5):702–4. https://doi.org/10.1378/chest.77.5.702.
39. Raymond GS, Miller RM, Muller NL, Logan PM. Congenital thoracic lesions that mimic neoplastic disease on chest radiographs of adults. AJR Am J Roentgenol. 1997;168(3):763–9. https://doi.org/10.2214/ajr.168.3.9057531.
40. Thomas GG, Clitherow NR. Herniation through the foramen of Morgagni in children. Br J Surg. 1977;64(3):215–7.
41. Paris F, Tarazona V, Casillas M, et al. Hernia of Morgagni. Thorax. 1973;28(5):631–6. https://doi.org/10.1136/thx.28.5.631.
42. Gaerte SC, Meyer CA, Winer-Muram HT, Tarver RD, Conces DJ, Jr. Fat-containing lesions of the chest. Radiographics 2002;22 Spec No(suppl_1):S61–78. https://doi.org/10.1148/radiographics.22.suppl_1.g02oc08s61.
43. Tarver RD, Conces DJ Jr, Cory DA, Vix VA. Imaging the diaphragm and its disorders. J Thorac Imaging. 1989;4(1):1–18. https://doi.org/10.1097/00005382-198901000-00007.
44. Wayne ER, Campbell JB, Burrington JD, Davis WS. Eventration of the diaphragm. J Pediatr Surg. 1974;9(5):643–51. https://doi.org/10.1016/0022-3468(74)90101-8.

4 Traumatic Skeletal Injuries

4.1 Introduction

Traumatic thoracic skeletal injury is fairly common in an emergency setting. The causes of thoracic trauma include traffic accidents, falls from heights, assaults, and blows from blunt objects. Chest CT is frequently performed to evaluate the presence and complications of thoracic skeletal injury. Such injuries may be missed on chest imaging since the interpreting radiologists may not be familiar with thoracic skeletal injuries, or may pay more attention to other organs such as the lungs, mediastinum, and cardiovascular system. However, accurate diagnosis of skeletal injury is important because the presence of a skeletal injury is associated with a patient's symptoms and can provide diagnostic clues for more severe associated injuries.

4.2 Rib Fractures

Rib fracture is the most common form of blunt thoracic injury. The sensitivity of chest radiography for rib fractures is limited; only two-thirds of rib fractures are observed on chest CT [1]. Diagnosis of associated complications such as pneumothorax, hemothorax, or flail chest is clinically important. Isolated rib fractures generally have relatively low morbidity and mortality, and do not necessarily alter patient management or outcome in uncomplicated cases [2].

4.2.1 Imaging Findings

The stage (acute vs. chronic), location, and type of rib fractures should be described in radiologic reports. In acute-stage traumatic rib fractures, the margin of the fractured segments is sharp, and no callus formation is seen (Fig. 4.1). As rib fractures heal, they show osteosclerosis (Fig. 4.1), callus formation, and bony remodeling. Since old rib fractures are not related to a current trauma, differentiating between acute and old rib fractures helps to understand the severity of the current trauma.

There are five types of rib fractures: stress, buckle, nondisplaced, displaced, and segmental fractures [3]. Stress rib fractures are overuse injuries that can result from repetitive contraction of chest wall muscles or the diaphragm at the point where it attaches to the ribs. This type of fracture is commonly caused by chronic cough or repetitive motion in athletes (e.g., weightlifters, pitchers, golfers, and rowers). Buckle rib fracture (Fig. 4.2) occurs when there is disruption of either the inner or the outer cortex, with no observable fracture of the other cortex; it is often missed. When a fracture remains anatomically aligned, it is classified as non-displaced (Fig. 4.3). On the other hand, when there is a substantial abnormality in alignment, a rib fracture is classified as displaced (Fig. 4.4). Segmental fractures are high-grade injuries with at least two separate complete fractures located in the same rib.

T. J. Kim et al., *Emergency Chest Radiology*, https://doi.org/10.1007/978-981-33-4396-2_4

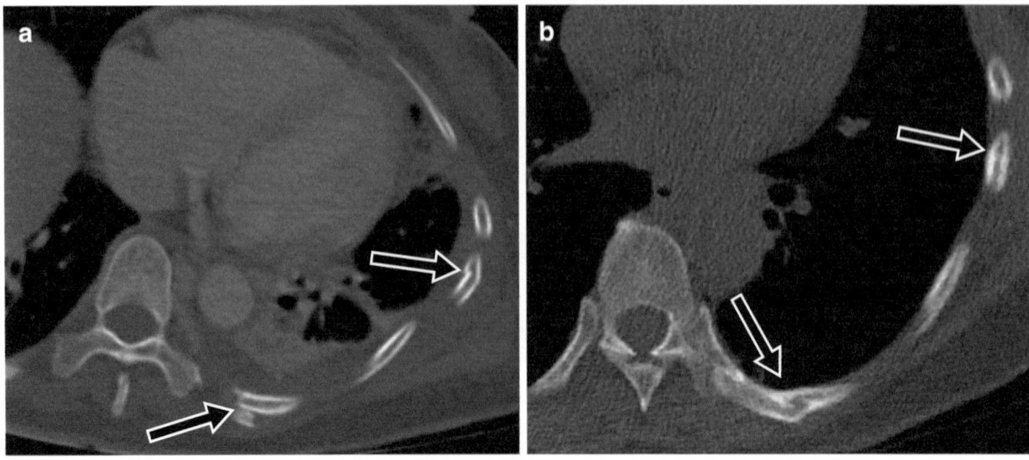

Fig. 4.1 Acute and chronic rib fractures. (**a**) Chest CT shows acute fractures at the left seventh and ninth ribs (arrows). Note that the margins of the fractured segments are sharp and no callus formation is seen. (**b**) Chest CT was performed 16 months after (**a**). As the rib fractures heal, they show osteosclerosis, callus formation, and bony remodeling (arrows)

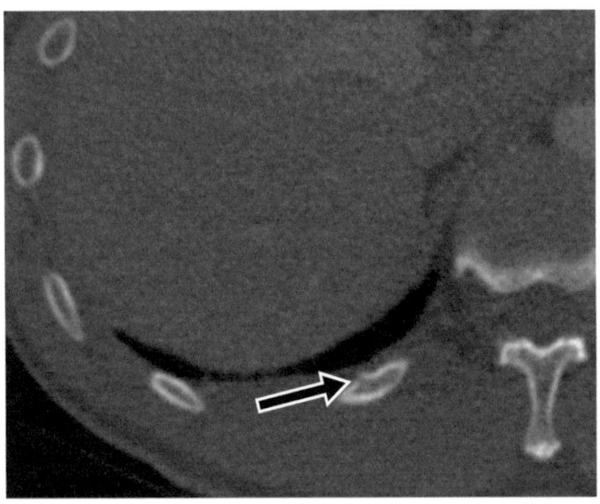

Fig. 4.2 Buckle fracture. Chest CT shows buckle fracture. Only the inner cortex is disrupted (arrow)

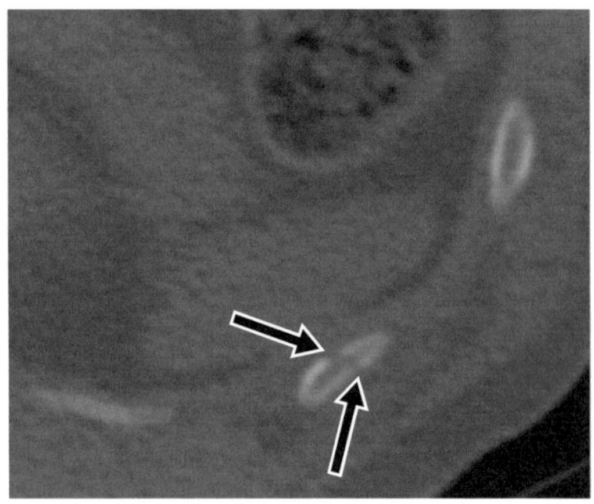

Fig. 4.3 Non-displaced fracture. Chest CT shows acute non-displaced fracture (arrows). Note that the fractured ribs remain anatomically aligned

Segmental fractures may remain anatomically aligned but often become partially or significantly displaced at one or both fracture sites. Segmental fractures (Fig. 4.5) are important to note as segmental rib fractures affecting three or more contiguous rib levels are associated with increased risk for flail chest.

4.2.2 Complications

Key complications associated with rib fracture include pain, hemothorax, pneumothorax, extrapleural hematoma, pulmonary contusion, pulmonary laceration, cardiovascular injury, flail chest, and abdominal solid-organ injury. Older patients are at especially high risk of complications. Treatment for the vast majority of patients with rib fractures is supportive care, including pain control and pulmonary rehabilitation. Associated traumatic injuries in the lungs and pleura are described in detail in Chaps. 1 and 13.

Extrapleural hematoma develops when an intact parietal pleura prevents blood from draining into the pleural space [4]. Up to 81% of patients with extrapleural hematoma have associated rib fracture [5]. Chest CT findings enable differentiation between extrapleural hematoma and hemothorax, which warrant different treatment approaches. Unlike hemothorax, fluid collection with high attenuation causes inward displacement of the extrapleural fat on chest CT (Fig. 4.6). Most cases of extrapleural hematoma associated with rib fractures show slightly convex or linear contours. In these cases, the hematoma probably has a venous origin and no surgical management is required. However, when the size of the hematoma is large and its contour shows biconvexity, the hematoma probably has an arterial origin and may require surgical management.

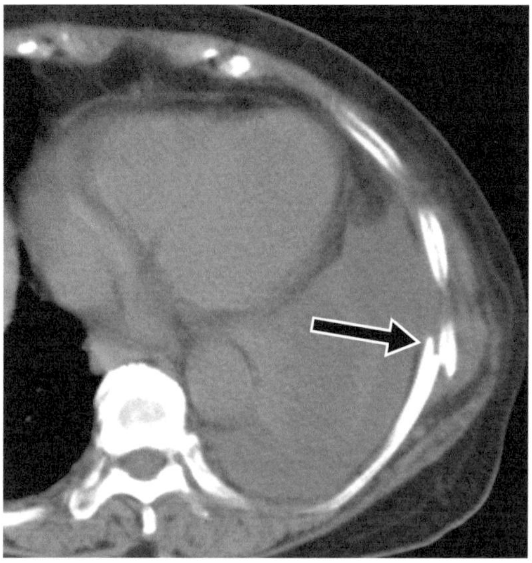

Fig. 4.4 Displaced fracture. Chest CT shows acute displaced fracture (arrow) with hemothorax. Note that there is a substantial abnormality in alignment

Among vascular injury, the intercostal arteries and veins are particularly susceptible to injury from concomitant rib fracture, as they are located in the costal groove along the inferior aspect of the ribs. Active intercostal arterial or venous hemorrhage may lead to hemothorax or extrapleural hematoma, depending on the location and degree of regional pleural and muscular disruption.

Flail chest is the most severe form of blunt thoracic injury. The diagnosis of flail chest is made clinically. Clinically, a flail segment is associated with paradoxical respiratory motion. Flail chest serves as a marker for significant intrathoracic injury, since more than one-half of affected patients have associated injuries that require surgical treatment [6, 7]. These patients often require mechanical ventilation for prolonged periods [8].

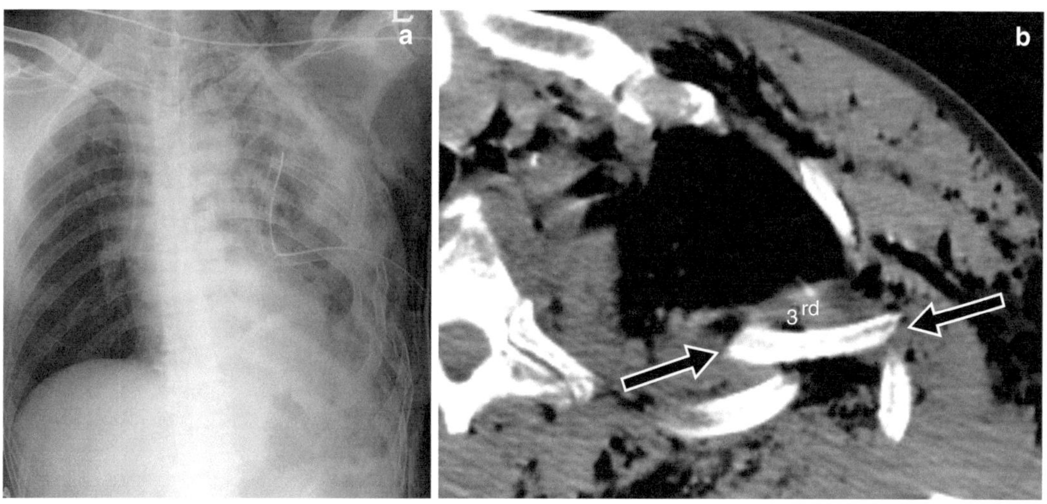

Fig. 4.5 Segmental fractures. (**a**) Chest radiograph shows multiple left rib fractures and subcutaneous emphysema. (**b**) Segmental fracture refers to two separate complete fractures located in the same rib. Note that there are two fracture sites (arrows) in the left third rib which result in the fractured segment. (**c**, **d**) Segmental rib fractures affecting three or more contiguous rib levels (arrows) are associated with increased risk of flail chest

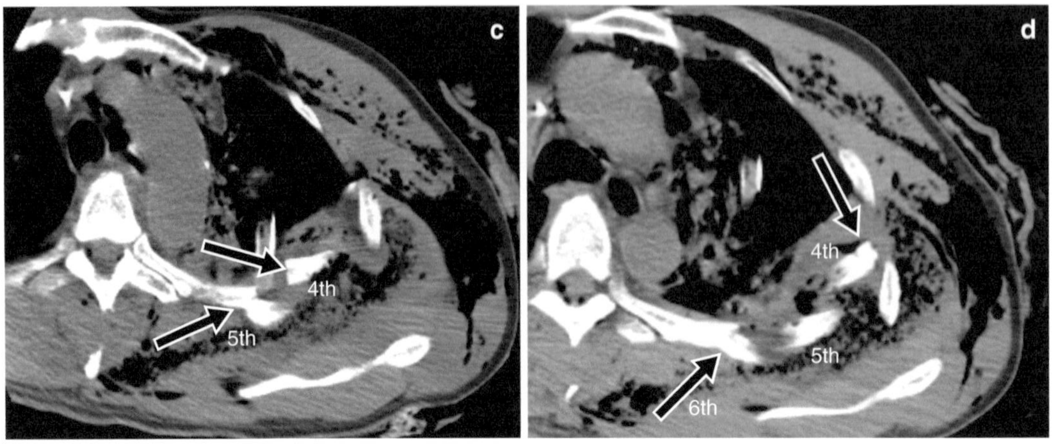

Fig. 4.5 (continued)

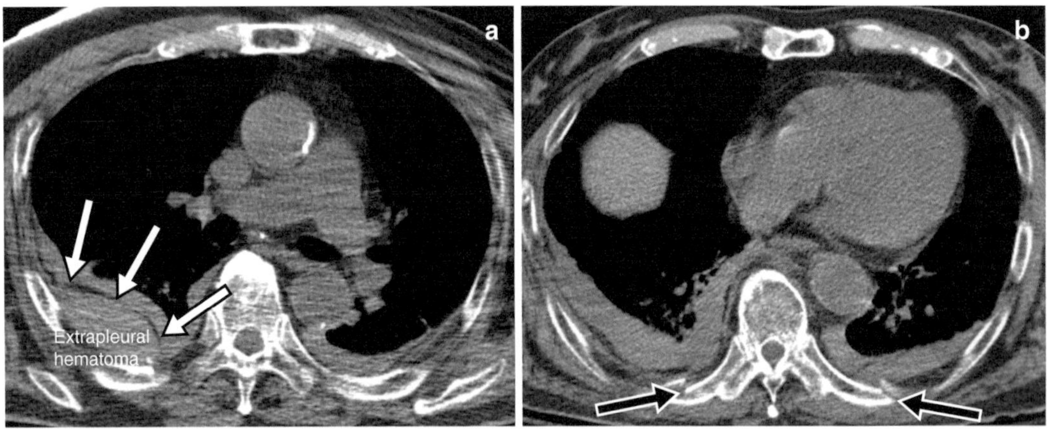

Fig. 4.6 Extrapleural hematoma and hemothorax associated with rib fractures. (**a**) Unlike hemothorax, extrapleural hematoma causes inward displacement of the extrapleural fat (white arrows) visible on chest CT. (**b**) Chest CT shows bilateral hemothorax associated with bilateral acute rib fractures (black arrows). The average attenuation value of the hemothorax was 67 Hounsfield units, which is higher than that of simple fluid (0–10 Hounsfield units)

Flail chest is accompanied by pulmonary contusion in most cases (Fig. 4.7). The respiratory impairment that occurs in such cases is due to the underlying pulmonary parenchymal injury rather than chest wall instability [9].

Lower rib fractures (9th–12th) are associated with abdominal solid organ injury (liver [right ribs], spleen [left ribs], and kidneys) (Figs. 4.8 and 4.9). Fractures of the first through third ribs are considered to be high-energy trauma because these ribs are well-protected by the scapulae, clavicles, and musculature [7]. These fractures may be associated with brachial plexus injury or subclavian vascular injuries.

4.2.3 Costochondral Junction Fracture

Patients with multiple consecutive rib fractures often have costochondral junction fractures (Fig. 4.10). Costochondral junction fractures contribute to rib cage instability and may manifest clinically as late as weeks or months after the acute trauma. They are common in cases of high-energy blunt chest trauma, but they are easily missed even on chest CT [10]. In one recent study, the incidence of costochondral junction fractures was 20% (114 of 574) in patients with thoracic trauma; however, the initial detection rate was

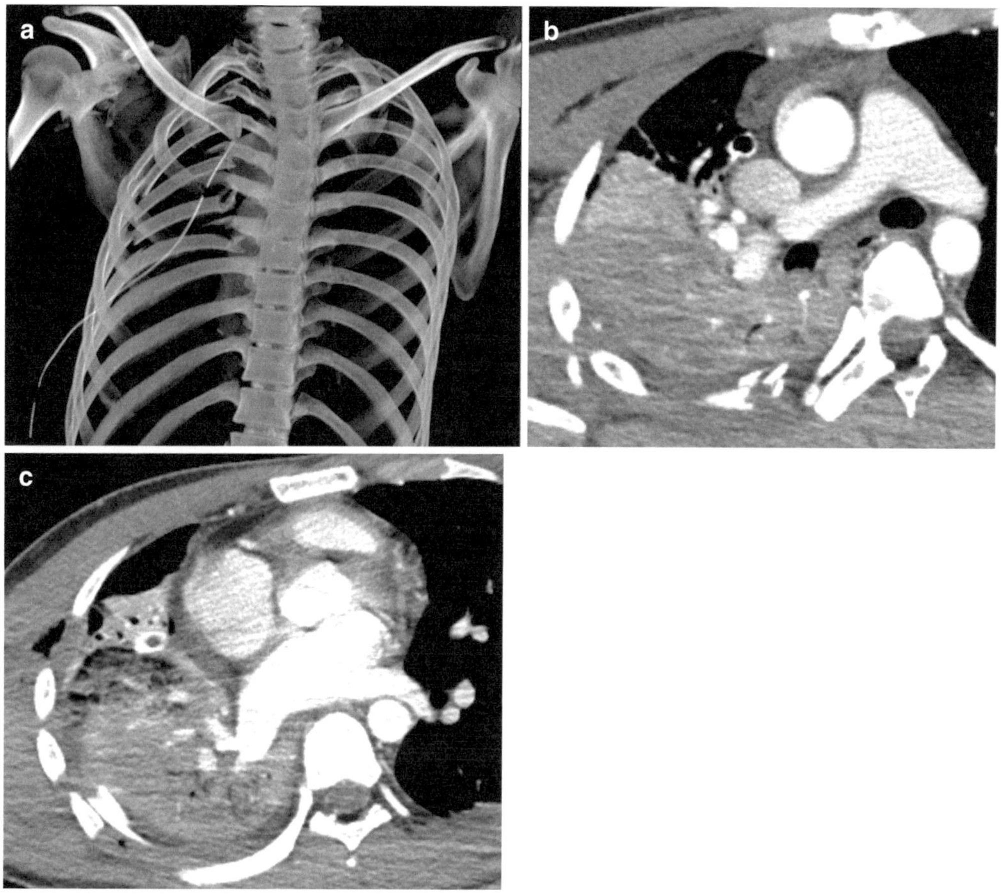

Fig. 4.7 Flail chest. (**a**) CT scan with 3D reconstruction shows multiple consecutive segmental fractures from the right second to right seventh ribs, which suggests the possibility of flail chest. (**b**, **c**) Chest CT images show contusion mixed with atelectasis in the right lung

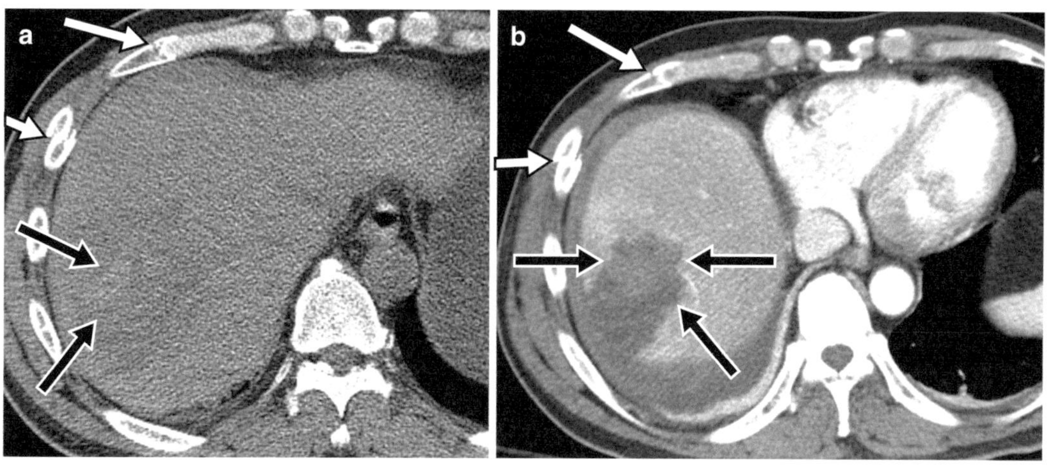

Fig. 4.8 Liver laceration. (**a**) Non-contrast chest CT shows multiple acute right lower ribs fractures (white arrows) from the right fifth to eighth ribs. In addition to the rib fractures, there is a high-attenuating lesion in the liver (black arrows), which raises concern for liver laceration and hematoma. (**b**) Contrast-enhanced chest CT confirms the presence of a liver laceration (black arrows) in addition to the right rib fractures (white arrows)

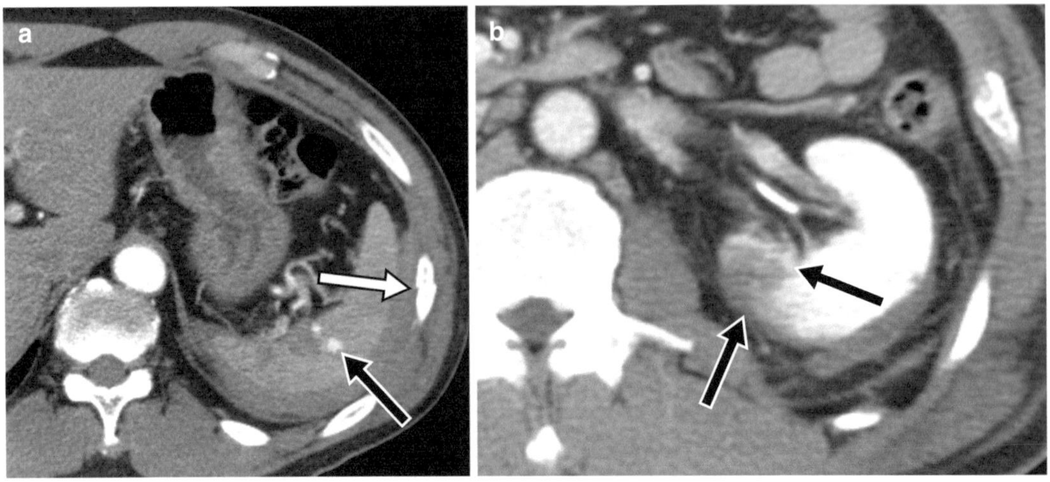

Fig. 4.9 Spleen and kidney injury. (**a**) There are multiple rib fractures (white arrow) from the left third to left tenth ribs. In addition, a small pseudoaneurysm (black arrow) was suspected in the spleen. (**b**) There is also a small laceration in the left kidney (black arrows)

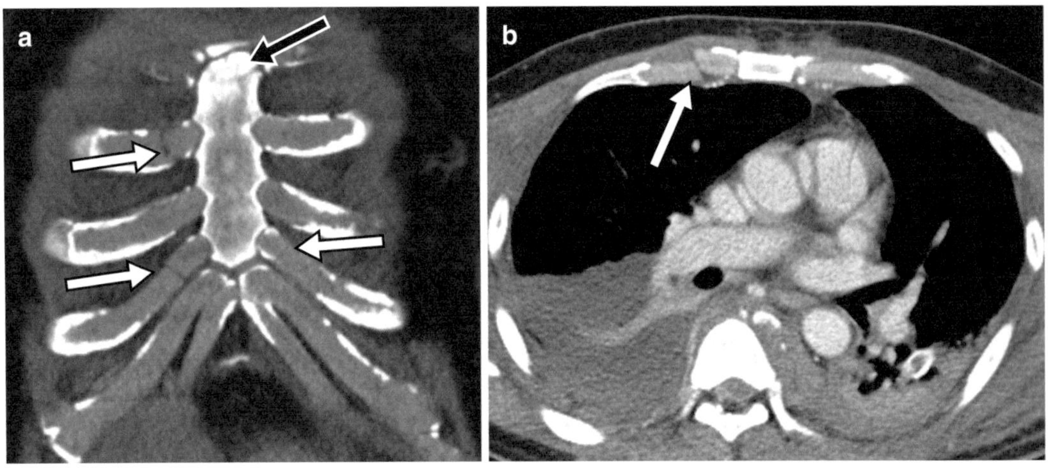

Fig. 4.10 Costochondral fracture. (**a**) There are multiple fractures in the bilateral costal cartilage (white arrows) and sternum (black arrow). (**b**) There is a fracture at the right third costal cartilage (white arrow) with mild displacement

only 40% (45 of 114) [10]. Aortic and hepatic injuries were more common in patients with costochondral junction fractures than in patients without costochondral junction fractures [10].

4.2.4 CPR-Related Rib Fractures

Rib fractures are often seen in patients who survived after cardiopulmonary resuscitation (CPR) (Fig. 4.11). In a retrospective analysis of 40 patients who survived CPR, CT detected rib fractures in 65% of patients ($n = 26$) [11]. These fractures are commonly anterior, on the left side, and are more numerous in the elderly. The diagnosis of such fractures in CPR survivors may be important, as approximately half of CPR survivors with rib fractures experience complications, and the presence of rib fractures in these patients may impair ventilation and compromise recovery.

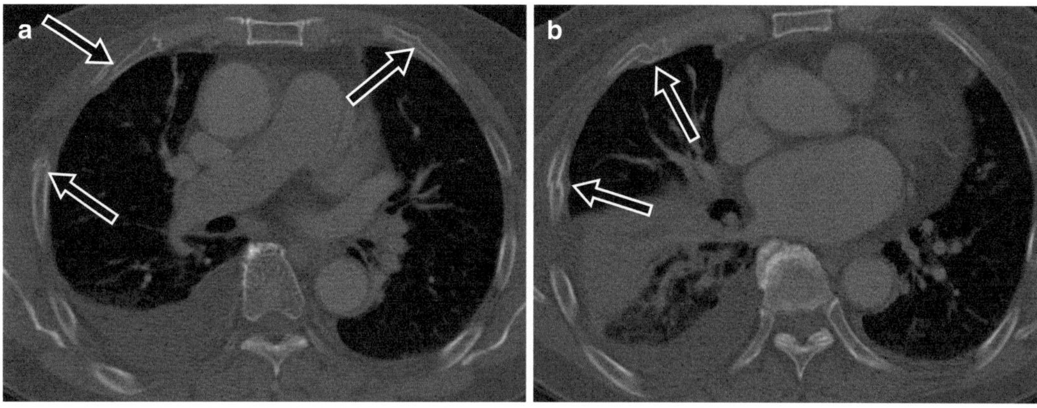

Fig. 4.11 CPR-related rib fractures. (**a**, **b**) Chest CT shows multiple bilateral anterolateral acute rib fractures (arrows) that were caused by cardiac compression

4.3 Clavicle Fractures

Clavicle fractures are easy to diagnose and are nearly always seen on radiography (Fig. 4.12). Additional thoracic injuries are more prevalent in patients with a clavicle fracture (76% vs. 47%) than in those without [12]. Same-level falls and bicycle accidents were the most common mechanisms of injury [13]. Clavicle fractures most commonly occur within the middle third of the clavicle and exhibit some degree of displacement [14]. Whereas many midshaft clavicle fractures can be treated nonsurgically, surgical intervention may be required in cases of neurovascular compromise or significant fracture displacement [14]. Most fractures of the medial or lateral end of the clavicle can be treated nonsurgically if fracture fragments remain stable.

4.4 Sternum Fractures

The most common cause of sternal fracture is motor vehicle crash [15]: approximately 90% of sternal fractures are secondary to motor vehicle accidents (due to seat belt or airbag trauma or, if unrestrained, due to collision with the steering wheel) [16]. Most sternal fractures are diagnosed only on chest CT, and most of those without concomitant injury are of minimal clinical significance. In a study which investigated 292 patients with sternal fractures, less than 2.0% of patients diagnosed only by CT received clinical diagnoses of cardiac contusion, and none required surgical intervention [17]. Acute sternum fracture may cause adjacent retrosternal hematoma on chest CT (Fig. 4.13). The fracture line is sometimes difficult to identify on axial CT. In these cases, the presence of retrosternal hemorrhage or identifying the fracture line on coronal/sagittal CT images may be the clue that leads to diagnosis. A study that assessed cardiovascular injury associated with sternal fracture showed that sternal fracture, either with or without a retrosternal hematoma, is not a marker for blunt cardiac injury [18]. Adequate pain control is the appropriate treatment for isolated sternal fractures.

4.5 Sternoclavicular Dislocation

Injuries to the sternoclavicular joint are uncommon in comparison with other shoulder girdle injuries [19]. The strong ligamentous support of the sternoclavicular joint requires a tremendous direct or indirect force to produce an injury [19]. Sternoclavicular dislocation produces anterior chest wall pain, impairment of shoulder movement, and, in some cases, visible deformity over the sternoclavicular joint [20]. The most frequent mechanism of injury is compression over the lateral aspect of the shoulder. Most sternoclavicular

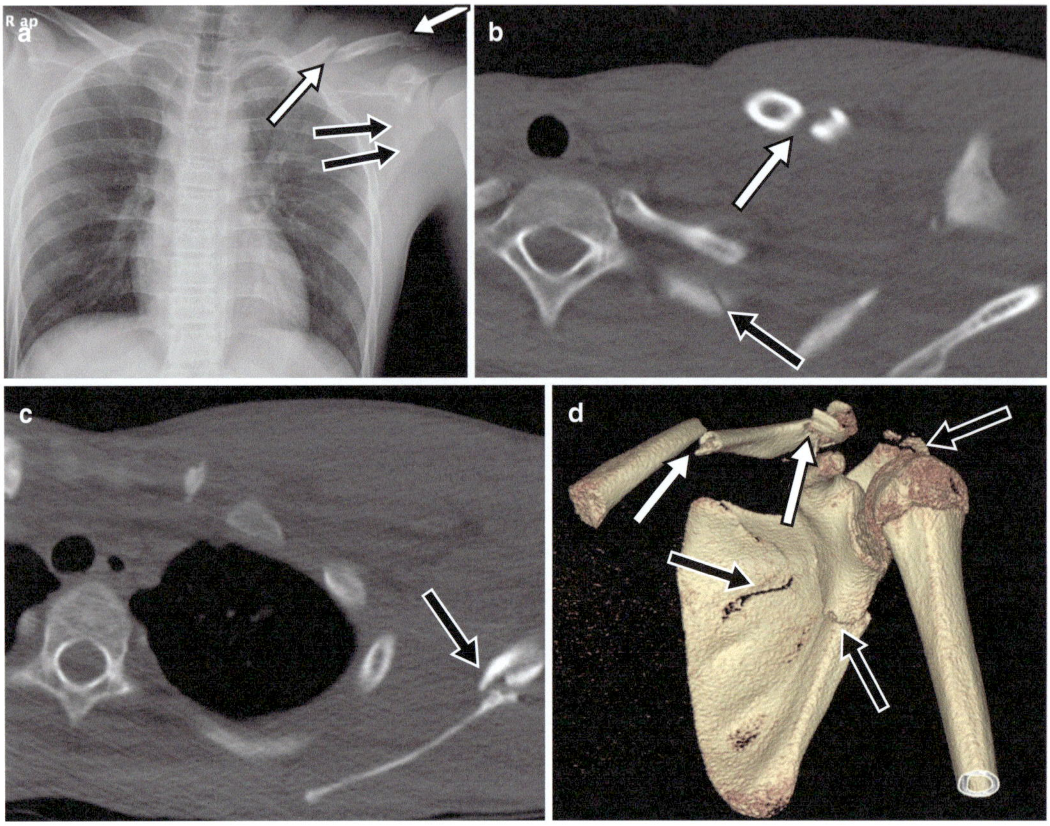

Fig. 4.12 Clavicle and scapula fractures. (**a**) Chest radiograph shows fractures of the clavicle (white arrows) and scapula (black arrows). Note that scapula fractures can be easily missed on chest radiograph. (**b**) There is a mid-shaft fracture in the clavicle (white arrow) and a left second rib fracture (black arrow). (**c**) A scapular fracture line (arrow) is noted. (**d**) 3D reconstructed CT image shows left clavicle fractures at the middle and distal portion (white arrows) and scapular fractures involving the body, lateral border, and acromion (black arrows)

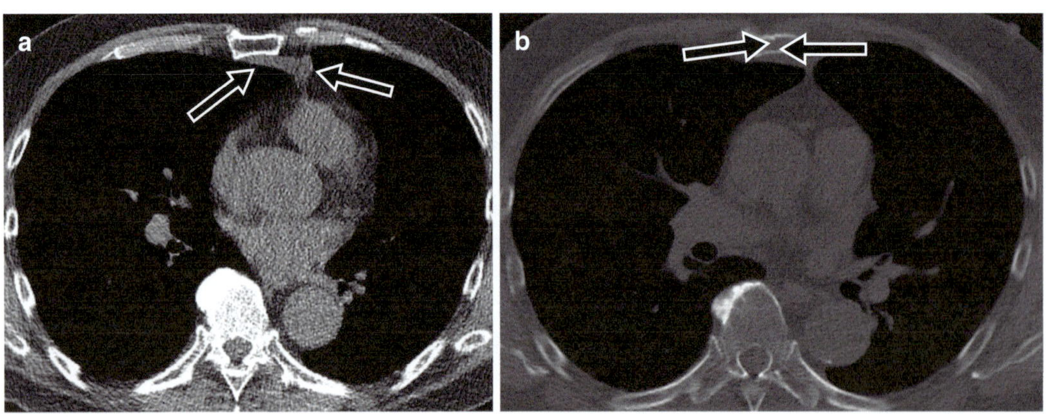

Fig. 4.13 Sternal fracture. (**a**) Chest CT shows a small retrosternal hematoma (arrows). (**b**) A sternal fracture is identified (arrows) on bone window setting

dislocations are anterior and have no major clinical significance [21] (Fig. 4.14). Posterior dislocation is rare but of greater concern due to its frequent association with mediastinal injuries (Fig. 4.15). The sternoclavicular joint is located adjacent to the subclavian vessels, brachial plexus, vagus nerve, recurrent laryngeal nerve, trachea, esophagus, larynx, and lungs [22]. Thus, complications of posterior dislocation of the sternoclavicular joints are common and include brachial plexus and vascular injury, pneumothorax, esophageal rupture, and death [23]. These lesions are seldom diagnosed by chest radiograph. Multidetector CT with multiplanar reconstruction and three-dimensional reconstructions allow accurate diagnosis and better visualization of the displaced clavicle and critical neurovascular and airway structures.

4.6 Scapular Fractures

Scapular fractures indicate that significant force was applied. Approximately 90% of patients with scapular fractures have associated injuries [24, 25], including ipsilateral subclavian, axillary, or

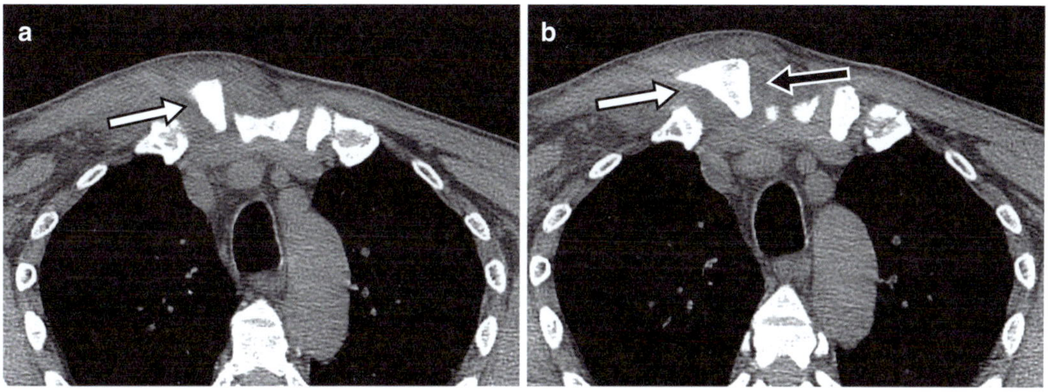

Fig. 4.14 Sternoclavicular dislocation (anterior). (**a**, **b**) Chest CT images show anterior dislocation of the right sternoclavicular joint (white arrow). Note accompanying mild soft tissue edema and fluid collection (black arrow)

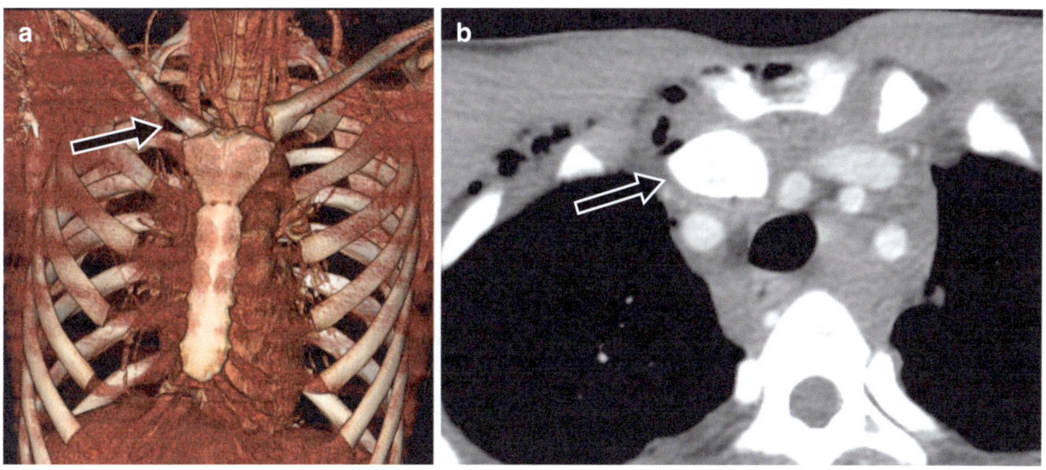

Fig. 4.15 Sternoclavicular dislocation (posterior). (**a**) 3D reconstructed CT image shows posterior dislocation of the right sternoclavicular joint (arrow). (**b**, **c**) Owing to the posterior dislocation of the right sternoclavicular joint (arrows), there is a narrowing in the left innominate vein. Subcutaneous emphysema is also noted

Fig. 4.15 (continued)

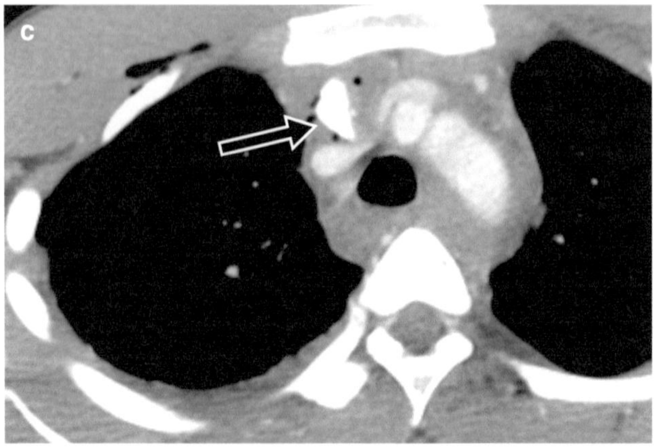

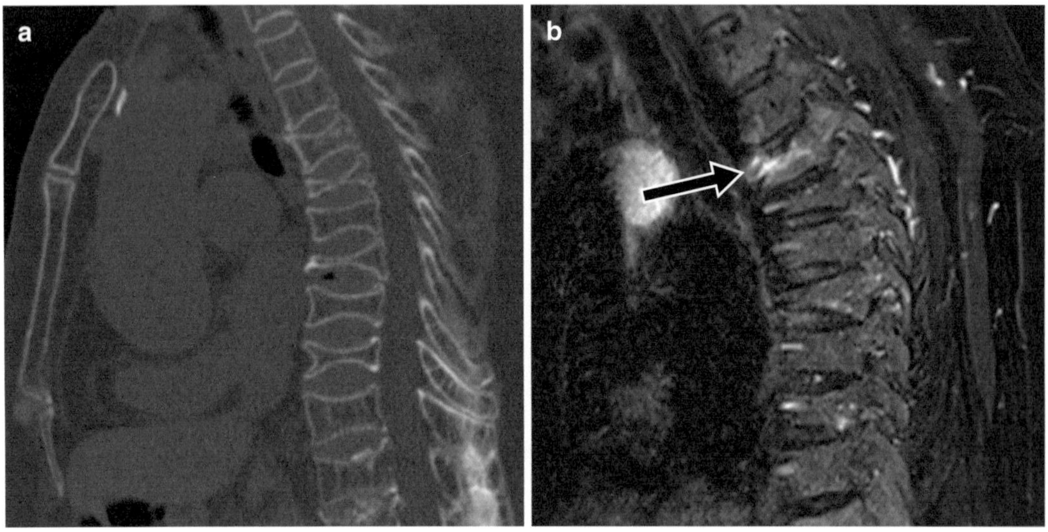

Fig. 4.16 Compression fracture. (**a**) Sagittal CT image shows multilevel compression fracture of T-L spine. (**b**) On spine MRI, high T2 signal intensity in the T4 vertebral body (arrow) indicates an acute compression fracture of the T4 vertebral body with retropulsion. Other vertebral bodies have old compression fractures

bronchial artery injury, pneumothorax, hemothorax, pulmonary injuries, and spinal injuries.

Scapular fractures may be overlooked at initial clinical evaluation due to more severe coexisting injuries (Fig. 4.12). The condition is also commonly missed on chest radiograph (missed in 43% of chest radiographs, although visible in 72% retrospectively [26]). Minimally to moderately displaced extra-articular fractures are generally managed nonoperatively [27]. Most fractures with glenoid involvement are treated operatively [25].

4.7 Spinal Fractures

In a recent analysis of data from 11,477 patients who underwent chest CT at trauma centers, thoracic spinal fracture was relatively uncommon (1.9%, $n = 217$). Most thoracic spinal fractures were associated with other thoracic injuries, and mortality was more closely related to these other injuries than to the thoracic spinal fracture itself [28].

In terms of fracture morphology, wedge compression and burst fractures secondary to hyperflexion and axial load mechanisms are the

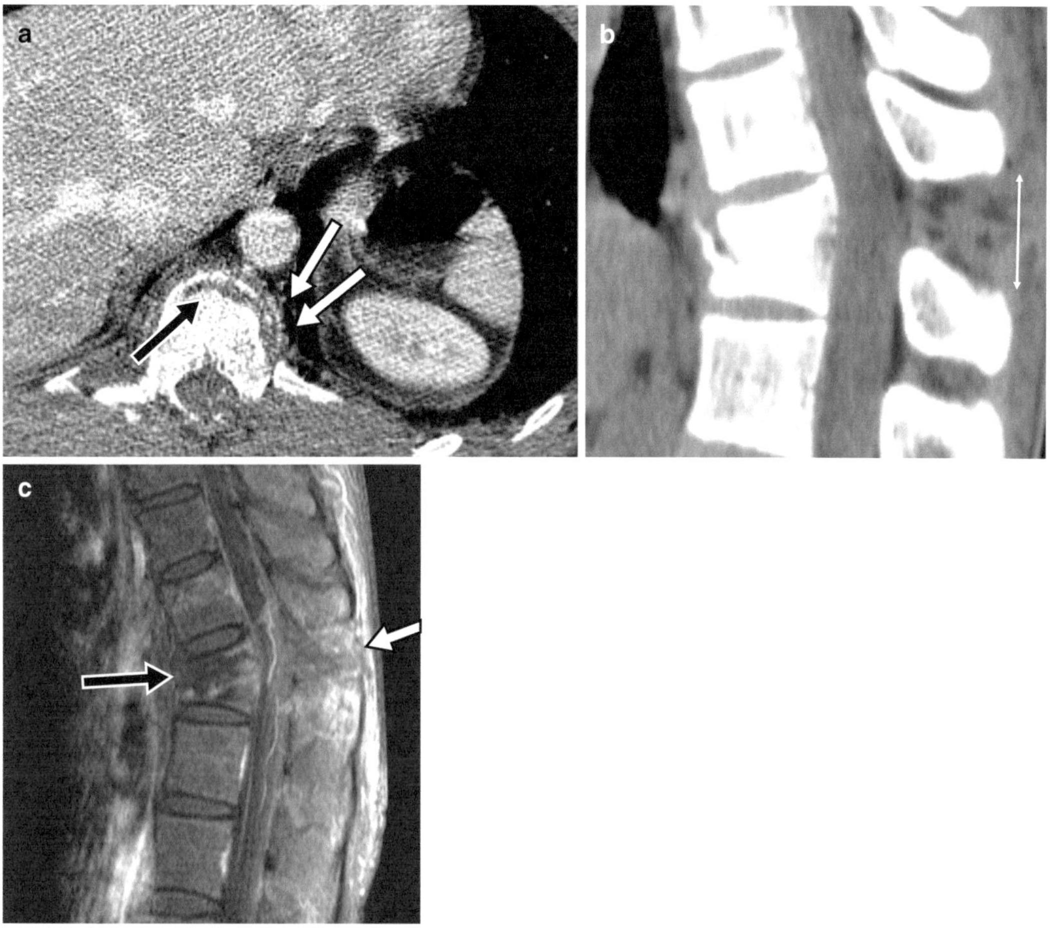

Fig. 4.17 Burst fracture. (**a**) On chest CT, a vertebral body fracture at the T12 level (black arrow) was detected. Note the air densities along the left paraspinal muscle (white arrows). (**b**) On spine CT, there is a burst fracture in the T12 vertebral body. Widening of the T11 and T12 interspinous space (arrow) suggests a combined posterior ligamentous complex injury. (**c**) Spine MRI confirms the burst fracture at the T12 vertebral body (black arrow) and interspinous ligament injury (white arrow)

predominant types of spinal fractures [28]. Compression injuries are defined on imaging as a visible loss of vertebral body height or disruption of the vertebral endplate [29] (Fig. 4.16). Burst fracture is a specific form of compression fracture of the vertebral body wherein a fragment arising from the posterior margin of the vertebral body is displaced into the spinal canal [30] (Fig. 4.17). The retropulsed fragment may result in neurologic injury to the spinal cord, conus medullaris, or cauda equina. Thoracic spinal injury with retropulsion may cause significant neurologic injury because the spinal canal in the thoracic area is narrow and blood supply to the cord is sparse.

The posterior ligamentous complex (PLC) is composed of the supraspinous ligament, interspinous ligament, ligamentum flavum, and facet capsule and is a critical predictor of spinal fracture stability [31]. It serves as the posterior tension band of the spinal column and protects the spine from excessive flexion, rotation, translation, and distraction. A lack of PLC integrity usually requires surgical intervention because of its poor healing potential. Without surgery, an injured PLC can result in progression of deformity after thoracolumbar burst fractures [31]. Spine MRI is the imaging method of choice for detecting PLC injury; it is not easy to visualize PLC injury on chest CT. However, PLC injury may be suspected when there are CT findings of facet joint widening, empty ("naked") facet joints, interspinous distance widening (Fig. 4.17), spinous process avulsion fracture, and vertebral body or facet subluxation or dislocation [32].

4.8 Summary

Rib fracture is the most common location for blunt thoracic injury. In patients with rib fractures, it is important to diagnose associated complications. Key complications associated with rib fracture include pain, hemothorax, pneumothorax, extrapleural hematoma, pulmonary contusion, pulmonary laceration, cardiovascular injury, flail chest, and abdominal solid organ injury. Costochondral junction fractures and CPR-related rib fractures are easily overlooked in clinical practice. In addition to the ribs, it is important to carefully examine the clavicle, sternum, sternoclavicular joint, scapula, and spine.

Key Points

- Segmental fractures are defined as the presence of at least two separate complete fractures located in the same rib.
- Segmental rib fractures affecting three or more contiguous rib levels are associated with increased risk of flail chest.
- The presence of retrosternal hematoma can be a diagnostic clue indicating sternal fracture.
- Posterior sternoclavicular dislocation is rare but of greater concern than anterior sternoclavicular dislocation because it is frequently associated with mediastinal injuries.
- Scapular fractures are easily overlooked on chest radiographs.
- Thoracic spinal injury with retropulsion may cause significant neurologic injury because the spinal canal in the thoracic area is narrow and the blood supply to the cord is sparse.

References

1. Murphy CE, Raja AS, Baumann BM, et al. Rib fracture diagnosis in the panscan era. Ann Emerg Med. 2017;70(6):904–9. https://doi.org/10.1016/j.annemergmed.2017.04.011.
2. Henry TS, Kirsch J, Kanne JP, et al. ACR appropriateness criteria® rib fractures. J Thorac Imaging. 2014;29(6):364–6. https://doi.org/10.1097/rti.0000000000000113.
3. Talbot BS, Gange CP Jr, Chaturvedi A, Klionsky N, Hobbs SK, Chaturvedi A. Traumatic rib injury: patterns, imaging pitfalls, complications, and treatment. Radiographics. 2017;37(2):628–51. https://doi.org/10.1148/rg.2017160100.
4. Rashid MA, Wikström T, Ortenwall P. Nomenclature, classification, and significance of traumatic extrapleural hematoma. J Trauma. 2000;49(2):286–90. https://doi.org/10.1097/00005373-200008000-00016.
5. Chung JH, Carr RB, Stern EJ. Extrapleural hematomas: imaging appearance, classification, and clinical significance. J Thorac Imaging. 2011;26(3):218–23. https://doi.org/10.1097/RTI.0b013e3181ebeaba.
6. Athanassiadi K, Gerazounis M, Theakos N. Management of 150 flail chest injuries: analysis of risk factors affecting outcome. Eur J Cardiothorac Surg. 2004;26(2):373–6. https://doi.org/10.1016/j.ejcts.2004.04.011.
7. Kaewlai R, Avery LL, Asrani AV, Novelline RA. Multidetector CT of blunt thoracic trauma. Radiographics. 2008;28(6):1555–70. https://doi.org/10.1148/rg.286085510.
8. Ciraulo DL, Elliott D, Mitchell KA, Rodriguez A. Flail chest as a marker for significant injuries. J Am Coll Surg. 1994;178(5):466–70.
9. Yeh DD, Lee J. Chapter 76: Trauma and blast injuries. In: Broaddus VC, editor. Murray & Nadel's textbook of respiratory medicine, vol. 2. 6th ed; 2016. p. 1356.
10. Nummela MT, Bensch FV, Pyhältö TT, Koskinen SK. Incidence and imaging findings of costal cartilage fractures in patients with blunt chest trauma: a retrospective review of 1461 consecutive whole-body CT examinations for trauma. Radiology. 2018;286(2):696–704. https://doi.org/10.1148/radiol.2017162429.
11. Kim EY, Yang HJ, Sung YM, et al. Multidetector CT findings of skeletal chest injuries secondary to cardiopulmonary resuscitation. Resuscitation. 2011;82(10):1285–8. https://doi.org/10.1016/j.resuscitation.2011.05.023.
12. van Laarhoven J, Hietbrink F, Ferree S, et al. Associated thoracic injury in patients with a clavicle fracture: a retrospective analysis of 1461 polytrauma patients. Eur J Trauma Emerg Surg. 2019;45(1):59–63. https://doi.org/10.1007/s00068-016-0673-6.
13. Kihlström C, Möller M, Lönn K, Wolf O. Clavicle fractures: epidemiology, classification and treatment of 2 422 fractures in the Swedish Fracture Register; an observational study. BMC Musculoskelet

Disord. 2017;18(1):82. https://doi.org/10.1186/s12891-017-1444-1.
14. van der Meijden OA, Gaskill TR, Millett PJ. Treatment of clavicle fractures: current concepts review. J Shoulder Elbow Surg. 2012;21(3):423–9. https://doi.org/10.1016/j.jse.2011.08.053.
15. Sacks D, Baxter B, Campbell BCV, et al. Multisociety consensus quality improvement revised consensus statement for endovascular therapy of acute ischemic stroke. Int J Stroke. 2018;13(6):612–32. https://doi.org/10.1177/1747493018778713.
16. von Garrel T, Ince A, Junge A, Schnabel M, Bahrs C. The sternal fracture: radiographic analysis of 200 fractures with special reference to concomitant injuries. J Trauma. 2004;57(4):837–44. https://doi.org/10.1097/01.ta.0000091112.02703.d8.
17. Perez MR, Rodriguez RM, Baumann BM, et al. Sternal fracture in the age of pan-scan. Injury. 2015;46(7):1324–7. https://doi.org/10.1016/j.injury.2015.03.015.
18. Rashid MA, Ortenwall P, Wikström T. Cardiovascular injuries associated with sternal fractures. Eur J Surg. 2001;167(4):243–8. https://doi.org/10.1080/110241501300091345.
19. Yeh GL, Williams GR Jr. Conservative management of sternoclavicular injuries. Orthop Clin North Am. 2000;31(2):189–203. https://doi.org/10.1016/s0030-5898(05)70140-1.
20. Sangster GP, González-Beicos A, Carbo AI, et al. Blunt traumatic injuries of the lung parenchyma, pleura, thoracic wall, and intrathoracic airways: multidetector computer tomography imaging findings. Emerg Radiol. 2007;14(5):297–310. https://doi.org/10.1007/s10140-007-0651-8.
21. Mirvis SE. Imaging of acute thoracic injury: the advent of MDCT screening. Semin Ultrasound CT MR. 2005;26(5):305–31. https://doi.org/10.1053/j.sult.2005.08.001.
22. Sernandez H, Riehl J. Sternoclavicular Joint dislocation: a systematic review and meta-analysis. J Orthop Trauma. 2019;33(7):e251–5. https://doi.org/10.1097/bot.0000000000001463.
23. Groh GI, Wirth MA, Rockwood CA Jr. Treatment of traumatic posterior sternoclavicular dislocations. J Shoulder Elbow Surg. 2011;20(1):107–13. https://doi.org/10.1016/j.jse.2010.03.009.
24. Ideberg R, Grevsten S, Larsson S. Epidemiology of scapular fractures. Incidence and classification of 338 fractures. Acta Orthop Scand. 1995;66(5):395–7. https://doi.org/10.3109/17453679508995571.
25. Zlowodzki M, Bhandari M, Zelle BA, Kregor PJ, Cole PA. Treatment of scapula fractures: systematic review of 520 fractures in 22 case series. J Orthop Trauma. 2006;20(3):230–3. https://doi.org/10.1097/00005131-200603000-00013.
26. Harris RD, Harris JH Jr. The prevalence and significance of missed scapular fractures in blunt chest trauma. AJR Am J Roentgenol. 1988;151(4):747–50. https://doi.org/10.2214/ajr.151.4.747.
27. Cole PA, Gauger EM, Schroder LK. Management of scapular fractures. J Am Acad Orthop Surg. 2012;20(3):130–41. https://doi.org/10.5435/jaaos-20-03-130.
28. Bizimungu R, Sergio A, Baumann BM, et al. Thoracic spine fracture in the panscan era. Ann Emerg Med. 2020; https://doi.org/10.1016/j.annemergmed.2019.11.017.
29. Patel AA, Dailey A, Brodke DS, et al. Thoracolumbar spine trauma classification: the Thoracolumbar Injury Classification and Severity Score system and case examples. J Neurosurg Spine. 2009;10(3):201–6. https://doi.org/10.3171/2008.12.spine08388.
30. Atlas SW, Regenbogen V, Rogers LF, Kim KS. The radiographic characterization of burst fractures of the spine. AJR Am J Roentgenol. 1986;147(3):575–82. https://doi.org/10.2214/ajr.147.3.575.
31. Radcliff K, Su BW, Kepler CK, et al. Correlation of posterior ligamentous complex injury and neurological injury to loss of vertebral body height, kyphosis, and canal compromise. Spine (Phila Pa 1976). 2012;37(13):1142–50. https://doi.org/10.1097/BRS.0b013e318240fcd3.
32. Khurana B, Sheehan SE, Sodickson A, Bono CM, Harris MB. Traumatic thoracolumbar spine injuries: what the spine surgeon wants to know. Radiographics. 2013;33(7):2031–46. https://doi.org/10.1148/rg.337135018.

5 Traumatic and Nontraumatic Esophageal Emergency

5.1 Introduction

Esophageal injury is rare, but when it does occur it is associated with significant morbidity and mortality in the setting of trauma. Esophageal injuries can be iatrogenic or traumatic. Endoscopic examination and surgical procedures are the most common causes of iatrogenic esophageal injuries. The mechanisms of traumatic esophageal injuries include blunt and penetrating injuries. Foreign body ingestion, spontaneous rupture (e.g., Boerhaave syndrome), and ingestion of acid/caustic substances can also cause esophageal injuries. Esophageal perforation leads to transmural disruptions of the esophagus and leakage of esophageal and gastric contents into the mediastinum. This leads to inflammation of the mediastinum (e.g., mediastinitis) and subsequent sepsis, contributing to increased morbidity and mortality. Therefore, early and accurate diagnosis is mandatory for proper management of patients with esophageal perforation. Foreign body impaction in the esophagus is discussed in Chap. 14: Foreign Bodies in the Thorax.

5.2 Esophageal Perforation

5.2.1 Mechanism of Injury

Most esophageal perforations are iatrogenic and occur following esophageal instrumentation. Iatrogenic esophageal perforations are typically caused by endoscopy of the upper gastrointestinal tract or surgical procedures such as thoracotomy, neck explorations, or anterior cervical diskectomy. The prevalence of esophageal injury is increasing with the widespread use of endoscopy in diagnostic and therapeutic procedures [1, 2]. Radiofrequency ablation of the left atrium may cause thermal injury to the anterior wall of the esophagus, leading to esophageal necrosis and perforation (Fig. 5.1) [3]. The most common cause of non-iatrogenic esophageal perforation is spontaneous rupture, followed by foreign body ingestion (Fig. 5.2), trauma (Fig. 5.3), and malignancy (Table 5.1) [4].

The mechanisms of traumatic esophageal injuries and modalities show substantial geographic differences. In penetrating esophageal injuries, gunshot wounds are much more common in the United States, while stab wounds are more prevalent in other countries [5]. Gunshot wounds can cause severe shearing, stretching, and blast injury to surrounding structures, which lead to tissue ischemia and necrosis, contributing to delayed or missed diagnosis, both of which significantly increase the morbidity and mortality rates. Stab wounds usually cause less damage to surrounding structures, but it may be difficult to identify the focal or minimal extent of a stab wound. Esophageal perforations in blunt thoracic trauma are uncommon, occurring in less than 1% of cases. Perforation can occur in blunt trauma due to a sudden increase in intra-abdominal pressure, leading to sudden stretching of the esophagogastric

T. J. Kim et al., *Emergency Chest Radiology*, https://doi.org/10.1007/978-981-33-4396-2_5

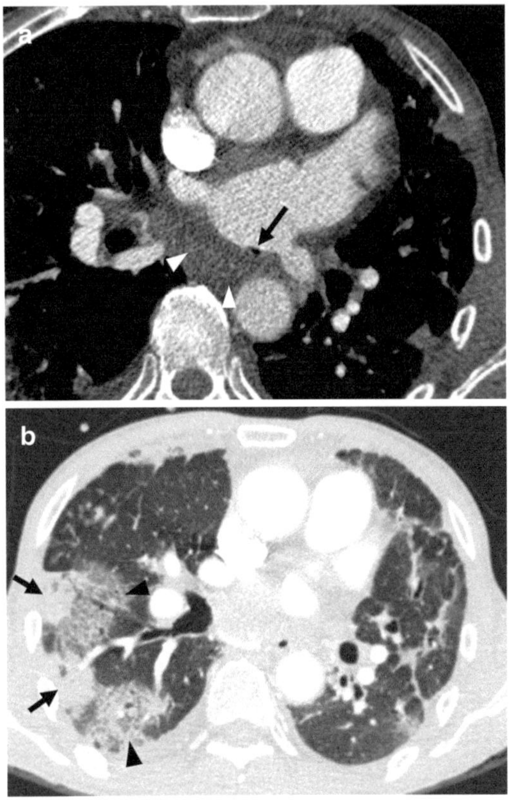

Fig. 5.1 Atrioesophageal fistula with mediastinitis and septic pneumonia in a 68-year-old man who underwent radiofrequency ablation due to intractable atrial fibrillation. (**a**) Mediastinal window image of a CT scan obtained at the level of the left atrium shows a focal air density (arrow) in the posterior aspect of the left atrium, suggesting an atrioesophageal fistula. Also note the diffuse increase in periesophageal soft tissue attenuation (arrowheads), indicating mediastinitis due to esophageal perforation. (**b**) Lung window image of a CT scan obtained at the level of the left atrium shows multiple nodular consolidations (arrows) with ground-glass opacity (arrowhead) in the periphery of the right lung, suggesting septic pneumonia. (Courtesy of Dr. Hye-Jeong Lee, Severance Hospital, Yonsei University School of Medicine)

junction and shearing forces that result in tearing of the esophageal wall. The esophagus, unlike other hollow viscera, does not have a serosal layer, and its absence promotes progression of esophageal injury and subsequent perforation. Spontaneous esophageal rupture not otherwise associated with a pre-existing condition accounts for approximately 15% of nontraumatic esophageal perforation. Possible mechanisms include

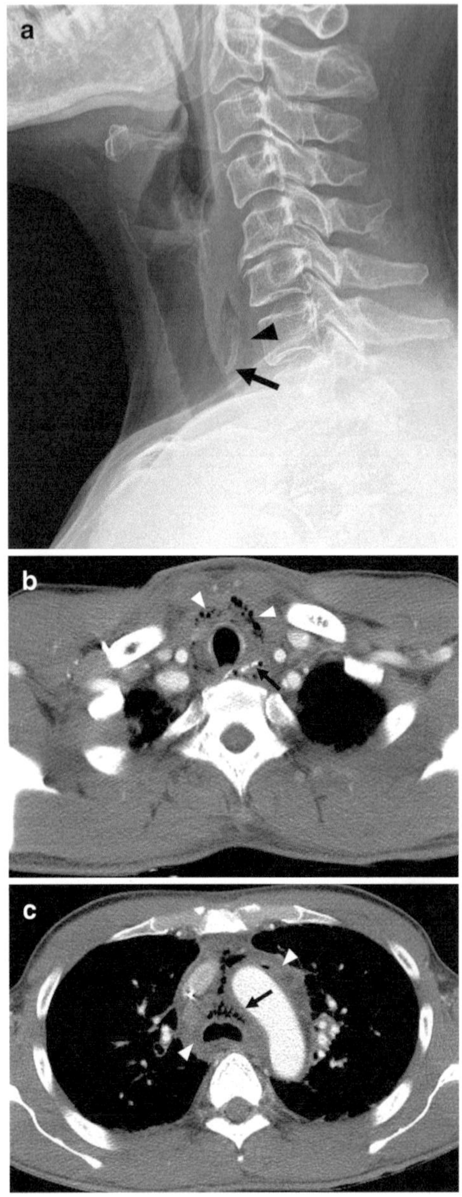

Fig. 5.2 Esophageal perforation due to foreign body ingestion in a 45-year-old woman. (**a**) Lateral radiograph of the neck shows a tubular radiopaque foreign body (arrow) in the retroesophageal area. Also note free gas collection (arrowhead) around the foreign body, suggesting esophageal perforation. (**b**) Mediastinal window image of a CT scan obtained at the level of the thoracic inlet shows a foreign body (arrow) in the cervical esophagus. Also note increased gas collection around the esophagus (arrowheads). (**c**) Mediastinal window image of a CT scan obtained at the level of the aortic arch demonstrates extension of gas in the mediastinum (arrow) and increased attenuation of the mediastinum with or without fluid collection, indicating mediastinitis (arrowheads)

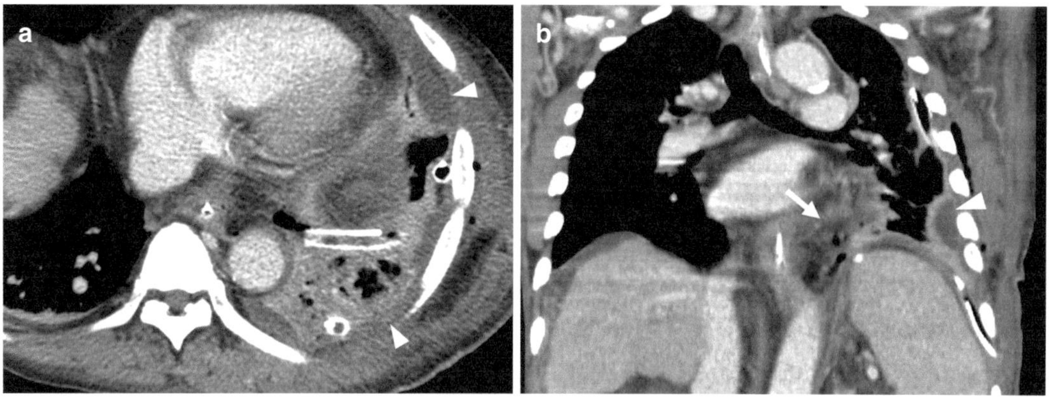

Fig. 5.3 Esophageal perforation due to a fall in a 54-year-old man. (**a**) Mediastinal window image of a CT scan obtained at the level of the left ventricle shows left pleural effusion (arrowhead) and atelectasis of the left lower lobe secondary to esophageal perforation. (**b**) Coronal reformatted CT image shows dirty infiltration and air collection in the mediastinum (arrow) secondary to esophageal perforation and loculated pleural effusion (arrowhead)

Table 5.1 Etiology and frequency of esophageal perforation

Etiology	Frequency (%)
Iatrogenic	59
Spontaneous	15
Foreign body ingestion	12
Trauma	9
Operative injury	2
Malignancy	1
Others	2

Adapted from Brinster CJ, Singhal S, Lee L, et al. Evolving options in the management of esophageal perforation. Ann Thorac Surg 2004; 77:1475

forceful vomiting, retching, or elevated intra-abdominal pressure, as seen in Boerhaave syndrome (Fig. 5.4) [6]. Because the esophagus is inherently surrounded and protected by nearby mediastinal structures, the presence of esophageal perforation is considered to be a marker for potentially critical injuries of the adjacent structures, including tracheal, vascular, pulmonary, diaphragmatic, and spinal injuries.

5.2.2 Imaging Diagnosis

Chest radiography is generally a baseline imaging modality in the trauma setting. A chest radiograph may demonstrate subcutaneous emphysema in the neck, unexplained or sustained pneumomediastinum, left-sided pneumothorax, and left-sided pleural effusion, which warrant complete investigation for suspected esophageal perforation and other combined injuries (Fig. 5.4a).

Evaluation of an esophageal injury can be performed with esophagography. Water-soluble contrast agents (i.e., gastrografin) are first used to avoid the negative effects of barium spillage into the mediastinum, which may cause mediastinitis; if no leak is identified, a follow-up study using barium sulfate should be performed [7]. One study reported that esophagography using barium detected esophageal perforation in 4 of 18 patients, which were initially missed with esophagography using water-soluble agents [8]. Diluted CT contrast media may be used in cases that carry risks of mediastinitis due to leakage and pneumonitis due to aspiration tendency. It should also be noted that esophagography has a false-negative rate of up to 10% in patients with esophageal perforation because of inflammation and edematous swelling of the esophagus. Compared to CT, esophagography is difficult to perform in uncooperative, neurologically impaired, or critically ill patients. CT is useful for evaluating nontransmural esophageal perforation, which is undetectable on esophagography. In addition, CT can be useful for evaluating nonpenetrating esophageal injury, where endoscopy is generally not indicated because air insufflation during endoscopy may exacerbate the injury. CT is useful to establish the full extent of an injury

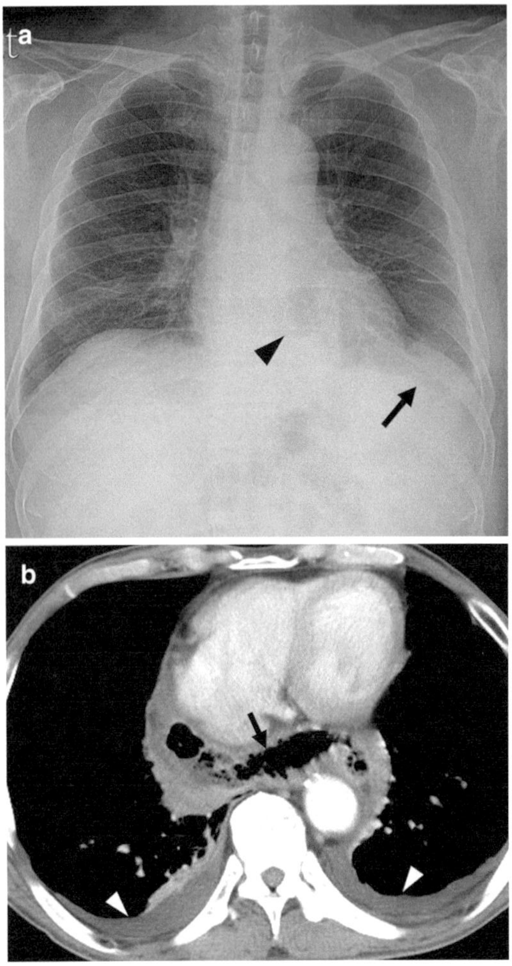

Fig. 5.4 Boerhaave's syndrome in a 70-year-old man who presented with substernal chest pain and vomiting after heavy drinking. (**a**) Chest radiograph shows retrocardiac air densities (arrowhead), indicating free gas due to esophageal perforation. Also note the left pleural effusion (arrow). (**b**) Mediastinal window image of a CT scan obtained at the level of the left ventricle shows free gas and fluid collection in the mediastinum (arrow) due to esophageal perforation, with bilateral pleural effusion (arrowheads). The presence of an esophageal rupture was confirmed at surgery

and guide subsequent therapeutic decisions. CT can demonstrate the site of esophageal perforation and may also uncover indirect signs of esophageal perforation, such as gas and/or fluid collection around the esophagus, esophageal wall thickening, and thickening of the esophageal mucosa at the site of perforation (Figs. 5.3 and 5.4). Air or air-fluid collection in the mediastinum, pleural effusion, pneumopericardium, and pneumoperitoneum may also be seen [9–11]. CT scan additionally be used to evaluate simultaneous injuries of nearby structures, such as the aorta and major airways.

5.2.3 Boerhaave's Syndrome

Boerhaave's syndrome is a spontaneous perforation of the esophagus that results from a sudden increase in intraesophageal pressure combined with negative intrathoracic pressure such as severe straining or vomiting. It is most prevalent in males with alcoholism, and is also associated, though less frequently, with childbirth, seizure, prolonged coughing or laughing, and weightlifting. The tears in Boerhaave's syndrome are vertically oriented, 1–4 cm in length, and typically occur along the left posterolateral wall of the esophagus, 3–6 cm above the esophagogastric junction. Boerhaave's syndrome should be differentiated from a Mallory-Weiss tear, which is a partial-thickness tear of the esophageal wall. Most cases of Mallory-Weiss tear have a benign course and are treated with supportive care. The classic radiographic findings of Boerhaave's syndrome include pneumomediastinum, pleural effusion, and pneumothorax with a left-sided predilection, and subcutaneous emphysema in the neck and chest wall. Naclerio's V sign, representing pneumomediastinum due to esophageal perforation, may be seen. CT may show esophageal perforation directly or indirectly by demonstrating periesophageal air collection at a supradiaphragmatic level (Fig. 5.4) [12]. CT with oral contrast medium may show direct contrast spillage into the mediastinum or pleural cavity.

5.3 Esophageal Intramural Dissection

5.3.1 Mechanism of Injury

Esophageal intramural dissection is also called intramural rupture, intramural tear, or esophageal apoplexy. It is different from the mucosal tear seen in Mallory-Weiss syndrome and from transmural tear in esophageal perforation. The lesion in the esophageal intramural dissection is typically long and usually spares the lower thoracic esophagus, in contrast to Mallory-Weiss tear or Boerhaave's syndrome, both of which are usually short tears and involve the distal esophagus just above the esophagogastric junction. Patients often present with sudden-onset severe chest pain, odynophagia, dysphagia, and hematemesis. A recent history of instrumentation is the most important risk factor, followed by foreign body impaction and forceful vomiting. If the hematoma accumulates in the false lumen resulting from the intramural dissection, it is called a dissecting intramural hematoma. Intramural hematoma of the esophagus may be eccentric or concentric depending on the extent of the hematoma along the esophageal wall [13]. Spontaneous intramural hematoma has also been reported in patients with coagulopathy or anticoagulant drug therapy. Intramural dissection of the esophagus has an excellent prognosis and can be managed conservatively [14, 15].

5.3.2 Imaging Diagnosis

Chest radiography is usually normal but may demonstrate widening ofthe mediastinum and a hyperlucent elongated mass in the retrocardiac area. Esophagography and CT can demonstrate a mucosal flap with submucosal collection of contrast material or gas, giving the esophagus a typical double-barreled appearance, similar to the true and false lumens seen in aortic dissection (Fig. 5.5). Dissection frequently occurs posterior to the true lumen with longitudinal directionality, and, therefore, the full extent of dissection may be best appreciated on coronal or sagittal reformatted images. Pneumomediastinum, pneumothorax, and intramural hematoma may be accompanied. Intramural dissection of the esophagus may progress to overt esophageal perforation (Fig. 5.5). CT is the modality of choice for evaluating intramural hematoma and may demonstrate an eccentric or concentric hyperattenuating lesion extending along the esophageal wall. The attenuation values of the hematoma vary

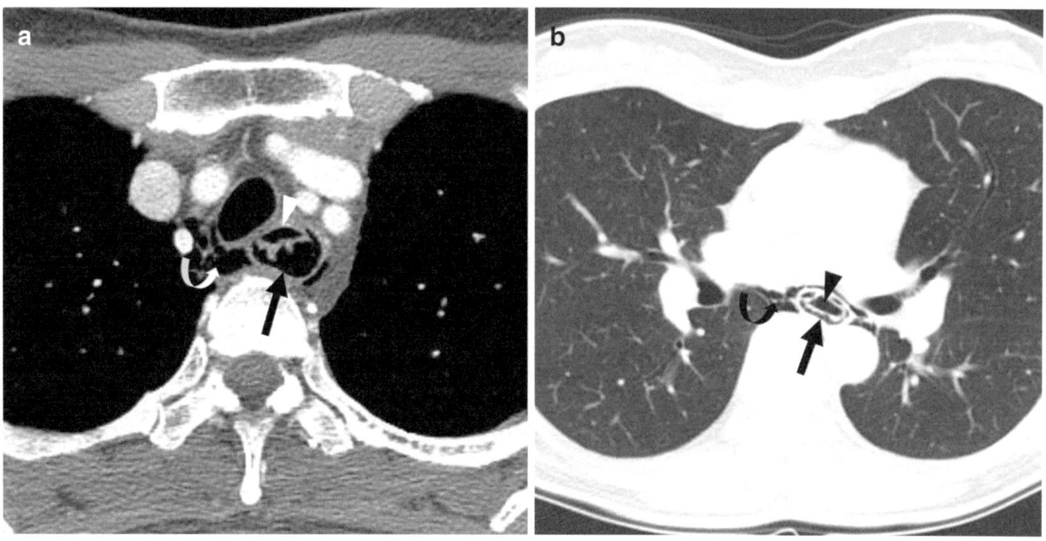

Fig. 5.5 Intramural dissection of the esophagus in a 45-year-old man who underwent a diagnostic esophagogastroscopy. (**a**) Mediastinal window image of a CT scan obtained at the level of the arch vessels shows an intramural dissection, which lead to anterior displacement of the true esophageal -lumen (arrowhead) due to gas collection in the false esophageal lumen (arrow). Also note pneumomediastinum (curved arrow), a finding indicative of esophageal perforation. (**b**) Lung window image of a CT scan obtained at the level of the pulmonary trunk demonstrates concentric intramural dissection of the esophagus. Note a true lumen (arrowhead), a false lumen (arrow), and pneumomediastinum (curved arrow)

depending on its stage. CT is also useful for excluding other diseases associated with severe chest pain, such as aortic dissection or myocardial infarction, from the differential diagnosis.

5.4 Esophageal Hernia (Paraesophageal)

5.4.1 Pathophysiology

Herniation of abdominal contents through the esophageal hiatus is common, especially in the elderly and obese individuals. With a provocative maneuver that increased intra-abdominal pressure, about half of patients were found to have herniation of the stomach into the chest on barium esophagography [16]. There are four types of hiatal hernia. Type 1, sliding hernia, is the most common, accounting for more than ~90% of all hiatal hernias (Fig. 5.6) [17]. In type I hernia, thinning and widening of the hiatus occurs, resulting in herniation of the esophagogastric junction into the posterior mediastinum. It is usually asymptomatic but may manifest symptoms related with gastroesophageal reflux. Obviously, there is no potential for incarceration. The less common types of hiatal hernia, types II, III, and IV, are called paraesophageal hernias, and together account for 5–15% of all hiatal hernias. The main clinical significance of paraesophageal hernia lies in the potential for mechanical obstruction. Type II hernia results from a defect in or weakness of the phrenoesophageal ligament, allowing a portion of the stomach to herniate through the hiatus while the esophagogastric junction remains fixed to the preaortic fascia and the median arcuate ligament (Fig. 5.7). Type III, or mixed, hiatal hernia is the second most common type. As a type III hernia increases in size, the stomach may roll up into the thorax. Because the stomach is fixed at the esophagogastric junction, the herniated stomach may rotate around its longitudinal axis, resulting in an organoaxial volvulus and strangulation (Fig. 5.8). Type IV hernia is associated with a large defect in the phreno-

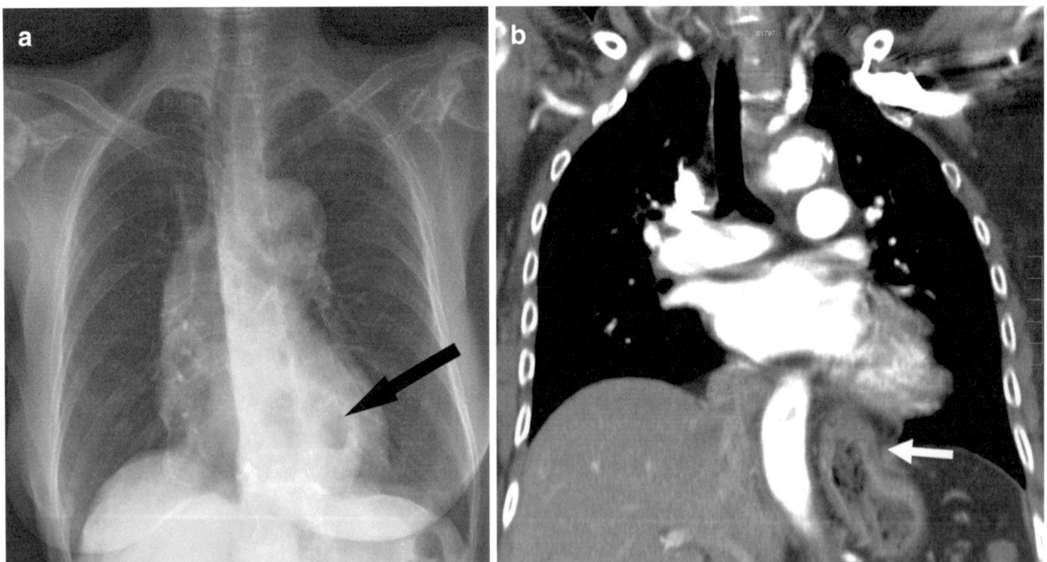

Fig. 5.6 Hiatal hernia (type I: sliding hernia) in an asymptomatic 78-year-old woman. (**a**) Chest radiograph shows an air-fluid level (arrow) in the retrocardiac area, a finding consistent with esophageal hiatal hernia (sliding type). (**b**) Coronal reformatted CT image shows a herniated stomach (arrow) through the widened hiatus. The esophagogastric junction is above the hiatus (not shown)

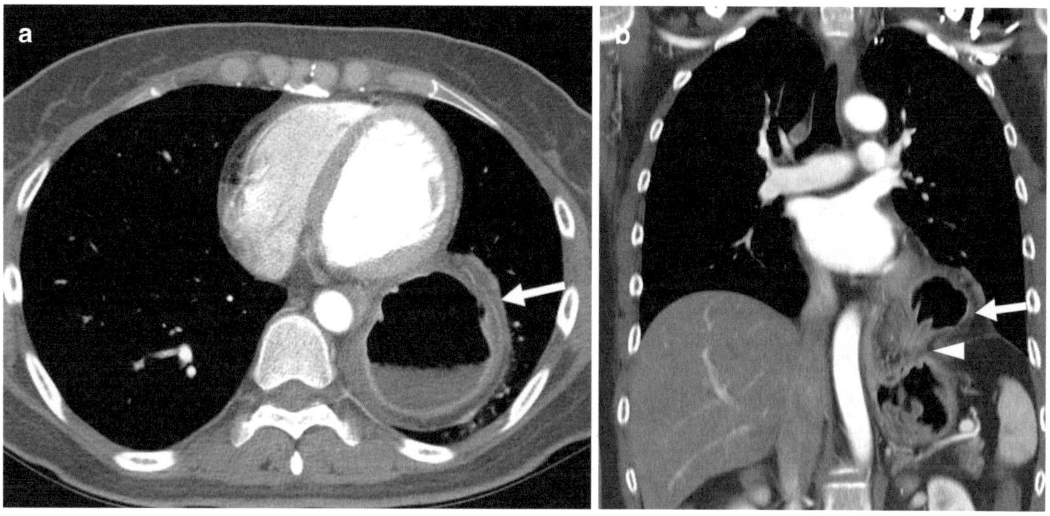

Fig. 5.7 Hiatal hernia (type II: paraesophageal hernia) in a 51-year-old woman with intermittent postprandial discomfort. (**a**) Mediastinal window image of a CT scan obtained at the level of the left ventricle shows a herniated stomach with an air-fluid level, suggesting gastric obstruction (arrow). (**b**) Coronal reformatted CT image depicts a narrowing point (arrow head) at the esophageal hiatus. Also note the distended, herniated stomach, suggesting gastric obstruction (arrow). Hernia repair was performed using a laparoscopic approach

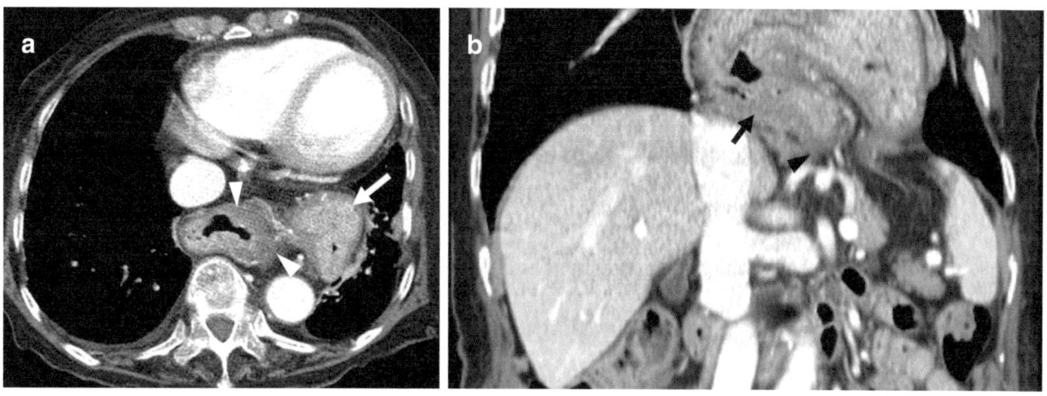

Fig. 5.8 Gastric volvulus in a 57-year-old woman with a type III hiatal hernia. (**a**) Mediastinal window image of a CT scan obtained at the level of the left ventricle shows the herniated fundus (arrow) and antrum (arrowheads) of the stomach into the left thorax. Note the poor contrast enhancement of the gastric wall (arrowhead) compared to that of the fundus (arrow), indicating ischemic changes due to the volvulus (arrow). (**b**) Coronal reformatted CT image demonstrates a herniated stomach through the esophageal hiatus (arrowhead). Note the poor bowel wall enhancement in the gastric antrum (arrow). The reversed positions of the greater and lesser curvatures (organoaxial gastric volvulus) were confirmed at surgery

esophageal membrane, allowing herniation of other abdominal organs, such as the colon, spleen, small bowel, and pancreas, along with the stomach. All symptomatic paraesophageal hiatal hernias should be repaired, particularly in those with acute obstructive symptoms or those that have undergone volvulus [18].

5.4.2 Imaging Diagnosis

In sliding hiatal hernia, chest radiographs may identify soft tissue opacity with or without air-fluid level in the retrocardiac area (Fig. 5.6). This opacity typically changes position or shape on follow-up imaging because the esophagogastric junction is able to move freely through the hiatus. In paraesophageal hernia, visceral gases other than those of stomach may be seen in cases of colon or small bowel herniation. Esophagography is useful for evaluating the size and reducibility of the hernia and precisely localizing the esophagogastric junction in relation to the esophageal hiatus. Barium is generally recommended for patients with paraesophageal hernia with gastric obstruction, given the increased aspiration risk in these patients and the risk of aspiration pneumonitis related with ionic water-soluble contrast agents [19].

CT can distinguish sliding from paraesophageal hernias by demonstrating cephalad migration of the esophagogastric junction or gastric fundus in relation to the esophageal hiatus. These differences, as well as the hernia site and any herniated organs, can best be appreciated on coronal or sagittal reformatted images (Figs. 5.6 and 5.7) [20]. CT is especially useful in urgent patients with suspected complications such as volvulus (Fig. 5.8). CT can confirm the diagnosis of gastric volvulus by showing herniation of the distal stomach into the left hemithorax and demonstrating the reversed position of the greater and lesser curvatures [21]. Ischemic changes in gastric volvulus can be seen as a lack of contrast enhancement of the gastric wall, with or without pneumatosis (Fig. 5.8).

5.5 Acute Phlegmonous Esophagitis

5.5.1 Pathophysiology

Phlegmonous infection may involve any part of the gastrointestinal tract, although the stomach is the most frequently involved segment [22]. Acute phlegmonous esophagitis is a rare and life-threatening condition characterized by bacterial infection of the submucosal and muscularis layers of the esophagus, causing intramural purulent discharge [23]. The pathogenesis of acute phlegmonous esophagitis is unclear but several predisposing factors, such as a mucosal defect or underlying chronic condition, especially diabetes mellitus, immune suppression, alcoholism, and malignancy have been suggested [24]. The most common pathogens involved are *Streptococcus* species, followed by *Staphylococcus*, *Escherichia coli*, *Haemophilus influenza*, *Proteus,* and *Clostridia* [25]. Histopathologically, the submucosal layer is thickened and infiltrated by neutrophils and plasma cells, with hemorrhage, necrosis, and thrombosis of submucosal blood vessels [22]. Patients may present with chest pain, odynophagia, dysphagia, and septicemia. Acute phlegmonous esophagitis usually progresses rapidly and has a high mortality rate due to subsequent perforation, mediastinitis, and sepsis. The mortality rate of phlegmonous enteritis is reportedly up to 42% [25]. Treatment of acute phlegmonous esophagitis includes infection control, including administration of systemic antibiotics, adequate nutritional support, preservation of digestive tract continuity, and timely surgical intervention if necessary [26]. Surgical resection is mandatory if there is extensive esophageal necrosis, esophageal stricture progression, and esophageal perforation [27].

5.5.2 Imaging Diagnosis

CT is the mainstay of diagnostic evaluation of acute phlegmonous esophagitis. CT demonstrates an intramural, circumferential, low-attenuation area of the esophagus surrounded by an enhancing peripheral rim [28], which corresponds to the histopathological findings of thickening and abscess formation in the submucosal and muscularis layers of the esophagus (Fig. 5.9). Clinically, the differentiation of acute phlegmonous esophagitis from dissecting intramural hematoma is difficult because the two conditions have similar CT findings and clinical presentations. High attenuation on pre-contrast CT images, eccentric location, and the absence of signs and symptoms related to acute infection may help differentiate dissecting intramural hematoma from acute phlegmonous esophagitis.

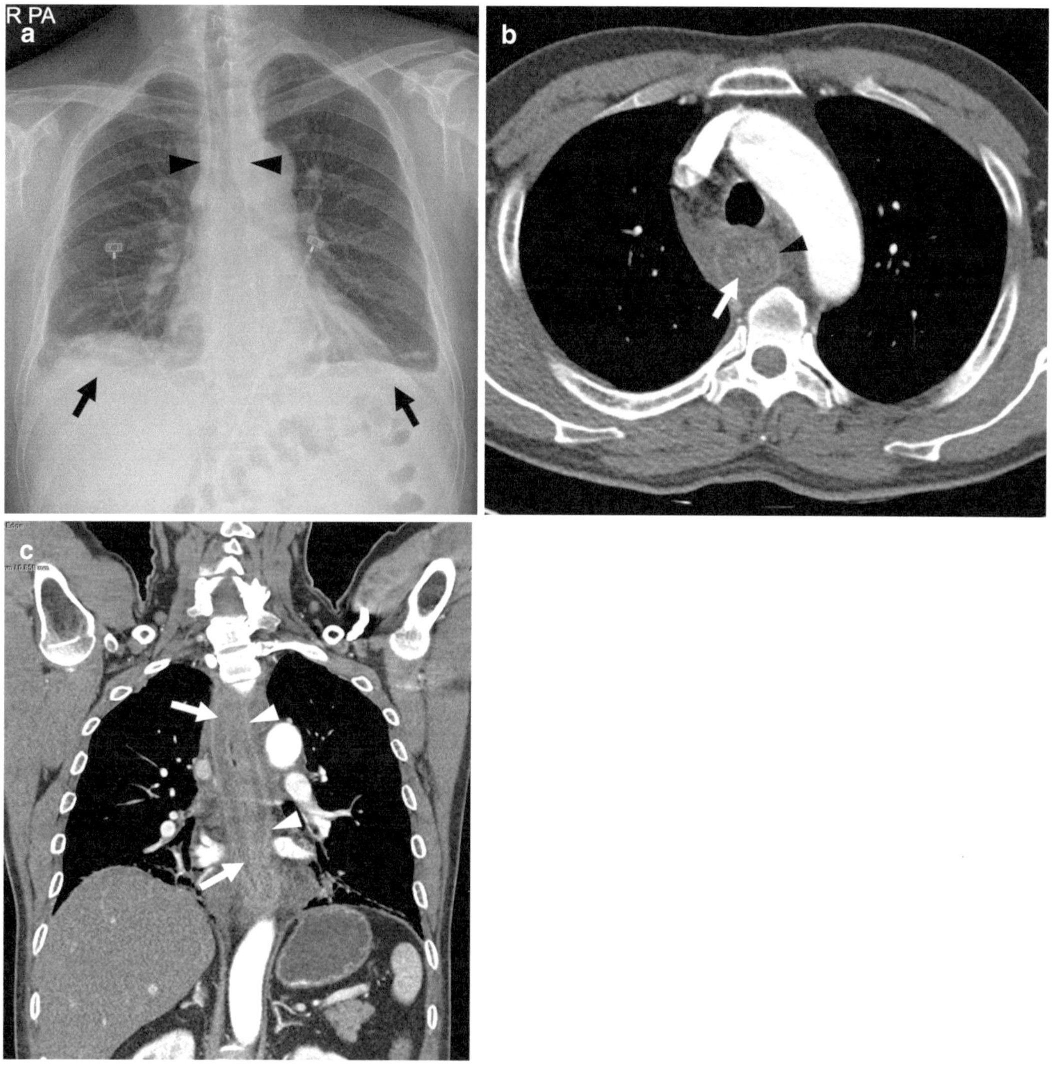

Fig. 5.9 Acute phlegmonous esophagitis in a 53-year-old man with odynophagia and fever. (**a**) Chest radiograph shows thickening of the bilateral paratracheal stripes (arrowheads), indicating mediastinitis. Also note bilateral pleural effusion (arrows). (**b**) Mediastinal window image of a CT scan obtained at the level of the aortic arch shows diffuse esophageal wall thickening with a circumferential, intramural low-attenuation area (arrow) surrounded by an enhanced peripheral rim (arrowhead). (**c**) Coronal reformatted CT image also demonstrates diffuse wall thickening with a low-attenuation area (arrows) and enhancing peripheral rim (arrowheads) along the entire esophagus, which are characteristic of acute phlegmonous esophagitis. Also note increased attenuation of the mediastinum along the esophagus, suggesting combined mediastinitis. The patient fortunately survived after broad-spectrum antibiotic treatment

5.6 Aortoesophageal Fistula

5.6.1 Pathophysiology

Aortoesophageal fistula (AEF) is a rare but life-threatening cause of upper gastrointestinal bleeding that can cause high-pressure aortic blood to enter the esophagus due to abnormal communication between the esophagus and the aorta [29]. It may develop secondary to esophageal or aortic conditions. The esophageal causes of AEF include foreign body ingestion, esophageal malignancy (Fig. 5.10), corrosive esophagitis, and postoperative complications

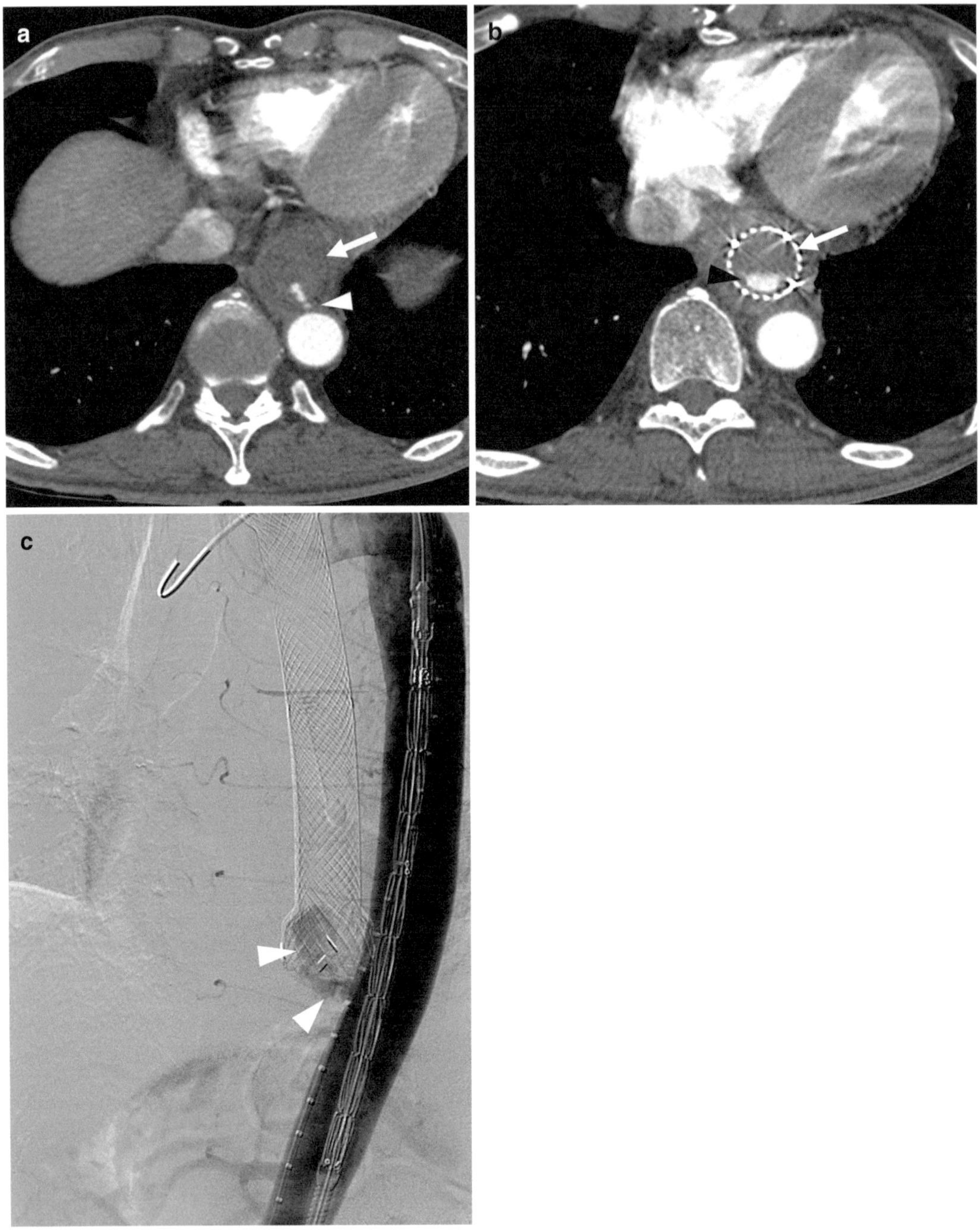

Fig. 5.10 Aortoesophageal fistula in a 64-year-old man who presented with massive hematemesis. The patient was undergoing combined chemoradiation therapy for esophageal carcinoma. (**a**) CT angiography of the thoracic aorta demonstrates contrast extravasation through a fistulous tract (arrowhead) between the descending thoracic aorta and the esophageal mass (arrow), a finding consistent with aortoesophageal fistula. (**b**) CT image at the level of the esophageal stent (arrow) shows collection of contrast media in the esophageal lumen (arrowhead). (**c**) Thoracic aortogram reveals contrast extravasation from the aorta to the esophagus (arrowheads). An aortic stent-graft placement was performed immediately

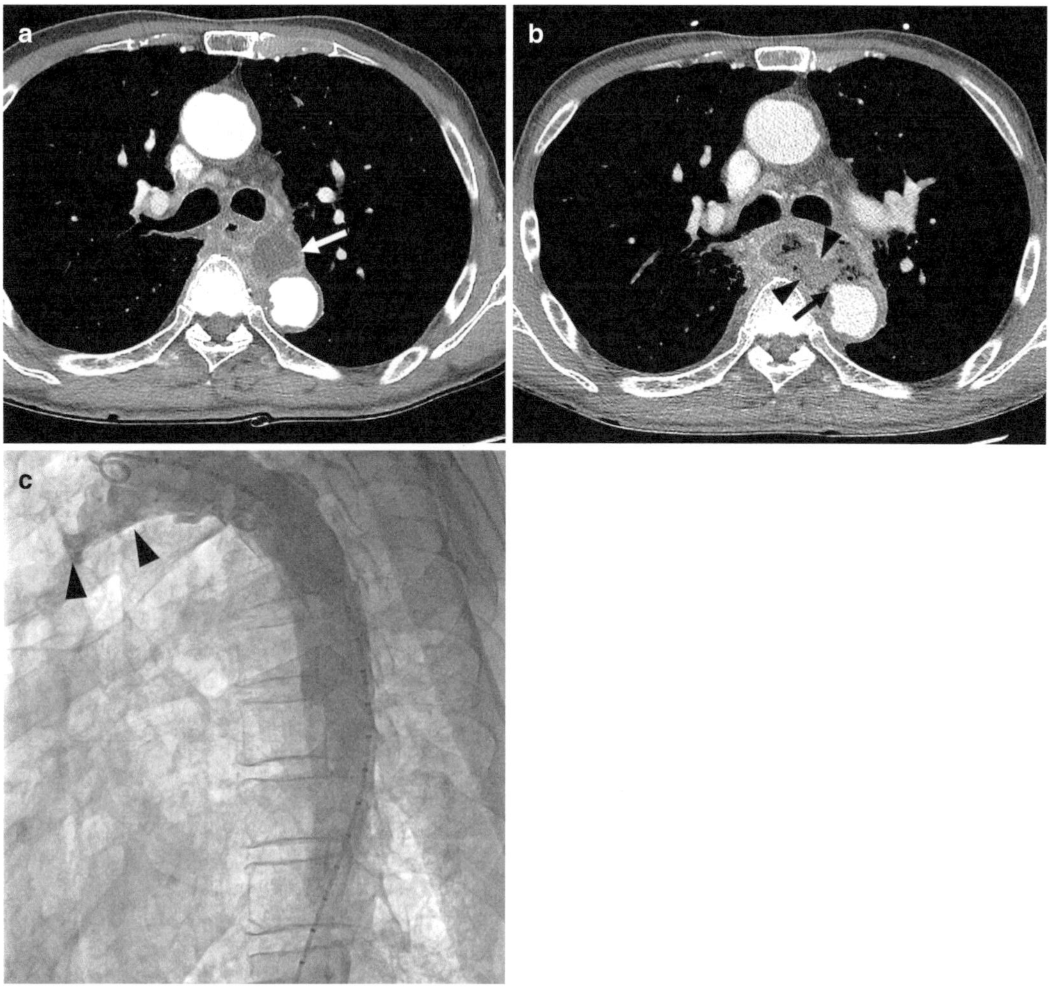

Fig. 5.11 Aorto-neoesophageal fistula due to mediastinal abscess in a 60-year-old man with a history of Ivor-Lewis operation due to esophageal cancer. (**a**) Mediastinal window image of a CT scan obtained at the level of the main bronchi shows a mediastinal abscess (arrow) adjacent to the descending thoracic aorta. (**b**) CT image obtained 2 weeks after (**a**) shows perforation of the neoesophagus (pulled-up stomach, arrowheads) with large abscess formation. Note an outpouching lesion (arrow) from the aorta, indicating aorto-neoesophageal fistula. The patient expired due to sepsis. (**c**) Thoracic aortogram confirms contrast leakage (arrowheads) from the thoracic aorta

(Fig. 5.11) [30]. The aortic causes of AEF include thoracic aortic aneurysm, ruptured atheromatous plaque, penetrating atherosclerotic ulcer, and complications of prosthetic aortic grafting (Fig. 5.12) and aortic reconstructive surgeries [30]. The diagnosis of AEF can be made at the time of presentation because the clinical presentation is so unique. Patients may present with the triad of midthoracic pain, sentinel arterial hemorrhage, and a symptom-free interval followed by exsanguination (Chiari's triad) [31]. The bright red arterial blood characteristically distinguishes the bleeding of AEF from that of other etiologies, such as esophageal variceal or gastric bleeding. Patients in stable condition may undergo diagnostic work-up such as endoscopy or CT angiography, but unstable patients should undergo immediate surgery as no survivors have been reported with nonsurgical management [29].

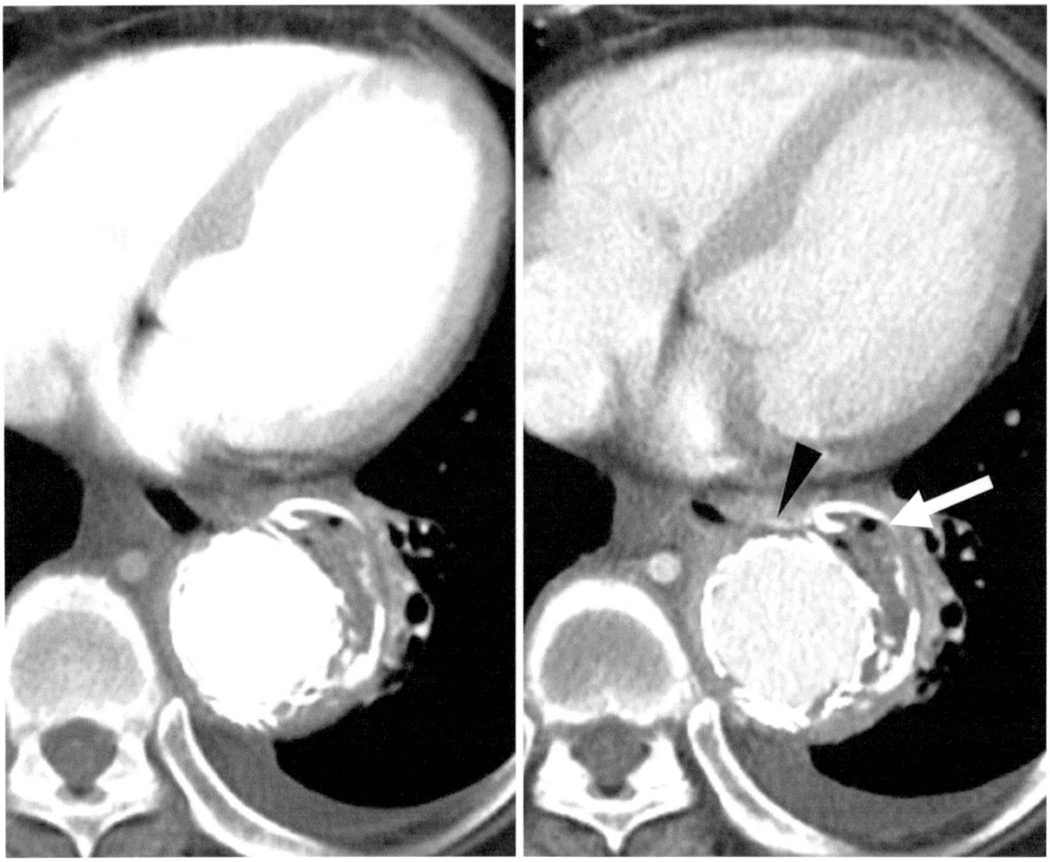

Fig. 5.12 Aortoesophageal fistula secondary to aortic stent-graft placement demonstrated on delayed-phase CT angiography in a 70-year-old man with thoracic aortic aneurysm. CT angiography of the thoracic aorta reveals gas collection (arrow) within the stent-graft, a finding suggestive of aortoesophageal fistula. Note the late opacification of the contrast extravasation (arrowhead) on delayed phase imaging (right), which is not definitely present on early arterial phase imaging (left)

5.6.2 Imaging Diagnosis

CT is the modality of choice for evaluating patients with suspected AEF given its acquisition speed and wide availability in the emergency setting. CT is useful in evaluating abnormalities related to AEF in both the esophagus and the aorta. Multiphase CT angiography is preferred, and the addition of a non-contrast scan may be helpful in differentiating contrast extravasation from high-attenuation material in the esophageal lumen, surgical material, or vascular calcification [32]. Arterial phase images should be obtained for optimal opacification of the aorta (Fig. 5.10), whereas delayed phase images may be useful for visualizing late opacification of the fistulous tract (Fig. 5.12) or adjacent structures and detecting esophageal malignancy as a possible etiology [32, 33]. CT may demonstrate an irregular outpouching of the aorta and effacement of the fat plane between the aorta and the esophagus at the site of an aortic aneurysm (Fig. 5.11) [32]. A definite fistulous tract may not be detected because of transient clot formation, so the presence of a high-attenuating esophageal or periesophageal mass adjacent to an aortic aneurysm or aortic stent graft may be indicative of AEF [29, 34]. Detection of subtle gas collection around the aorta can also be a useful sign that is suggestive of AEF (Fig. 5.12). Endoscopy may confirm the presence of a fistula or be used to directly visualize the pulsatile blood from the aorta, and can also be used to exclude other common causes of esophageal bleeding [30]. Magnetic resonance imaging is an alternative modality, but its use in evaluating AEF is limited due to availability, long scan time, and the requirement for patient cooperation.

5.7 Summary

Esophageal emergency is a rare but potentially life-threatening condition. The types of esophageal injury include esophageal perforation (including Boerhaave syndrome), esophageal intramural dissection, esophageal hernia with strangulation, acute phlegmonous esophagitis, and aortoesophageal fistula. These conditions may present nonspecific clinical manifestations, but the imaging findings are often characteristic. Awareness of various esophageal emergencies and their imaging features is crucial for ensuring an accurate diagnosis.

Key Points

- CT can demonstrate the site of esophageal perforation and may also uncover indirect signs of esophageal perforation, such as gas and/or fluid collection around the esophagus, esophageal wall thickening, and thickening of the esophageal mucosa at the site of perforation.
- In Boerhaave's syndrome, the classic radiographic findings include pneumomediastinum, pleural effusion, and pneumothorax with a left-sided predilection, and subcutaneous emphysema in the neck and chest wall. Naclerio's V sign, representing pneumomediastinum due to esophageal perforation, may be seen.
- CT is the modality of choice for evaluating intramural hematoma and may demonstrate an eccentric or concentric hyperattenuating lesion extending along the esophageal wall. The attenuation values of the hematoma varies depending on its stage.
- CT can confirm the diagnosis of gastric volvulus by showing herniation of the distal stomach into the left hemithorax and demonstrating the reversed position of the greater and lesser curvatures [21]. Ischemic changes in gastric volvulus can be seen as a lack of contrast enhancement of the gastric wall, with or without pneumatosis.
- In acute phlegmonous esophagitis, CT demonstrates an intramural, circumferential, low-attenuation area of the esophagus surrounded by an enhancing peripheral rim, which corresponds to the histopathological findings of thickening and abscess formation in the submucosal and muscularis layers of the esophagus.
- In aortoesophageal fistula, arterial phase images should be obtained for optimal opacification of the aorta, whereas delayed phase images may be useful for visualizing late opacification of the fistulous tract or adjacent structures and detecting esophageal malignancy as a possible etiology.

References

1. Costamagna G, Marchese M. Management of esophageal perforation after therapeutic endoscopy. Gastroenterol Hepatol (N Y). 2010;6(6):391–2.
2. Quine MA, Bell GD, McCloy RF, Matthews HR. Prospective audit of perforation rates following upper gastrointestinal endoscopy in two regions of England. Br J Surg. 1995;82(4):530–3. https://doi.org/10.1002/bjs.1800820430.
3. Ren JF, Lin D, Marchlinski FE, Callans DJ, Patel V. Esophageal imaging and strategies for avoiding injury during left atrial ablation for atrial fibrillation. Heart Rhythm. 2006;3(10):1156–61. https://doi.org/10.1016/j.hrthm.2006.06.006.
4. Brinster CJ, Singhal S, Lee L, Marshall MB, Kaiser LR, Kucharczuk JC. Evolving options in the management of esophageal perforation. Ann Thorac Surg. 2004;77(4):1475–83. https://doi.org/10.1016/j.athoracsur.2003.08.037.
5. Sudarshan M, Cassivi SD. Management of traumatic esophageal injuries. J Thorac Dis. 2019;11(Suppl 2):S172–6. https://doi.org/10.21037/jtd.2018.10.86.
6. Teh E, Edwards J, Duffy J, Beggs D. Boerhaave's syndrome: a review of management and outcome. Interact Cardiovasc Thorac Surg. 2007;6(5):640–3. https://doi.org/10.1510/icvts.2007.151936.

7. James AE Jr, Montali RJ, Chaffee V, Strecker EP, Vessal K. Barium or gastrografin: which contrast media for diagnosis of esophageal tears? Gastroenterology. 1975;68(5 Pt 1):1103–13.
8. Buecker A, Wein BB, Neuerburg JM, Guenther RW. Esophageal perforation: comparison of use of aqueous and barium-containing contrast media. Radiology. 1997;202(3):683–6. https://doi.org/10.1148/radiology.202.3.9051016.
9. Tonolini M, Bianco R. Spontaneous esophageal perforation (Boerhaave syndrome): diagnosis with CT-esophagography. J Emerg Trauma Shock. 2013;6(1):58–60. https://doi.org/10.4103/0974-2700.106329.
10. de Lutio di Castelguidone E, Merola S, Pinto A, Raissaki M, Gagliardi N, Romano L. Esophageal injuries: spectrum of multidetector row CT findings. Eur J Radiol. 2006;59(3):344–8. https://doi.org/10.1016/j.ejrad.2006.04.027.
11. Backer CL, LoCicero J 3rd, Hartz RS, Donaldson JS, Shields T. Computed tomography in patients with esophageal perforation. Chest. 1990;98(5):1078–80. https://doi.org/10.1378/chest.98.5.1078.
12. Ghanem N, Altehoefer C, Springer O, et al. Radiological findings in Boerhaave's syndrome. Emerg Radiol. 2003;10(1):8–13. https://doi.org/10.1007/s10140-002-0264-1.
13. Restrepo CS, Lemos DF, Ocazionez D, Moncada R, Gimenez CR. Intramural hematoma of the esophagus: a pictorial essay. Emerg Radiol. 2008;15(1):13–22. https://doi.org/10.1007/s10140-007-0675-0.
14. Younes Z, Johnson DA. The spectrum of spontaneous and iatrogenic esophageal injury: perforations, Mallory-Weiss tears, and hematomas. J Clin Gastroenterol. 1999;29(4):306–17. https://doi.org/10.1097/00004836-199912000-00003.
15. Cullen SN, McIntyre AS. Dissecting intramural haematoma of the oesophagus. Eur J Gastroenterol Hepatol. 2000;12(10):1151–62. https://doi.org/10.1097/00042737-200012100-00014.
16. Stilson WL, Sanders I, Gardiner GA, Gorman HC, Lodge DF. Hiatal hernia and gastroesophageal reflux. A clinicoradiological analysis of more than 1,000 cases. Radiology. 1969;93(6):1323–7.
17. Kahrilas PJ, Kim HC, Pandolfino JE. Approaches to the diagnosis and grading of hiatal hernia. Best Pract Res Clin Gastroenterol. 2008;22(4):601–16. https://doi.org/10.1016/j.bpg.2007.12.007.
18. Kohn GP, Price RR, DeMeester SR, et al. Guidelines for the management of hiatal hernia. Surg Endosc. 2013;27(12):4409–28. https://doi.org/10.1007/s00464-013-3173-3.
19. Morcos SK. Review article: Effects of radiographic contrast media on the lung. Br J Radiol. 2003;76(905):290–5. https://doi.org/10.1259/bjr/54892465.
20. Eren S, Ciris F. Diaphragmatic hernia: diagnostic approaches with review of the literature. Eur J Radiol. 2005;54(3):448–59. https://doi.org/10.1016/j.ejrad.2004.09.008.
21. Al-Balas H, Hani MB, Omari HZ. Radiological features of acute gastric volvulus in adult patients. Clin Imaging. 2010;34(5):344–7. https://doi.org/10.1016/j.clinimag.2010.02.001.
22. Hsu CY, Liu JS, Chen DF, Shih CC. Acute diffuse phlegmonous esophagogastritis: report of a survived case. Hepatogastroenterology. 1996;43(11):1347–52.
23. Kim HS, Hwang JH, Hong SS, et al. Acute diffuse phlegmonous esophagogastritis: a case report. J Korean Med Sci. 2010;25(10):1532–5. https://doi.org/10.3346/jkms.2010.25.10.1532.
24. Yun CH, Cheng SM, Sheu CI, Huang JK. Acute phlegmonous esophagitis: an unusual case (2005: 8b). Eur Radiol. 2005;15(11):2380–1. https://doi.org/10.1007/s00330-005-2842-6.
25. Kim GY, Ward J, Henessey B, et al. Phlegmonous gastritis: case report and review. Gastrointest Endosc. 2005;61(1):168–74. https://doi.org/10.1016/s0016-5107(04)02217-5.
26. Isik A, Firat D, Peker K, Sayar I, Idiz O, Soyturk M. A case report of esophageal perforation: complication of nasogastric tube placement. Am J Case Rep. 2014;15:168–71. https://doi.org/10.12659/AJCR.890260.
27. Wakayama T, Watanabe H, Ishizaki Y, et al. A case of phlegmonous esophagitis associated with diffuse phlegmonous gastritis. Am J Gastroenterol. 1994;89(5):804–6.
28. Shin HS, Kim SS, Kim JH. Acute phlegmonous esophagitis with mediastinitis complicated by an esophageal perforation: a case report. J Korean Soc Radiol. 2018;79(1):45–9.
29. Heckstall RL, Hollander JE. Aortoesophageal fistula: recognition and diagnosis in the emergency department. Ann Emerg Med. 1998;32(4):502–5. https://doi.org/10.1016/s0196-0644(98)70182-9.
30. Hollander JE, Quick G. Aortoesophageal fistula: a comprehensive review of the literature. Am J Med. 1991;91(3):279–87. https://doi.org/10.1016/0002-9343(91)90129-l.
31. Carter R, Mulder GA, Snyder EN Jr, Brewer LA III. Aortoesophageal fistula. Am J Surg. 1978;136(1):26–30. https://doi.org/10.1016/0002-9610(78)90195-2.
32. Sipe A, McWilliams SR, Saling L, Raptis C, Mellnick V, Bhalla S. The red connection: a review of aortic and arterial fistulae with an emphasis on CT findings. Emerg Radiol. 2017;24(1):73–80. https://doi.org/10.1007/s10140-016-1433-y.
33. Halvorsen RA Jr, Thompson WM. Computed tomographic staging of gastrointestinal tract malignancies. Part I. Esophagus and stomach. Invest Radiol. 1987;22(1):2–16.
34. Young CA, Menias CO, Bhalla S, Prasad SR. CT features of esophageal emergencies. Radiographics. 2008;28(6):1541–53. https://doi.org/10.1148/rg.286085520.

6 Acute Aortic Diseases: Evaluation with Computed Tomography and Magnetic Resonance Imaging

6.1 Introduction

Acute aortic syndrome (AAS) encompasses several nontraumatic life-threatening conditions of the thoracic aorta, including aortic dissection, intramural hematoma, and penetrating atherosclerotic ulcers. CT is the modality of choice for evaluation of acute aortic diseases. CT is also useful in ruling out acute coronary syndrome and pulmonary thromboembolism. Recent CT technologies enable simultaneous evaluation of the aorta and coronary arteries after a single injection of contrast material. Despite its limited availability, magnetic resonance imaging (MRI) can be used to evaluate the aorta with regard to the diagnosis of aortic dissection or aneurysm with or without the use of contrast material.

6.2 Imaging Techniques

6.2.1 CT Techniques

Multidetector CT scanners with 64 or more detector rows are recommended for aortic imaging, especially for electrocardiography (ECG)-gated scanning with uniform contrast enhancement in the aorta and its branches.

A non-contrast ECG-gated or non-gated CT scan should be performed to look for a rim of hyper-attenuation in the aortic intramural hematoma (IMH). In cases with impaired renal function, non-contrast CT may serve as the imaging modality. A virtual non-contrast scan taken with a dual-energy CT technique may replace non-contrast CT.

Motion-free images of the aortic root should be obtained with CT as the prevalence of aortic motion artifacts on non-gated CT has been reported to be higher than 50% [1]. ECG gating is preferred whenever possible to avoid motion artifacts in the ascending aorta (Fig. 6.1) [1]. High-pitch dual-source CT angiography (CTA) of the whole aorta without ECG gating is another option that eliminates motion artifacts in the ascending aorta [2].

Recently developed high-pitch and variable pitch CT techniques allow for simultaneous evaluation of the aorta and coronary arteries.

Premedication with a beta-blocker or nitroglycerin is generally unnecessary.

Arterial phase imaging is usually performed and pre-contrast and 1–2 min delayed phase imaging are optionally performed.

The contrast material should be given via the right arm to eliminate streak artifacts in the proximal segments of the branches of the aortic arch. Contrast injection should achieve adequate contrast attenuation of at least 250 HU uniformly throughout the aorta. Adequate contrast opacification of the aorta and its branches is achieved by an iodine delivery rate of 1.0–1.6 g/s (ideally up

T. J. Kim et al., *Emergency Chest Radiology*, https://doi.org/10.1007/978-981-33-4396-2_6

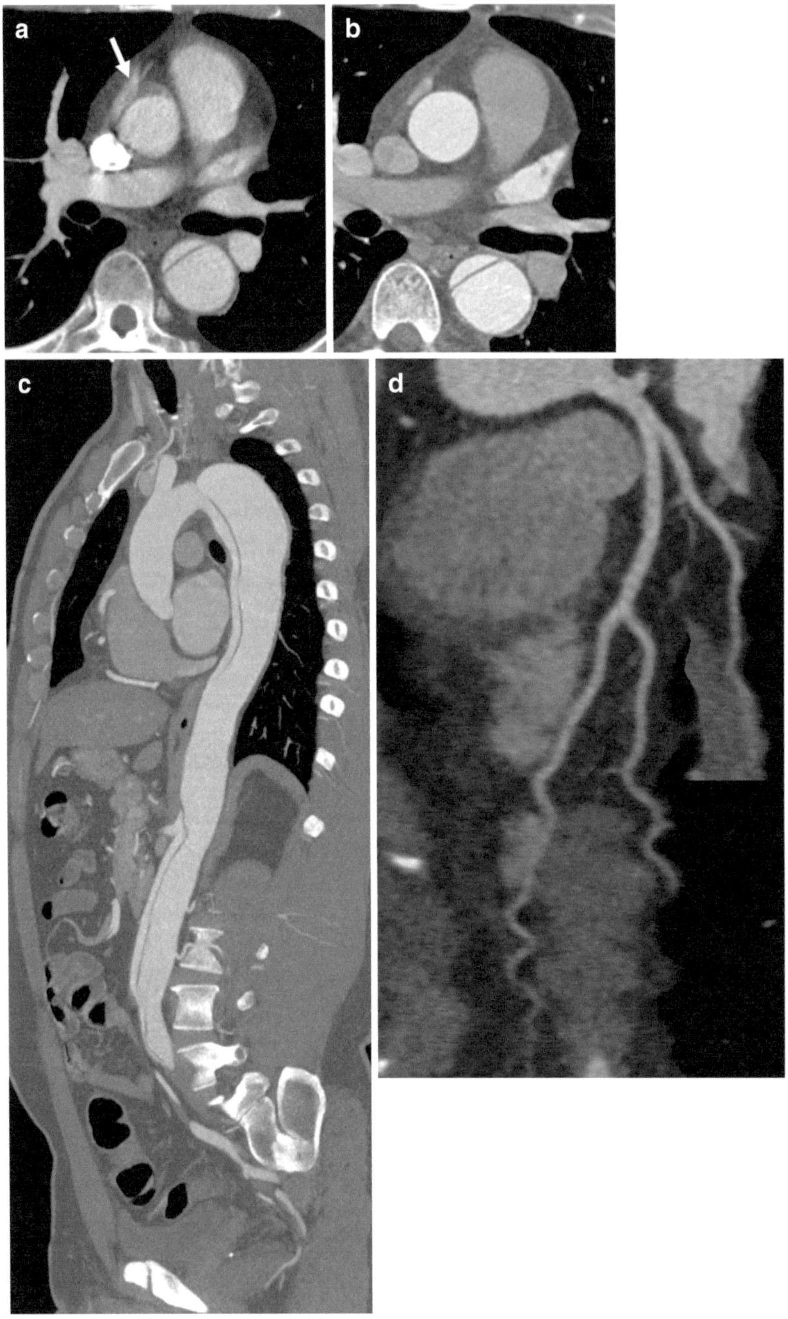

Fig. 6.1 Motion artifact mimicking Stanford type A aortic dissection (AD) in a 38-year-old male. (**a**) A pulsating motion artifact mimics dissection (arrow) of the ascending aorta on non-electrocardiography (ECG)-gated CT angiography (CTA). (**b**) ECG-gated high-pitch CTA shows a normal ascending aorta in the same patient. (**c**, **d**) High-pitch CTA enables acquisition of motion-free images of the whole aorta (**c**) and coronary arteries (**d**) during a single breath-hold. The dose–length product was 471 mGy·cm at 120 kVp. The patient's heart rate was 63 beats/min and 70 mL of contrast material and 30 mL of saline were injected at 4 mL/s

to 2 g/s, 3.5–6 mL/s, 60–120 mL, 350–400 mg I/mL) when using a tube voltage of 120 kVp. A low-tube voltage protocol (70, 80, 90, or 100 kVp) may provide a diagnostic performance comparable with that of the standard protocol (120 kVp) with reduced radiation dose and contrast material volume. According to Ippolito et al., the 100-kVp CT protocol (30 mL, 4 mL/s, 350 mg I/mL) showed a similar degree of attenuation in the thoracoabdominal aorta with reduced radiation dose compared with the standard protocol (120 kV, 80 mL) [3]. Non-ECG-gated 70 kVp high-pitch (pitch, 3.4) low-contrast volume (40 mL) thoracic CTA showed diagnostic image quality with an 85% reduction in radiation dose compared with CTA at 100 kVp, a pitch of 1.2, and 60 mL contrast material [4]. A combination technique consisting of a low concentration of contrast material and a low tube voltage with iterative image reconstruction (IR) is feasible and shows sufficient aortic contrast enhancement and image quality.

Scans should cover areas from the carotid bifurcation to the proximal femoral arteries (from the neck to femoral trochanter). Coverage may be limited to the thorax from the aortic arch to the diaphragmatic sulcus in the first instance.

6.2.2 MR Angiography with or without Contrast Enhancement

MRI may be adopted for aortic imaging in patients who are allergic to contrast material, those who are pregnant, or children. Fast imaging with a balanced steady state free precession (SSFP) technique enables detection of intimal flaps (Fig. 6.2). T1- and T2-weighted black blood fast spin-echo images are used for the evaluation of intramural hematoma (IMH). Cine MRI in axial, coronal, and oblique sagittal planes can be used for detection of aortic dissection (AD) and intimal tear. 3D-navigated SSFP has a sharp edge profile [5]. Non-ECG-gated or ECG-gated high-resolution contrast-enhanced-MR angiography (CE-MRA) can be used to measure the orthogonal diameter of the thoracic aorta [6, 7]. Phase-contrast MRI can be used to evaluate flow in the true lumen.

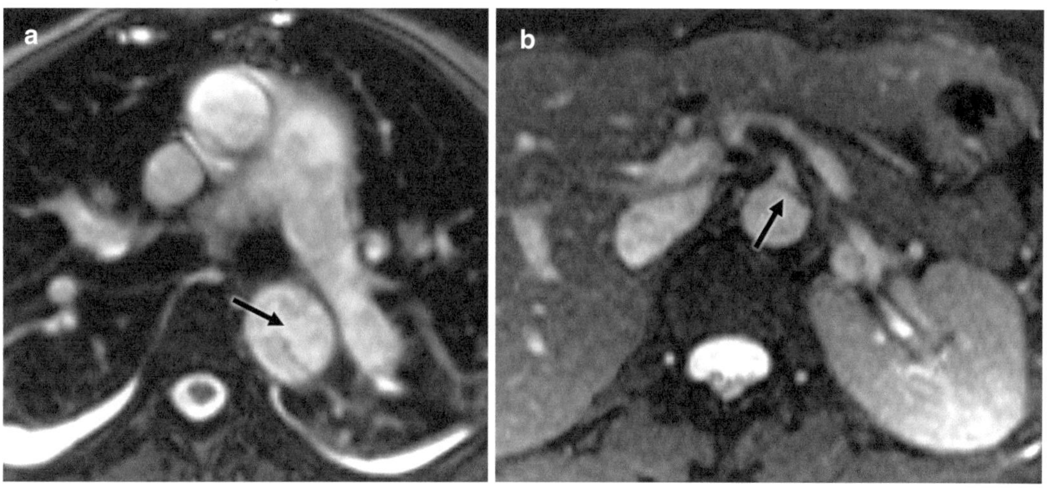

Fig. 6.2 MR imaging evaluation of Stanford type B AD in a pregnant 32-year-old female with Marfan syndrome. (**a**, **b**) Balanced steady-state free precession transverse images show aortic dissection with intimal defect (arrow) (**a**) in the descending aorta and true lumen collapse (arrow) in the abdominal aorta (**b**). (**c**) Cine MR image shows a normal ascending aorta. (**d**) Six-month follow-up CTA shows enlargement of the descending aorta with dissection

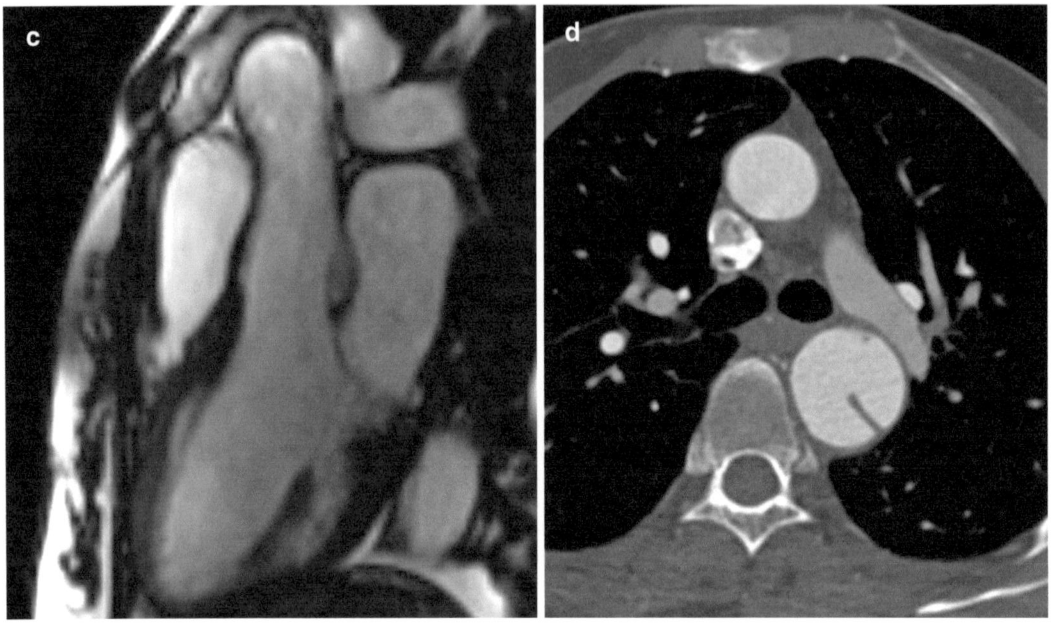

Fig. 6.2 (continued)

6.3 Diseases

6.3.1 Classic Acute Double-Lumen Dissection

Aortic dissection (AD) can be classified according to the location and extent of involvement. Stanford type A dissection involves the ascending aorta, whereas Stanford type B dissection is confined to the aortic arch and the descending aorta (Fig. 6.3). Acute AD is defined as AD diagnosed within 2 weeks, subacute AD from 2 to 6 weeks, and chronic AD more than 6 weeks after the onset of symptoms.

CT is the modality of choice for detection of AD. The sensitivity and specificity of CT for AAS approach 100% [8, 9]. The sensitivities of CT and MRI for diagnosis of AAS are 100% and 95–100%, respectively. Transesophageal echocardiography has a sensitivity of 86–100% [9]. CT, MRI, and transesophageal echocardiography are reliable tools for diagnosing AAS [9]. In one study with 1850 patients, a positive D-dimer test result had an overall sensitivity of 96.7% and a specificity of 64% for the diagnosis of AAS [10]. Transthoracic echocardiography is useful in assessing potential high-risk features or complications, such as pericardial effusion; however, it does not exclude AAS, as the sensitivity of transthoracic echocardiography is only 31–55% for dissections involving the descending aorta [11].

Motion artifacts in the ascending aorta should not be interpreted as AD. CT shows the extent of dissection, the degree of true lumen collapse, the involvement of visceral and extremity arteries, and resultant organ ischemia or infarction. Hemorrhage into the pericardium may occur (Fig. 6.4). Cardiac tamponade caused by rupture of the ascending aorta is the most common cause of death [12]. Hematoma along the pulmonary artery may compress the vessels.

Multichannel dissection occurs in around 4% of patients showing the Mercedes-Benz sign due to secondary dissection (Fig. 6.5) [13]. The cobweb sign represents thin linear filling defects (cobweb or tendrils) bridging the false lumen on CTA (Fig. 6.6) [14].

The true lumen is almost always narrower than the false lumen of a dissected aorta. The true lumen is the lumen connected to the left ventri-

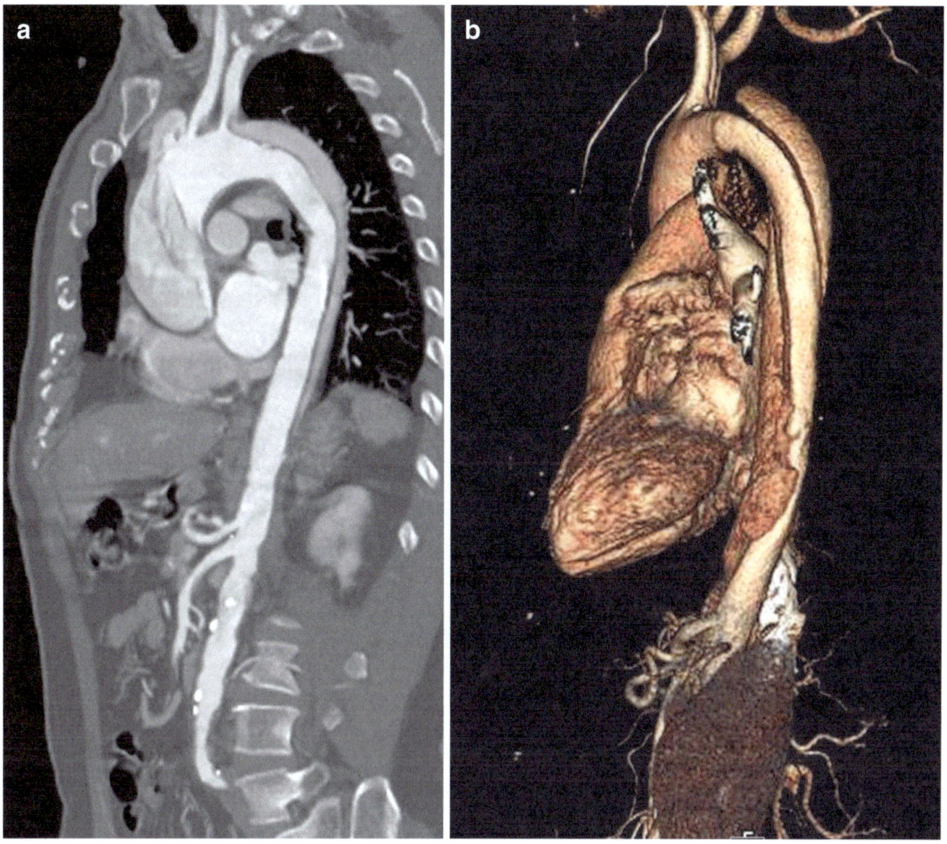

Fig. 6.3 Stanford classification of AD. (**a**) Type A AD involving the ascending aorta, aortic arch, and descending thoracic aorta (multiplanar reformatted image). (**b**) Type B AD involving the descending aorta (volume-rendered image)

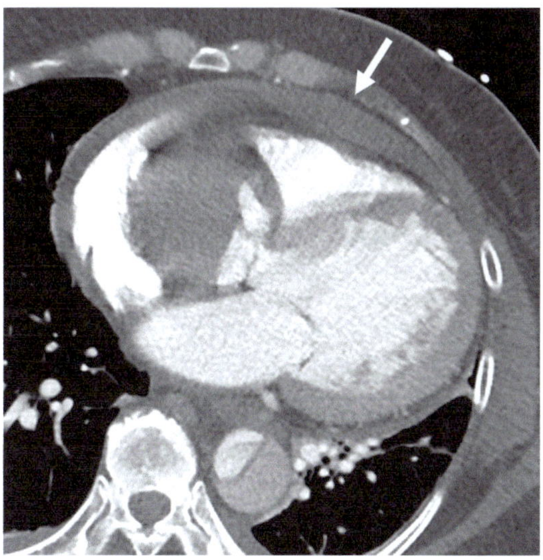

Fig. 6.4 Acute Stanford type A AD in a 60-year-old female. Note pericardial hemorrhage (arrow) and marked compression of the true lumen in the ascending aorta

cle; it is opacified earlier and more strongly than the false lumen on arterial-phase CTA. The beak sign represents an acute angle between the dissection flap and the outer wall of the false lumen. The true lumen is rarely severely compressed; it is hard to find a collapsed true lumen with substitution of the entire aortic lumen with the false lumen. Marked true lumen collapse in the aortic root and dissection in the sinus of Valsalva may decrease the coronary blood supply and cause myocardial ischemia (Fig. 6.7). Complete dissection of the intima results in a circumferential appearance of the intimomedial flap (Fig. 6.6). Intimointimal intussusception produces a windsock appearance.

Dissection may be focal or limited and the extent of dissection evolves from the penetrating aortic ulcer (PAU) (Fig. 6.8). The criteria for the

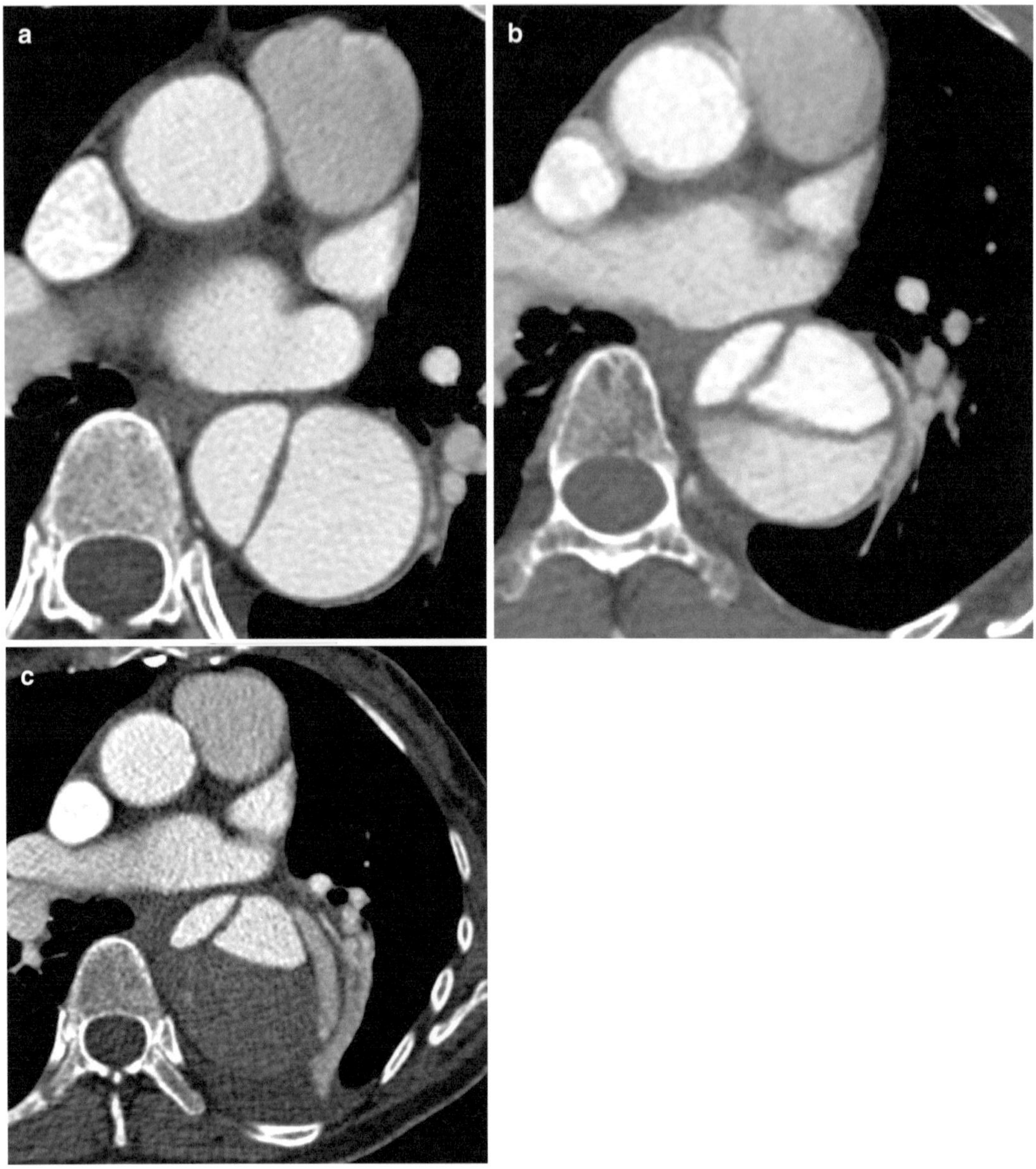

Fig. 6.5 Rapid progression of AD in a 37-year-old female with Marfan syndrome. (**a**) Double-lumen AD in the descending thoracic aorta after Bentall operation of the ascending aorta. (**b**) Follow-up CTA, taken 38 months later, shows 3-lumen AD in the descending aorta. (**c**) Seven days after the scan in (**b**), the lesion progressed to 4-lumen dissection with an enlarged aortic diameter

"limited intimal tear" (LIT) classification consist of a linear or stellate luminal contour abnormality without a dissection flap separating the true lumen from a false lumen [15]. Associated findings include focal linear filling defects corresponding to undermined edges of the tear, a small amount of local IMH under the lesion edges, and outpouching of the residual aortic wall at the base of the intimomedial defect [15]. An eccentric bulge may be the only imaging finding. ECG-gated CTA has the potential to detect subtle lesions with limited intimal tear [16]. In 2010, a multispecialty American College of Cardiology Foundation/American Heart

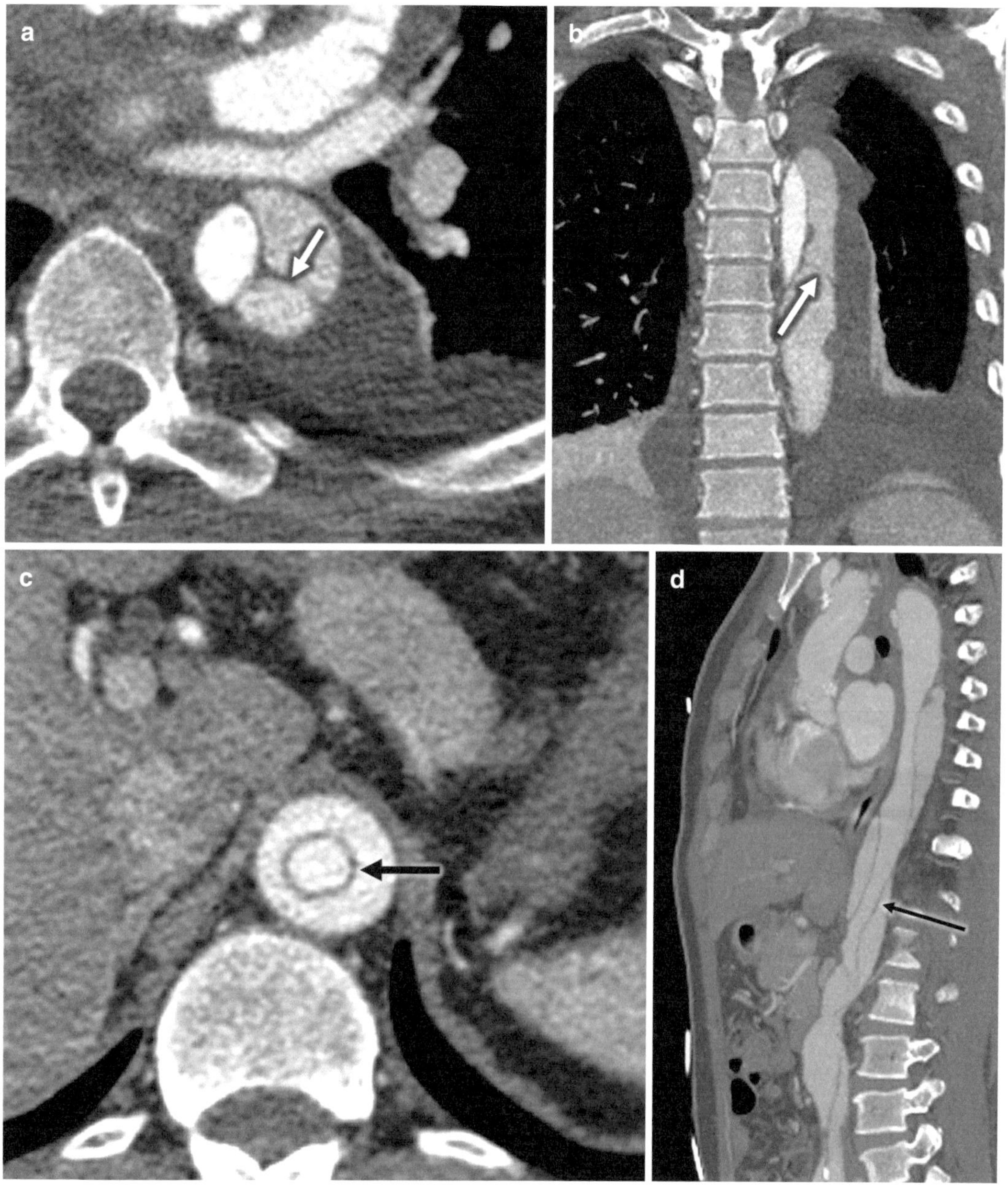

Fig. 6.6 Circumferential AD in a 51-year-old male with acute Stanford type A AD. (**a**, **b**) Follow-up CTA (**a**, transverse section; **b**, coronal section) 7 days after the initial surgical treatment, showing a linear structure (arrow, cobweb) in the false lumen of the descending aorta. (**c**, **d**) Transverse and oblique sagittal reformatted CT image at the 20-day follow-up shows the aortic true lumen (arrow) entirely surrounded by the false lumen in the proximal abdominal aorta

Association (ACCF/AHA) Task Force document classified this type of lesion as a "class 3 dissection variant (limited dissection)" [17]. Chin et al. identified 24 LITs (4.8% of 497 patients with AAS) [15]. Three patients presented with rupture. The in-hospital mortality rate was 4%, and five patients with LIT died subsequently at 1.5 years. CT detected all but one case of LIT. The condition was best visualized on volume-rendered images.

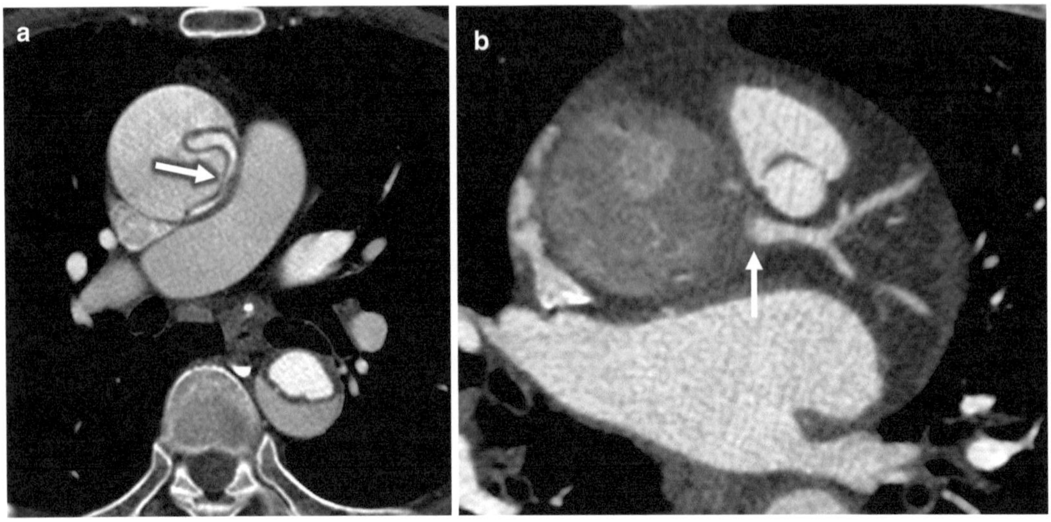

Fig. 6.7 Severe true lumen collapse in an 80-year-old male with acute type A AD. (**a**) ECG-gated CTA shows severe true lumen collapse (arrow) of the ascending aorta without motion artifact. (**b**) The ascending aortic lumen (arrow) abutting the left coronary ostium was also compromised

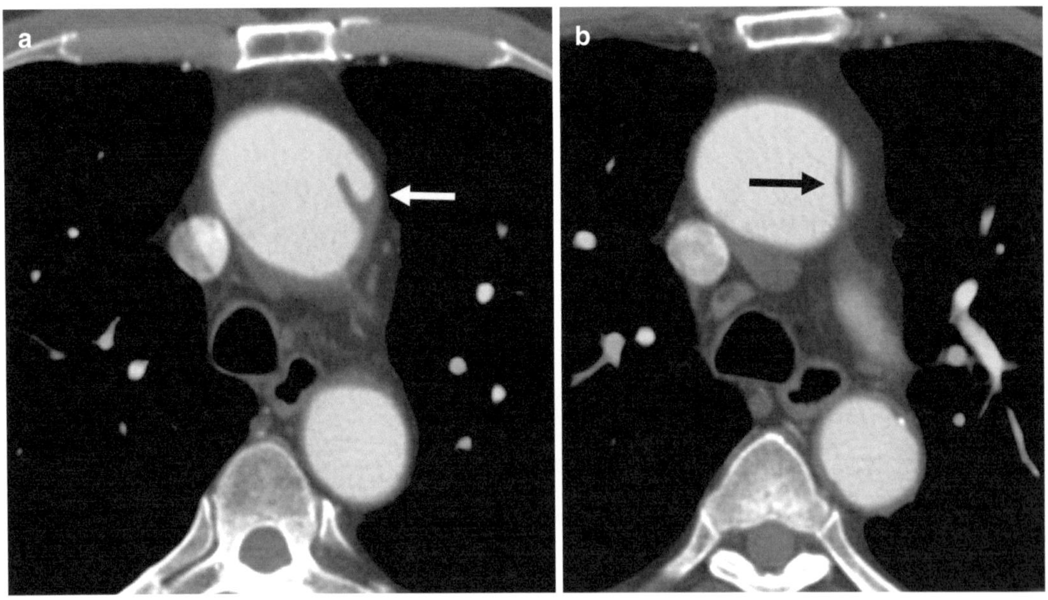

Fig. 6.8 Limited dissection of the ascending aorta in a 79-year-old male. (**a**, **b**) Contiguous transverse images show focal dissection (arrows) and bulging of the ascending aorta. (**c**) Volume-rendered image shows the discrete lesion (arrow)

Fig. 6.8 (continued)

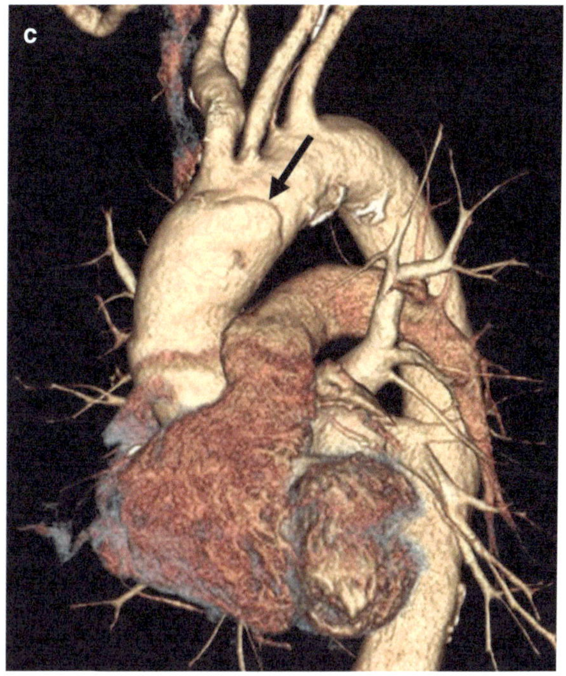

Ray et al. evaluated the predictors of intervention and mortality in patients with uncomplicated acute type B aortic dissection (UATBAD) in 294 patients [18]. Aortic diameter >44 mm was a predictor of mortality after adjustment for other significant risk factors. A false lumen with a diameter >22 mm, as well as those with maximum aortic diameter >44 mm on admission, were associated with decreased intervention-free survival. UATBAD patients with ascending aortic area >12.1 cm^2 or maximum ascending aortic diameter >40.8 mm were at high risk for development of subsequent arch and proximal progression and may require closer follow-up or earlier intervention (Figs. 6.9 and 6.10) [19]. Sailer et al. retrospectively assessed late adverse events in 83 patients with acute uncomplicated Stanford type B AD [13]. Adverse events were defined as aortic rupture, rapid aortic growth (>10 mm/year), aneurysm formation (≥6 cm), organ or limb ischemia, or new uncontrollable hypertension or pain. Five significant predictors for adverse events (40%, 33/83) were identified, including connective tissue disease, circumferential extent of false lumen in angular degrees, maximum aortic diameter, false lumen outflow, and number of intercostal arteries.

Coronary artery disease should be evaluated before surgical repair of AD with CCTA (Fig. 6.11). However, evaluation is often not possible because of the urgency of the situation. Arterial flow to the spinal cord can be evaluated with CT before and after graft replacement of the descending thoracic aorta. In a study by Kubota et al., the Adamkiewicz artery (AKA) showed significantly higher contrast-to-noise ratio and CT value with a 100-kVp than a 120-kVp protocol [20]. Intra-aortic CT angiography (IA-CTA) can be used to visualize the AKA in 90% of patients (27/30) [21]. In postoperative patients, anastomotic pseudoaneurysm, coronary ostial obstruction, graft infection, and the patency of visceral branches and intercostal arteries are evaluated.

The CTA report should describe the extent and location of AD (Stanford classification);

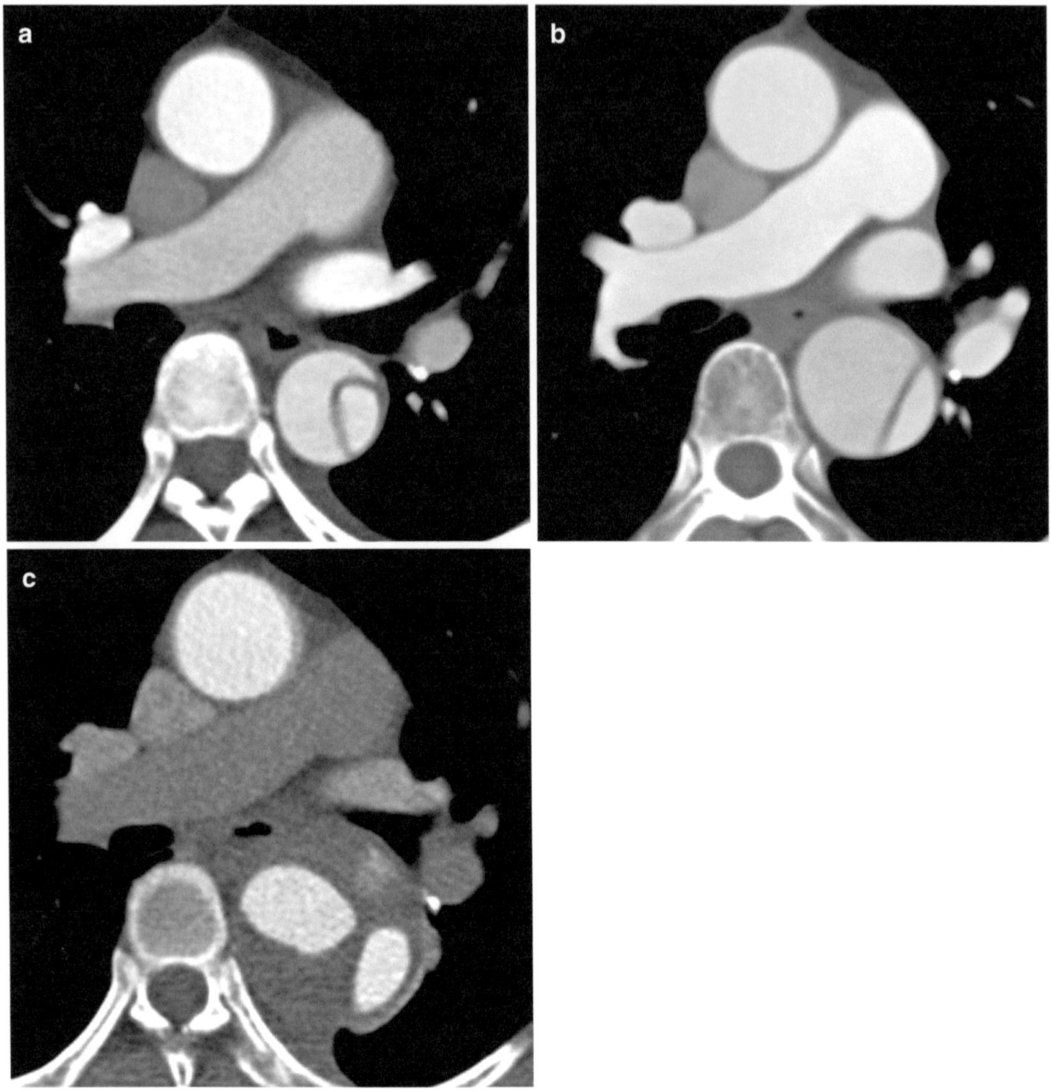

Fig. 6.9 Gradual progression of AD in a 56-year-old female. (**a**) Initial CTA showing Stanford type B AD measuring 26 mm. (**b**) Follow-up CTA, 3 years later, showing an increased aneurysmal diameter, measuring 37 mm. (**c**) After another 3 years, the aneurysm again increased to 51 mm

the site of entry and reentry tears; the maximal diameters of aneurysmal lesions (whole aorta and false lumen) in orthogonal planes perpendicular to the long axis of the aorta or the aortic flow; the degree of true lumen collapse; thrombus in the false lumen; involvement of the aortic valve and coronary, carotid, subclavian, mesenteric, celiac, renal, iliac, and femoral arteries; end-organ perfusion; and evidence of aortic rupture (periaortic hematoma, intrapericardial or pleural hemorrhage, and contrast extravasation) [17, 22].

Cine MRI may show turbulent jets in the aortic tear and reentry sites (Fig. 6.12). T1- and T2-weighted images may show increased/decreased signal intensity of mural hematoma because of methemoglobin/deoxyhemoglobin. The total number of pathologic findings is higher using 2D turbo spin echo (TSE) and balanced SSFP when compared to 3D CE-MRA [23].

Contrast-enhanced MR angiography (MRA) may replace CTA in select cases. The benefits of the smaller amount of contrast agent used for MR vs. CT and the absence of a radiation hazard are

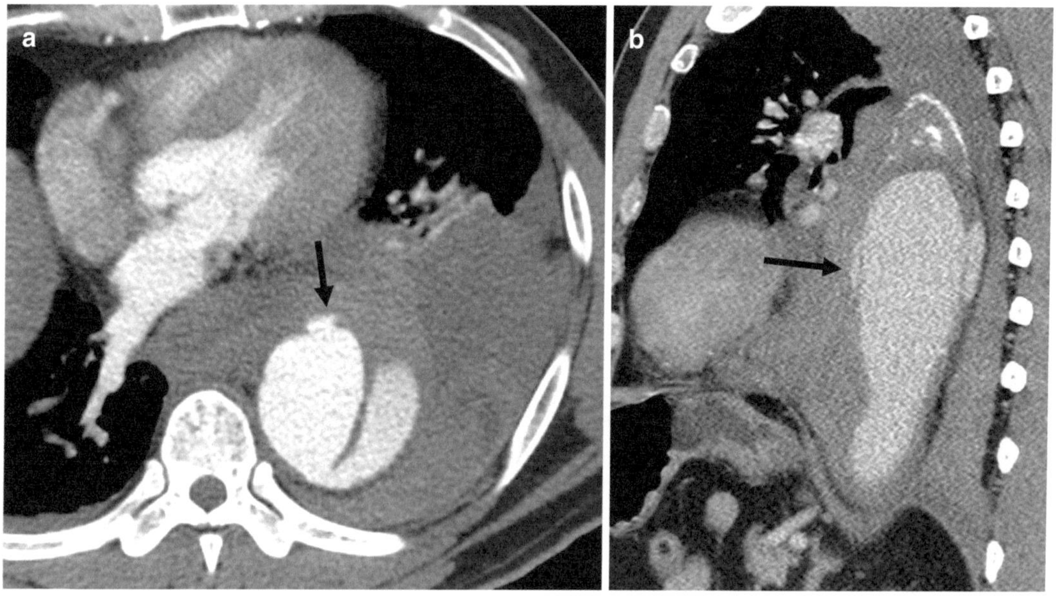

Fig. 6.10 Rupture of chronic AD of the descending aorta in a 53-year-old male. (**a**, **b**) Transverse (**a**) and sagittal (**b**) CT images show pleural hemorrhage and mediastinal hematoma. The aorta measures 61 mm. There is a focal contour deformity with pseudoaneurysm formation (arrow) in the anterior wall of the descending aorta, suggesting a point of rupture

especially appreciated in younger patients. MRA using a blood pool contrast agent has been shown to provide reliable and exact measurements before thoracic endovascular aortic repair (TEVAR), allowing noninvasive planning of the intervention despite lower image quality and without the disadvantages of ionizing radiation and nephrotoxicity. Unenhanced MRI with SSPF sequence can be an alternative modality for patients with contraindications for CT, such as renal impairment. Endoleaks that are occult on CT can be detected by MRI with blood pool contrast agents. Late-phase MRI 30 min after injection of contrast material can reveal additional endoleaks not seen 3 min after injection.

6.3.2 Penetrating Aortic Ulcer

Penetrating aortic ulcer (PAU) develops when an ulceration in the plaque penetrates through the internal elastic lamina into the media in the aortic wall (Fig. 6.13). Isolated PAU occurs in 2.3–7.6% of cases of AAS [24]. The terms used to describe different types of AAS are sometimes confusing and can overlap in meaning. PAU can be confused with ulcer-like projection (ULP) associated with IMH. The clinical and imaging features of AD and PAU can overlap [16]. Most cases with PAU (>90%) occur in the aortic arch or descending aorta, while atherosclerotic plaques are rarely seen in the ascending aorta [25]. According to a study by Nathan et al., most PAUs are located in the descending thoracic aorta (61.2%, 243 cases), followed by the abdominal aorta (29.7%, 118 cases), and the aortic arch (6.8%, 27 cases) [26]. CT shows an outpouching lesion and PAU may develop a localized IMH or a mural thrombus. PAU may progress into a pseudoaneurysm, which refers to a saccular lesion with a relatively narrow base lacking normal aortic wall tissue elements. A pseudoaneurysm is prone to rupture and needs treatment, especially when it is large. Larger ulcer diameter, greater ulcer depth, and increasing pleural effusion are associated with disease progression [27]. PAU is associated with a higher incidence of aortic rupture compared with aortic dissection [16]. According to Nathan et al., 57.7% of PAUs ($n = 224$) were isolated (without saccular aneurysm or IMH), 27.8% of PAUs ($n = 108$)

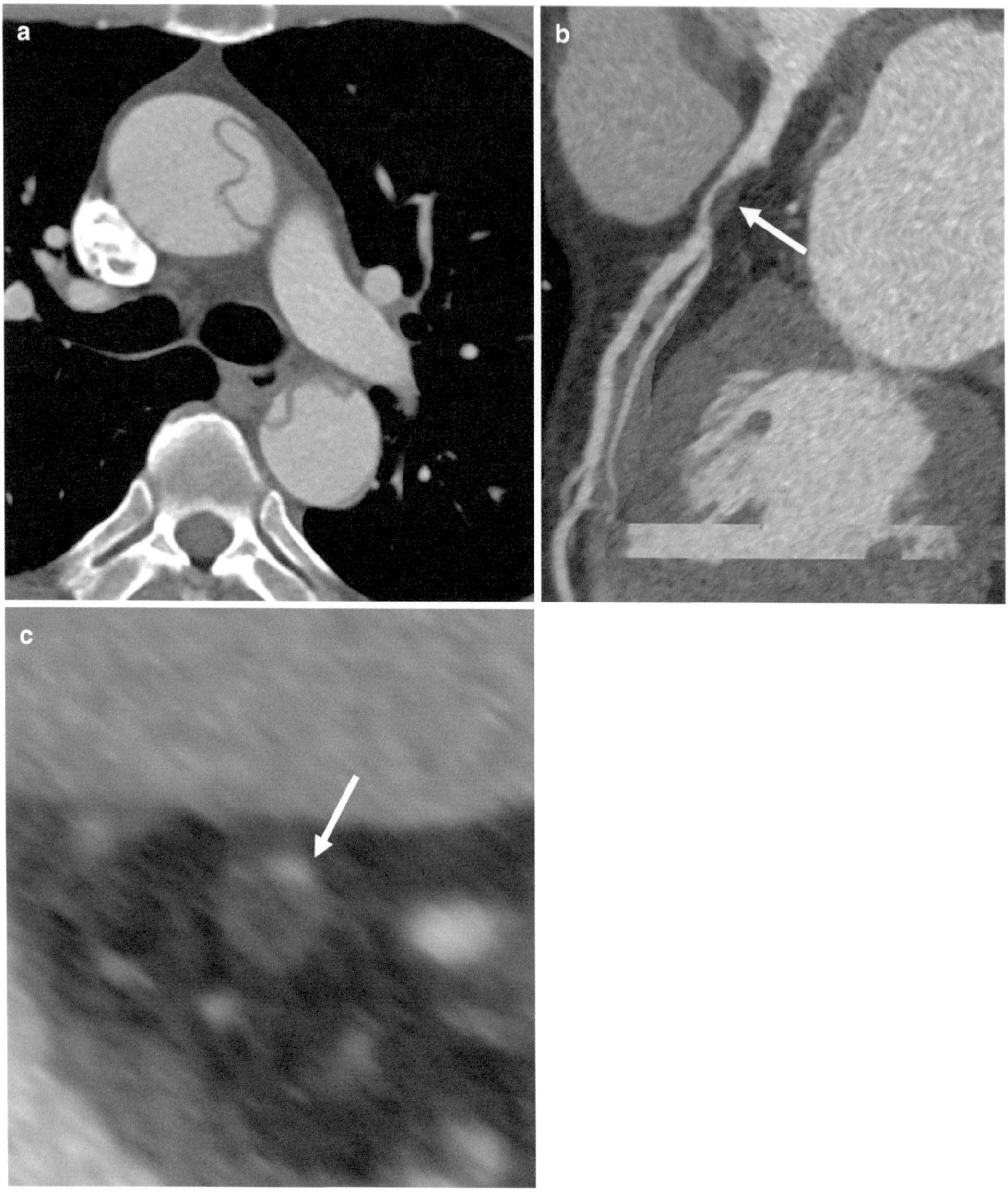

Fig. 6.11 Concomitant coronary artery disease in a 47-year-old male with acute Stanford type A AD. (**a**) CTA shows AD in the ascending thoracic and descending thoracic aorta. (**b**, **c**) Coronary CTA reveals severe noncalcific stenosis (arrows) in the proximal left anterior descending branch

had associated saccular aneurysms, and 14.4% of PAUs ($n = 56$) were associated with intramural hematoma. Rupture was present in 4.1% of cases ($n = 16$). Symptomatic PAU disease was more likely to progress than asymptomatic disease (42.9% vs. 16.7%, $P = 0.029$) [26].

6.3.3 Aortic Intramural Hematoma

Aortic intramural hematoma (IMH) refers to a mural hematoma that is isolated from the circulation. The cause of IMH is controversial. IMH may result from rupture of the vasa vasorum of the aortic wall or double-lumen dissection complicated with thrombosis in a false lumen. IMH of the aorta has a reported incidence of 5–20% among patients with acute aortic syndromes and a mortality rate of 21% [28]. IMH can be a variant of AD, and is synonymous with a "thrombosed type" or "non-communicating" AD [16]. IMH may evolve to double-lumen dissection or resolve and heal. IMH progresses to classic acute aortic dissection (AAD) in 28–47% of patients [29].

IMH may extend into the pericardial space, along the pulmonary arteries, and into the sinus of Valsalva and coronary arteries (Fig. 6.14) [29].

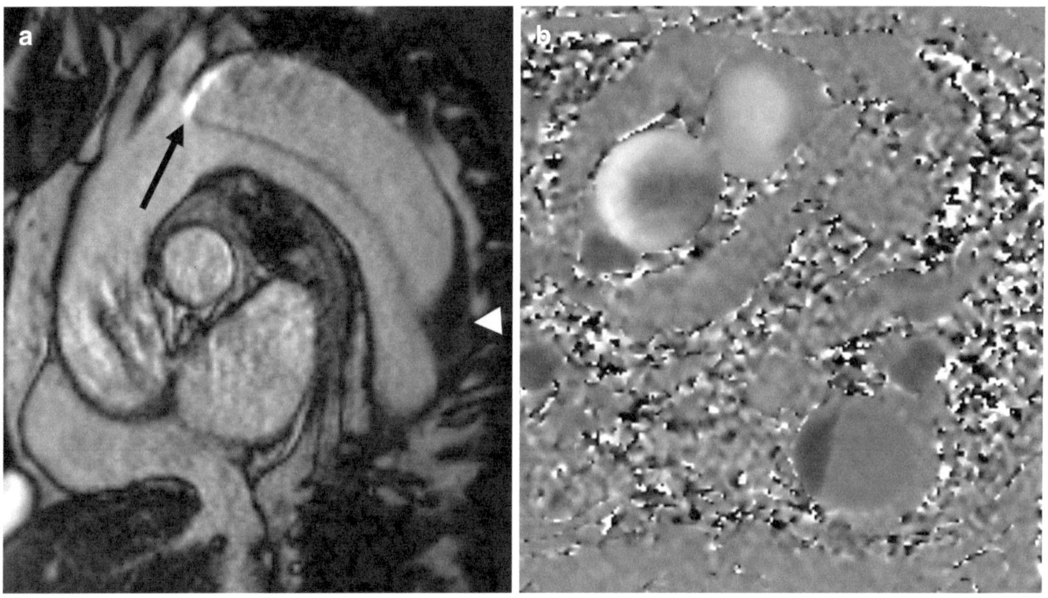

Fig. 6.12 Cine MR imaging follow-up of chronic Stanford type B AD in a 50-year-old male with hypertrophic cardiomyopathy. (**a**) Balanced steady-state free precession cine MR imaging in the oblique sagittal plane shows a small intimal defect (arrow) in the proximal descending aorta and a high-velocity jet and thrombosis (arrowhead) in the false lumen of the descending aorta. (**b**) Velocity-encoded cine MR imaging enables assessment of flow in the true and false lumens of the descending thoracic aorta

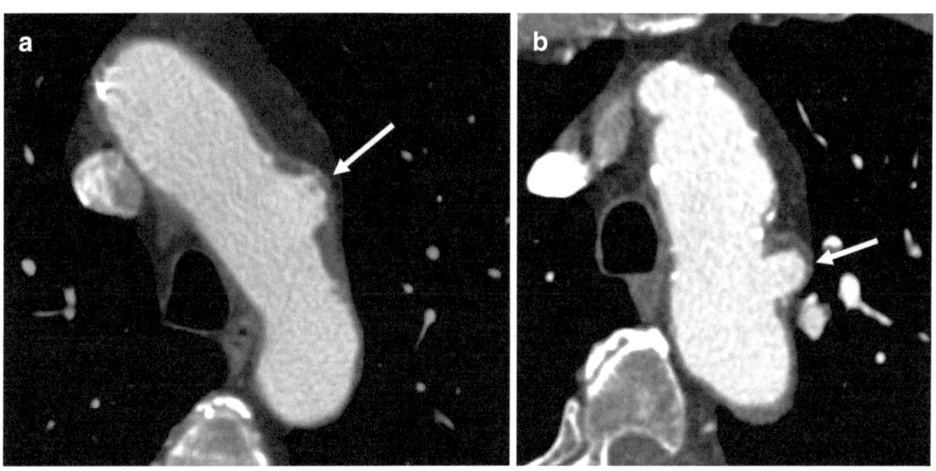

Fig. 6.13 Outpouching lesions of the thoracic aorta on CTA of varying severity in different patients. (**a**)–(**c**) Penetrating aortic ulcers (arrows) in varying degrees of protrusion. (**d**, **e**) Pseudoaneurysms. (**f**, **g**) Concealed rupture

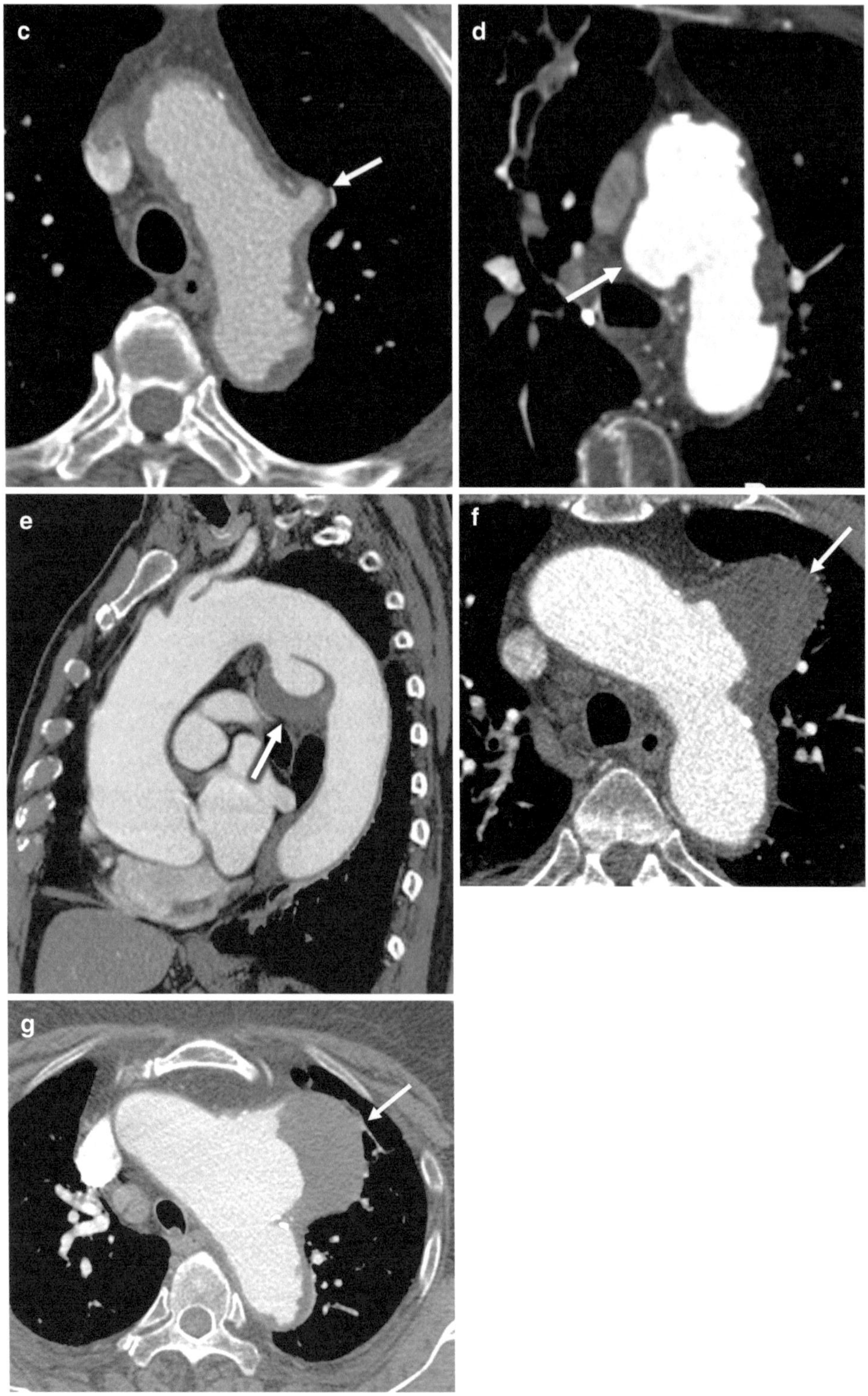

Fig. 6.13 (continued)

Stanford Type A IMH (ascending aorta) is associated with substantial mortality, whereas Stanford type B IMH (arch and descending aorta) are less likely to be associated with an adverse outcome [30]. An immediate open surgical procedure is needed for dissection of the ascending aorta, given the high mortality rate (26–58%) and proximity to the aortic valve and great vessels [9]. TEVAR may be optimal for treating type B IMH [9].

Harris et al. evaluated 2830 patients with AAS in the International Registry of Acute Aortic Dissection (IRAD) (1996–2011) to examine the differences between patients with IMH or classic AD based on the initial imaging test [31]. Of 2830 patients, 178 had IMH (64 type A [42%], 90 type B [58%], and 24 arch) [31]. Overall, in-hospital mortality did not significantly differ for type A IMH compared to AD (26.6% vs. 26.5%;

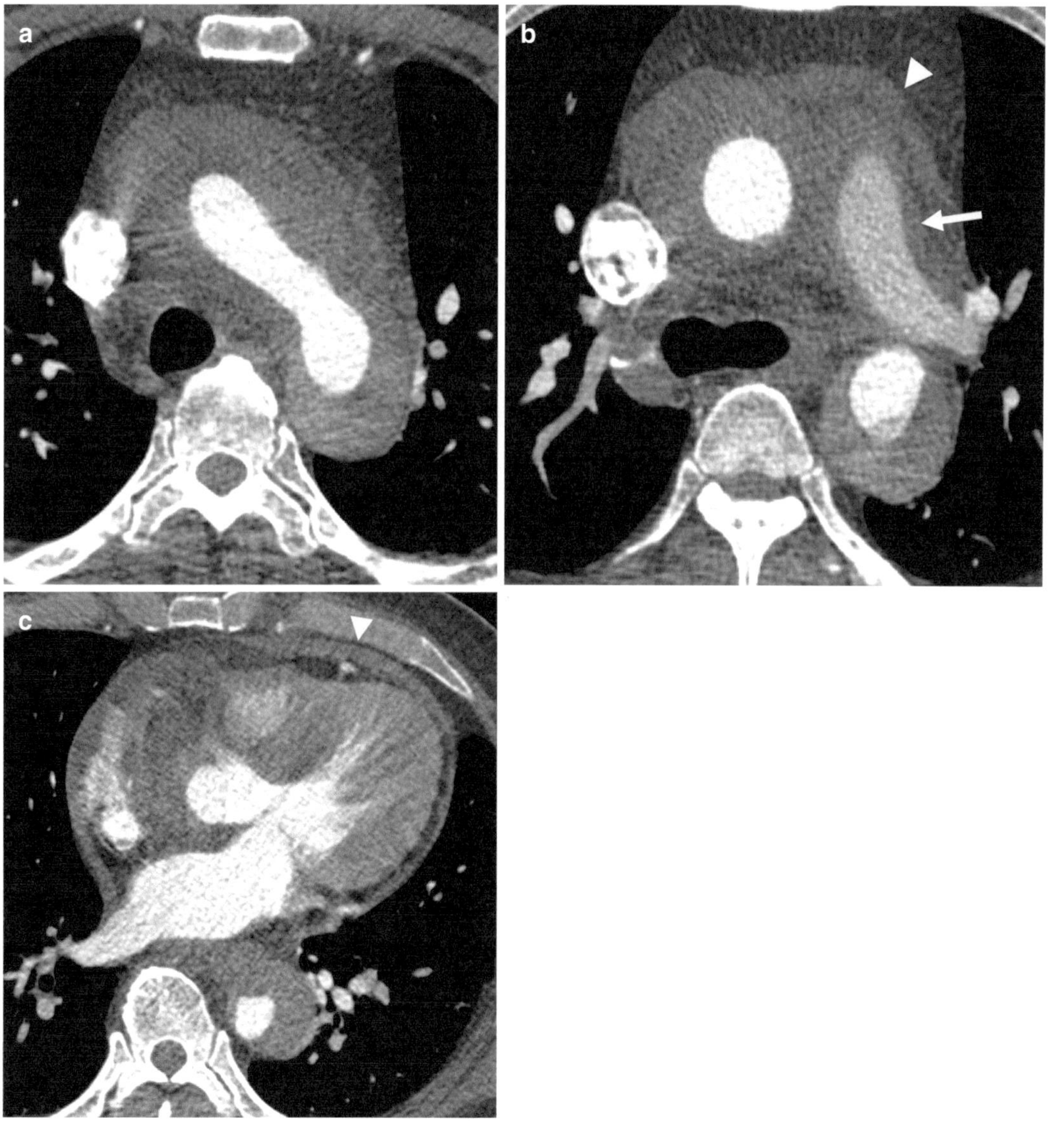

Fig. 6.14 Acute Stanford type A intramural hematoma in a 44-year-old male. (**a**)–(**c**) Transverse CT images show a 22-mm thick intramural hematoma (IMH) in the ascending aorta. Note hematoma extending along the main pulmonary artery (arrow) and pericardium (arrowhead)

$P = 0.998$). Type A IMH managed medically was associated with significant mortality (40.0%), although the mortality rate was less than that of classic AD (61.8%; $P = 0.195$). Patients with type B IMH had a lower in-hospital mortality rate than patients with classic AD, but the difference was not statistically significant (4.4% vs. 11.1%; $P = 0.062$). Acute IMH presents similarly to classic AD but is more frequently complicated with pericardial effusions and periaortic hematoma. In an earlier analysis of IRAD by Evangelista et al., of 1010 patients with AAS, 58 (5.7%) had IMH. Among the 51 patients whose initial diagnostic workup showed IMH only, 8 (16%) progressed to AD on a serial imaging study [30].

Li et al. investigated the prognostic significance of follow-up CT findings for initially medically treated type B aortic IMH in 238 patients. In a combined predictive model for 1-month aortic events, baseline maximal hematoma thickness (MHT) $\geq$ 11.8 mm, ULP, changes of MHT, newly developed ULP, and newly developed pleural effusion were independent predictors [32].

Differentiating IMH from mural thrombus or plaques is sometimes difficult. Pre-contrast CT shows increased attenuation of the aortic wall (high density) due to hematoma (Fig. 6.15). MRI may demonstrate varying degrees of intensity on T1- and T2-weighted images and cine MRI. MRI may detect small IMHs, which are not seen on CTA. Early after the development, the hematoma of IMH shows iso-intensity on T1-weighted imaging and high intensity on T2-weighted imaging. After the first 1–2 days, oxyhemoglobin is converted to methemoglobin, leading to a high signal on both T1- and T2-weighted MR images [24].

An ulcer-like projection is a localized blood-filled pouch protruding from the true lumen into the thrombosed false lumen of the aorta through an intimal defect [16]. An intramural blood pool (IBP) is defined as a focal or patchy contrast material collection within an IMH with a narrow or nondiscernible communication with the aortic lumen (Fig. 6.16) [29]. These lesions are most commonly present in the descending and abdominal aorta associated with acute IMH with a wall thickness greater than 10 mm. There is communication between the IBP and an emerging intercostal or lumbar artery. The prognostic significance of IBPs remains uncertain.

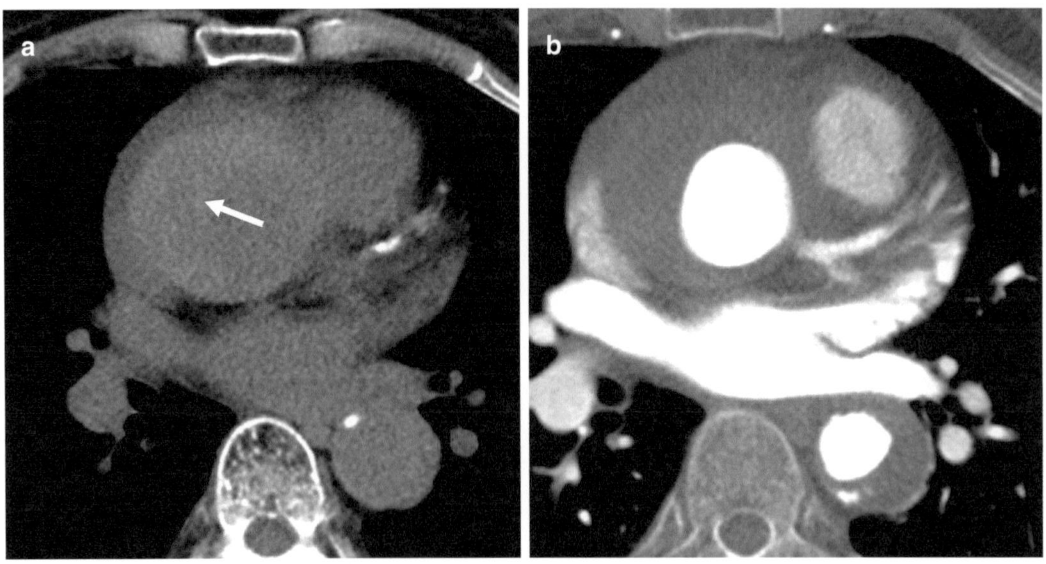

Fig. 6.15 Acute Stanford type A IMH in a 75-year-old female. (**a**) A high-attenuation ring or crescent (arrow) on pre-contrast CT. (**b**) Contrast-enhanced CT shows IMH in the ascending thoracic aorta

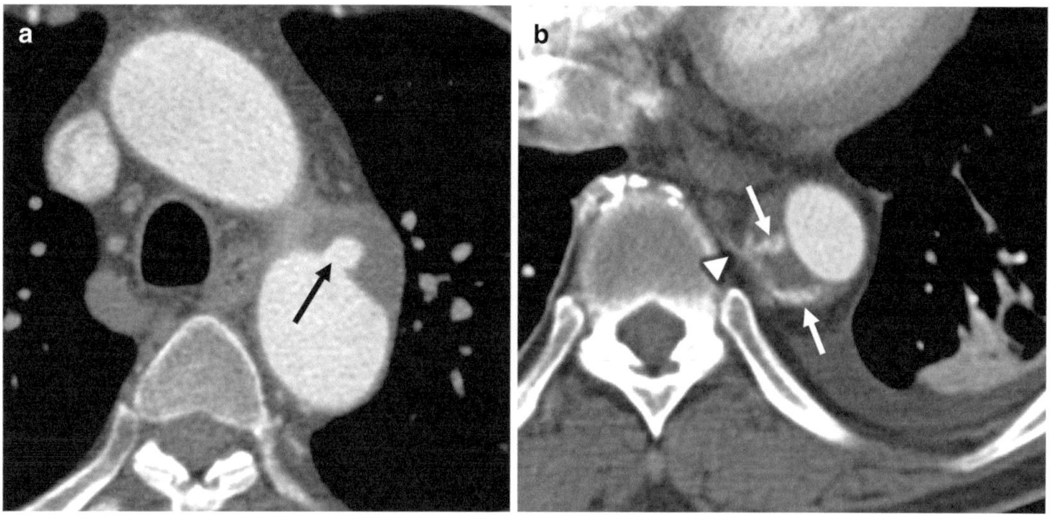

Fig. 6.16 An ulcer-like projection and intramural blood pool in a 52-year-old male with IMH of the descending thoracic aorta. (**a**) An ulcer-like projection (arrow). (**b**) Intramural blood pools (IBPs, arrows). Note the intercostal artery (arrowhead) connected to the IBP

Broken-crescent sign is defined as a focal defect within the hyper-attenuating crescentic IMH on unenhanced CT, corresponding to a smooth outbulging of the aortic lumen on CTA. Aortic IMH complicated with adventitial tear and partial outward oozing of IMH may cause a broken-crescent sign on CT. This sign is associated with a high risk of sudden aortic rupture [33].

6.3.4 Infectious Pseudoaneurysm

Mycotic aneurysms represent 0.7–2.6% of all aortic aneurysms [34]. Mycotic aneurysm is the most common form of infectious thoracic aneurysm (Fig. 6.17). Bacterial identification is not possible in approximately 25% of infected aneurysms [35]; the remaining 75% are associated with various microorganisms, most commonly *Staphylococcus*, *Enterococcus*, *Streptococcus*, and *Salmonella* species [36]. *Coxiella burnetii*, the etiologic agent of Q fever, has also been associated with vascular infection and aneurysm formation [37].

Periaortic nodularity, change in aorta size, air in the aortic wall, saccular aneurysm, and peri-aneurysmal fluid collection and soft tissue thickening are the radiological findings of infected aneurysms [38]. Areas of aortitis may appear as vessel wall edema, enhancement, or wall thickening on MRI [36].

6.3.5 Traumatic Pseudoaneurysm

Traumatic pseudoaneurysm, which is seen in patients who survived trauma, is most commonly found in the aortic isthmus. Tethering of the aorta by the ligamentum arteriosum during sudden deceleration is often the cause of traumatic pseudoaneurysm. The aneurysm appears as an irregular or ragged aortic contour, and aortic wall changes may be subtle (Fig. 6.18). Differential diagnoses include ductal diverticulum and pseudocoarctation of the aortic isthmus. In patients with a previous trauma, a triangular aneurysm in the aortic isthmus appears the same in ductal diverticulum and traumatic aneurysm.

Trauma to the aorta may result in aortic laceration, which is typically a transverse intimal tear or aortic transection in which the injury traverses the three layers of the vessel wall [39]. Aortic rupture is occasionally contained by the adventitia or periaortic tissue (aortic pseudoaneurysm), or it can cause a hematoma in the wall of the aorta (IMH). AD also occurs secondary to trauma

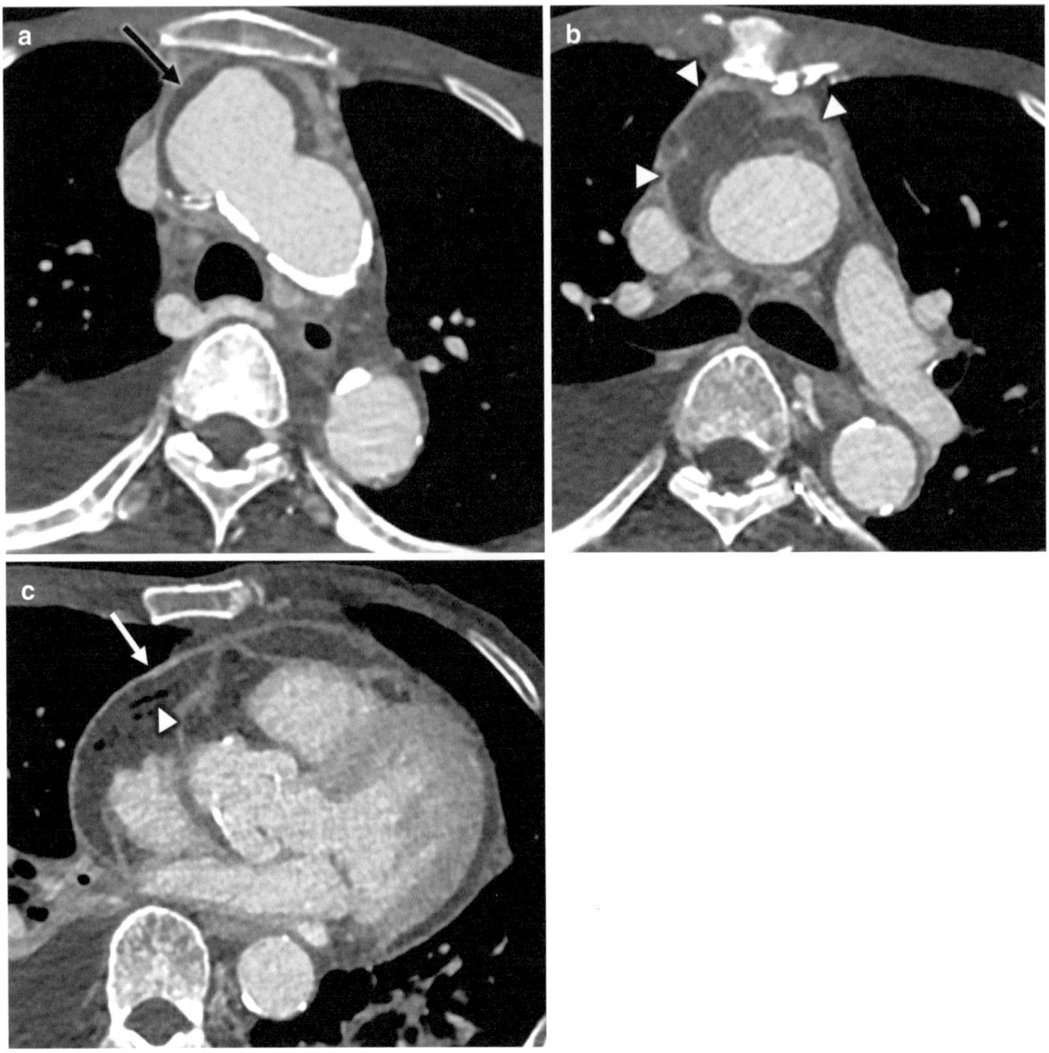

Fig. 6.17 Mycotic aneurysm of the ascending thoracic aorta and pericarditis due to *Streptococcus agalactiae* (Group B) infection in an 81-year-old male. (**a**, **b**) Two-min delayed-phase CT shows a pseudoaneurysm (arrows), abscess around the ascending aorta (arrowheads), and enhanced abscess wall. (**c**) Pericardial thickening (arrow) and gas bubbles (arrowhead) in the pericardial effusion, which are suggestive of infection

(Fig. 6.19). Penetrating aortic injuries secondary to either stab wounds or gunshot wounds have a very high mortality rate.

6.3.6 Rupturing Thoracic Aortic Aneurysm

Rupturing thoracic aortic aneurysm (RTA) is defined as thoracic diameter greater than 4 cm in patients presenting with aortic pain and imaging findings suggestive of transmural leakage, intraclot hemorrhage, periaortic hematoma, or active contrast medium extravasation [17]. TEVAR is the preferred treatment for rupturing descending thoracic aortic aneurysm. Preoperative imaging evaluation can help to determine the correct size of the aortic stent-graft and to localize the artery of Adamkiewicz [40].

Excessive aortic dilatation poses a significant risk for acute aortic events, and patients with aneurysm diameter ≥5.5 cm should be referred for prophylactic surgical intervention [41]. Impending rupture of an aortic aneurysm may appear as a cres-

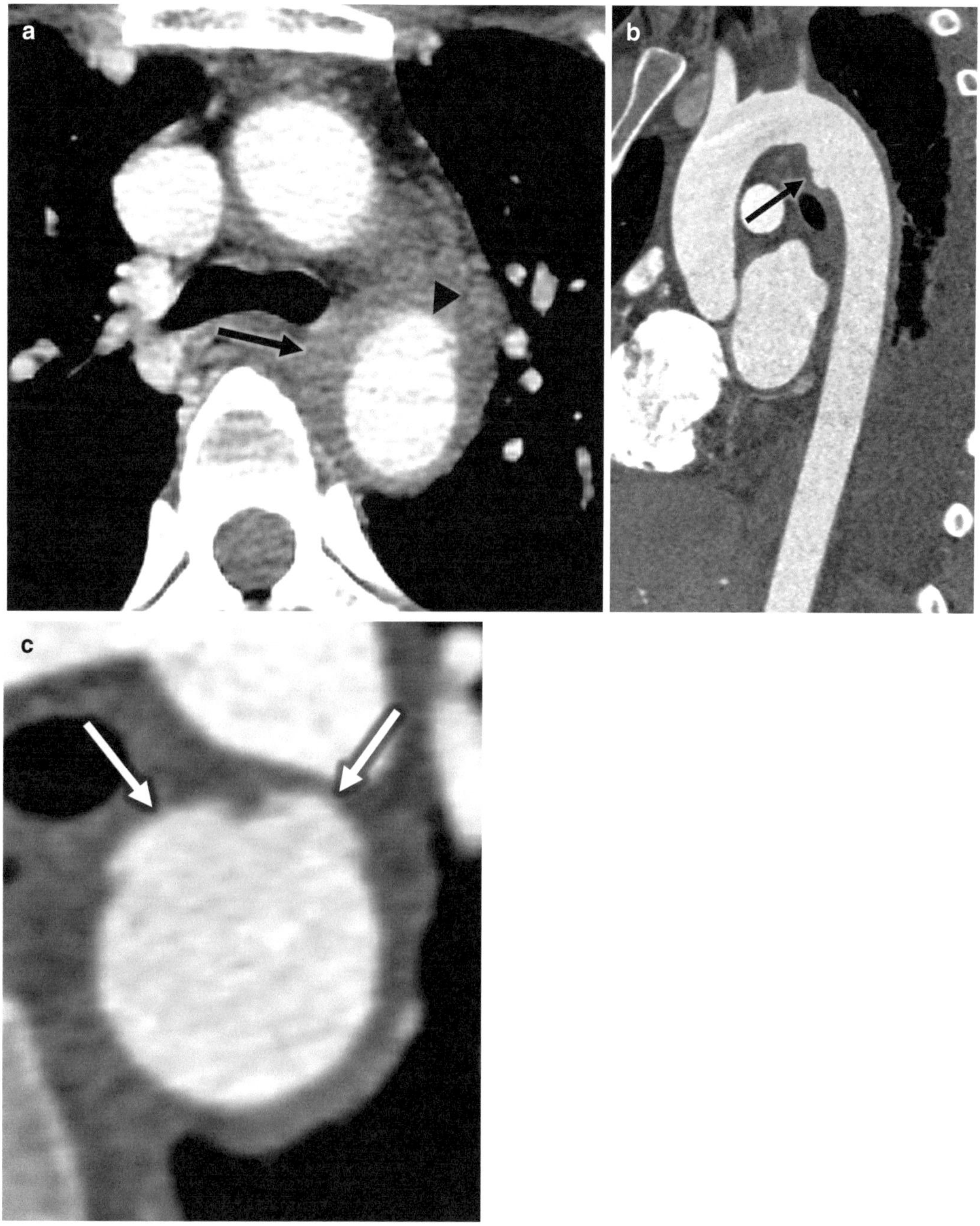

Fig. 6.18 Traumatic aortic injury in a 38-year-old female who survived an automobile accident. (**a**) Contrast-enhanced chest CT shows a subtle irregularity (arrowhead) in the anterior wall of the aortic isthmus, as well as IMH (arrow). (**b**) Oblique sagittal reformatted image reveals focal pseudoaneurysms (arrow). (**c**) Reformatted image demonstrates the irregular and ragged appearance (arrows) of the anterior wall of the aortic isthmus

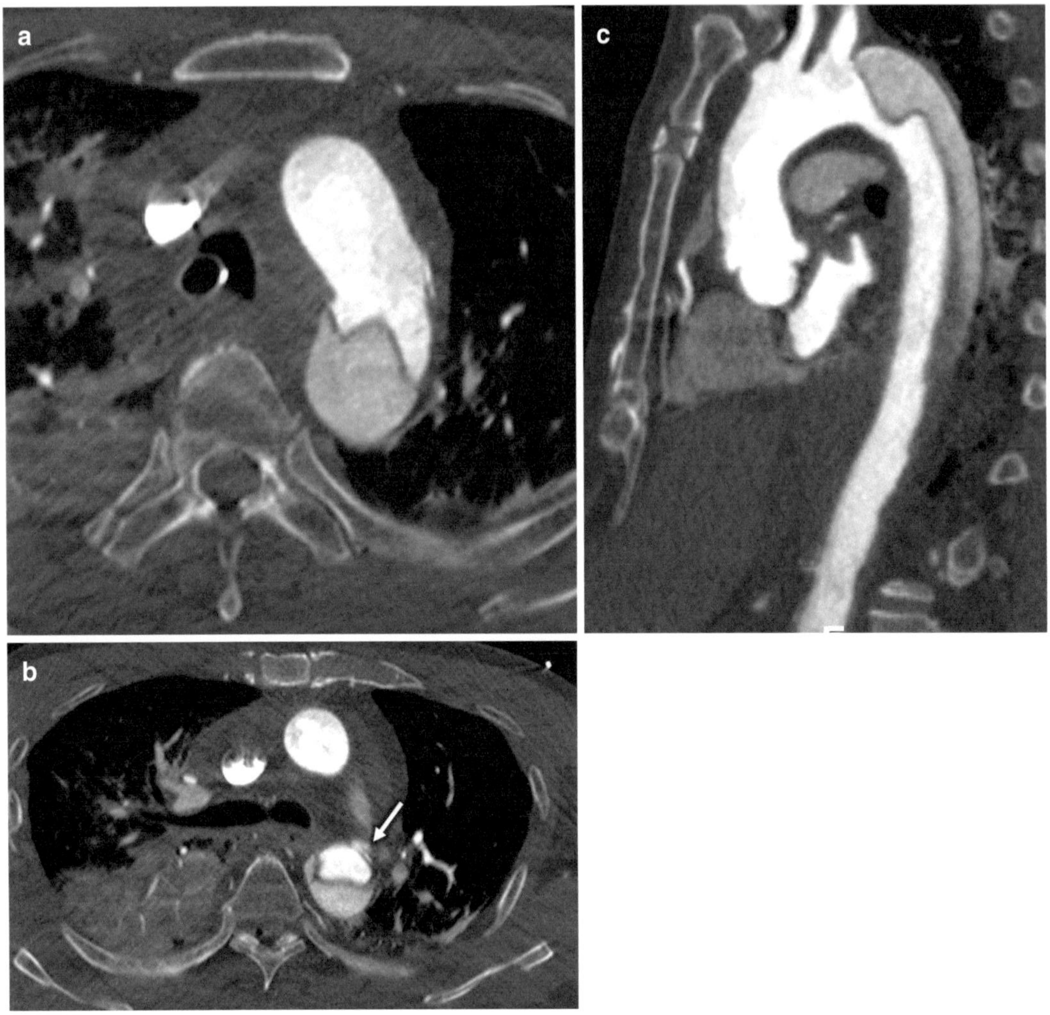

Fig. 6.19 Fatal traumatic aortic injury in an 88-year-old male who suffered a pedestrian road traffic accident. (**a**, **b**) Transverse CT images show dissection in the descending aorta and small pseudoaneurysms with a ragged appearance (arrow) in the anterior wall of the aortic isthmus. There is severe contusion of the right lung. (**c**) Oblique sagittal reformatted image shows AD involving the descending thoracic aorta and abdominal aorta

cent shape with high attenuation, representing acute hematoma within the wall or mural thrombus (Fig. 6.20) [8, 42]. Aortic aneurysms with unorganized loose thrombus, characterized by high thrombus signal intensity on T1-weighted MR imaging, may exhibit higher growth rates [43].

When an aneurysm ruptures, extravasation of contrast material, hematoma, and fluid collection occur around the rupture site. CT may show a large pseudoaneurysm, which is a concealed rupture. There may also be focal discontinuity of calcium in the wall of the aneurysm.

6.3.7 Aortoesophageal and Aortobronchial Fistula

Aortoesophageal fistula is a rare complication of foreign body ingestion, esophageal biopsy, or aortic aneurysm. CT may reveal gas and/or an abscess around the esophagus and aorta (Fig. 6.21). Aortic aneurysm or dissection may rupture into the esophagus, causing massive hematemesis. CT shows extravasation of contrast medium into the esophagus and stomach. The occurrence of aortoesophageal fistula increases after TEVAR, as it is one of the major complications of the procedure. CTA demonstrates para-aortic soft tissue shadowing and multiple gas bubbles surrounding the graft, suggesting aorto-

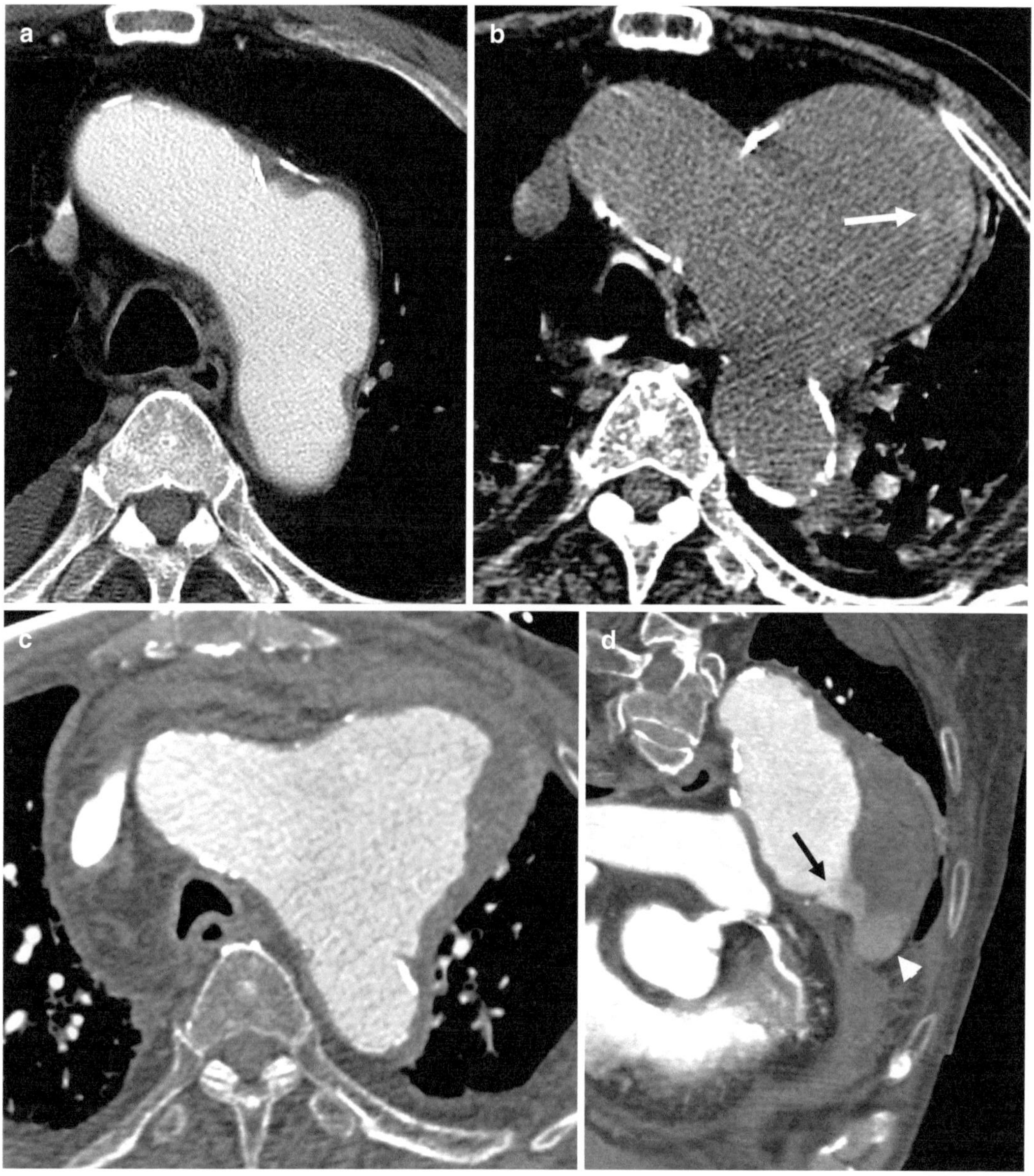

Fig. 6.20 Rupture of an aortic aneurysm in an 87-year-old male. (**a**) Initial CT, performed 5 years prior, showing aneurysmal change of the distal aortic arch and proximal descending aorta. (**b**) Non-contrast CT, performed 4 months prior, showing a markedly dilated aneurysm with a hyperattenuated crescent (arrow) in the mural thrombus. (**c**) CTA shows further increase in aneurysm size and mediastinal hematoma. (**d**, **e**) Obliquely reformatted image (**d**) and volume-rendered image (**e**) show a focal defect (arrow) in the wall of the aneurysm and extravasation (arrowhead) of contrast material

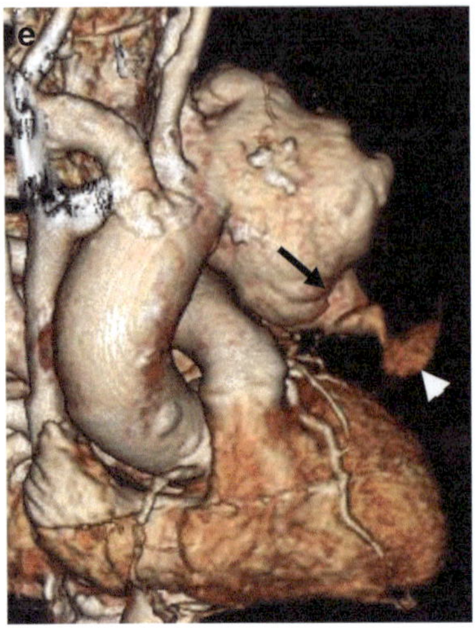

Fig. 6.20 (continued)

esophageal fistula [44]. In cases with aortobronchial fistula, CT shows intrapulmonary hematoma or consolidation around the aneurysms [45].

6.3.8 Miscellaneous Conditions

It is important to be aware of common pitfalls in diagnosing AAS on CT [46]. Takayasu's arteritis or Behçet disease may present aneurysmal changes, stenosis, and wall thickening of the thoracic aorta, pulmonary arteries, and neck vessels. IgG-related sclerotic disease may mimic IMH by showing diffuse concentric wall thickening of the thoracic aorta (Fig. 6.22). To differentiate IMH, pre-contrast CT and delayed CT (1–2 min) may be helpful in identifying high attenuation of IMH on pre-contrast CT and enhancement of fibrotic or inflammatory thickening of the aorta in cases with vasculitis or fibrosis. Subtle irregularities of the thickened fibrotic tissue around the aorta and a relative paucity of intrapericardial or pleural fluid may suggest a diagnosis of periaortic sclerotic disease.

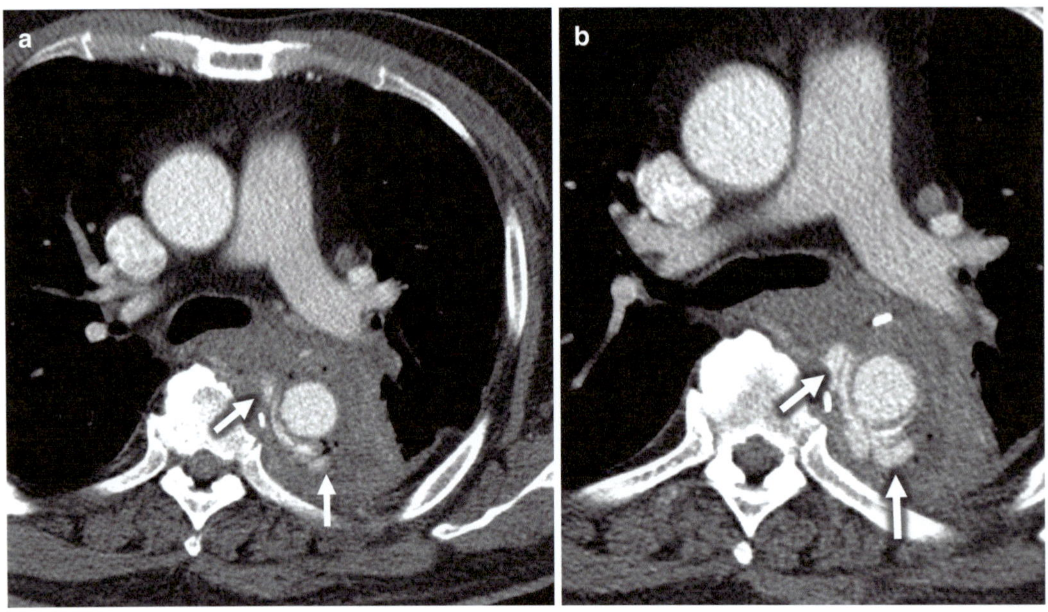

Fig. 6.21 Aortoesophageal fistula in a 66-year-old male with acute esophageal bleeding. The patient underwent graft replacement in the proximal descending aorta 6 years prior due to traumatic aortic injury. (**a**, **b**) Transverse CT images depict pseudoaneurysms (arrow), gas bubbles, and perigraft fluid collection. Surgery confirmed a fistula between the esophagus and graft

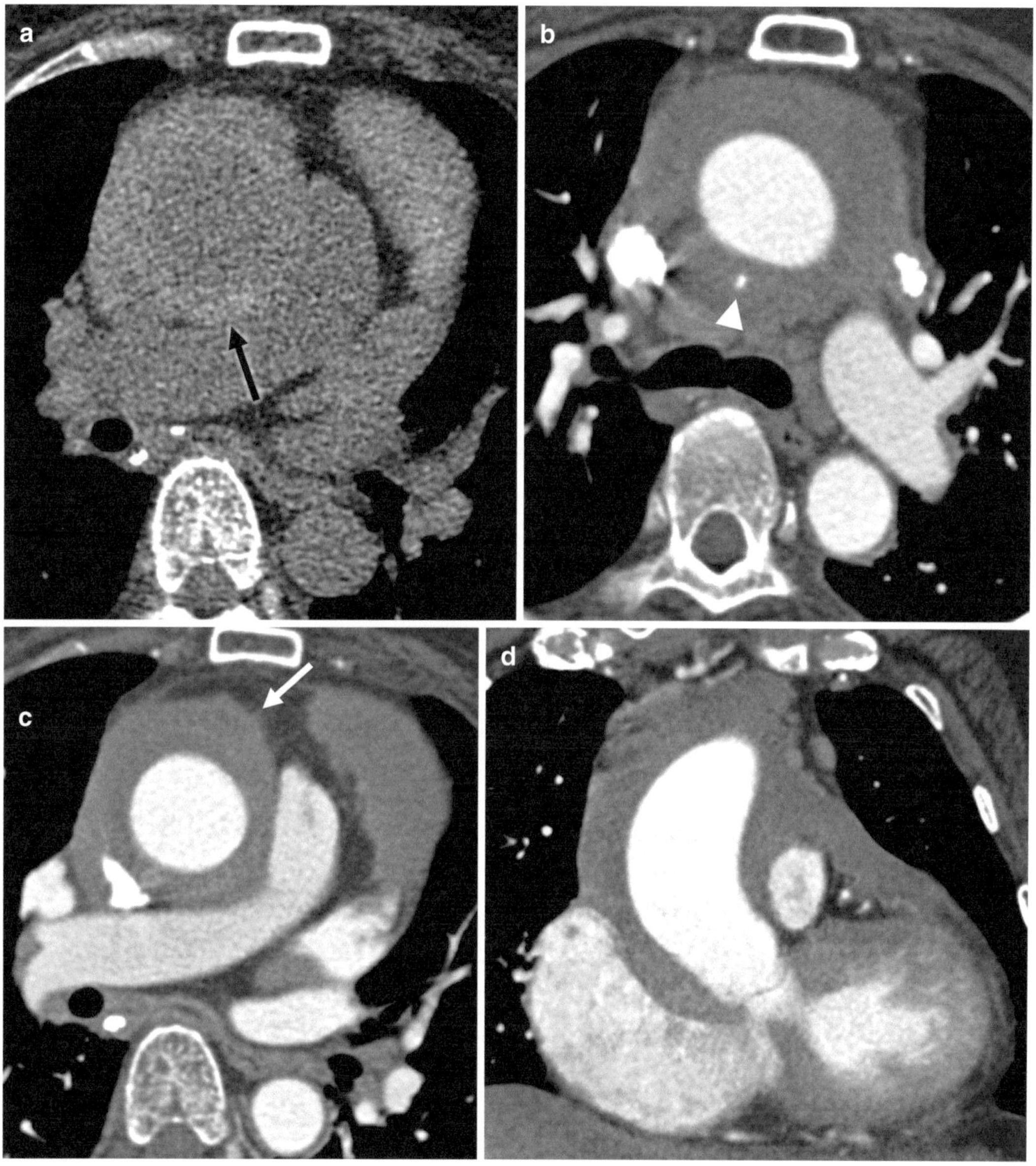

Fig. 6.22 IgG-related periaortic sclerotic disease mimicking IMH in a 67-year-old female. (**a**) Pre-contrast CT shows areas of increased attenuation (arrow) around the ascending aorta. (**b**)–(**d**) CTA demonstrates mild homogeneous enhancement of the thick periaortic fibrotic tissue. Note CT findings not typical of IMH, such as a focal calcification (arrowhead) in the middle of fibrotic tissue (**b**), the subtle irregular contour (arrows) of the fibrotic rind, and a thick pericardial mass

6.4 Summary

CT with optimized scanning and contrast injection techniques is the modality of choice for the evaluation of acute aortic diseases. MR angiography may replace CTA in selected cases of acute aortic disease. CT shows the extent of aortic dissection, the degree of true lumen collapse, the involvement of visceral and extremity arteries, and resultant organ ischemia or infarction. The clinical and imaging features of AD and PAU can overlap. Stanford Type A IMH (ascending aorta) is associated with substantial mortality, whereas Stanford type B IMH (arch and descending aorta) are less likely to be associated with an adverse outcome. Imaging findings of an infected aortic pseudoaneurysm, traumatic pseudoaneurysm, rupturing aortic aneurysm, aortoesophageal fistula, aortobronchial fistula, noninfectious aortitis, and periaortic sclerotic disease should be appreciated.

Key Points

- ECG-gated CTA is recommended to avoid motion artifacts in the ascending aorta.
- MRI may be adopted for aortic imaging in patients allergic to contrast material, those who are pregnant, or children.
- The sensitivities of CT and MRI for diagnosis of AAS are 100% and 95–100%, respectively.
- In patients with uncomplicated acute type B AD, aortic diameter >44 mm is a predictor of mortality after adjustment for other significant risk factors.
- Larger ulcer diameter, greater ulcer depth, and increasing pleural effusion are associated with PAU progression.
- Baseline MHT $\geq$ 11.8 mm, ULP, changes of MHT, newly developed ULP, and newly developed pleural effusion are independent predictors of aortic events in patients with IMH.
- Periaortic nodularity, change in aorta size, air in the aortic wall, saccular aneurysm, and perianeurysmal fluid collection and soft tissue thickening are the radiological findings of infected aortic pseudoaneurysm.
- Traumatic pseudoaneurysm of the aortic isthmus may produce a subtly ragged appearance of the anterior wall of the descending aorta.
- Impending rupture of an aortic aneurysm may be seen as a crescent of contrast with high attenuation within the aortic wall or mural thrombus.

References

1. Vardhanabhuti V, Nicol E, Morgan-Hughes G, et al. Recommendations for accurate CT diagnosis of suspected acute aortic syndrome (AAS)–on behalf of the British Society of Cardiovascular Imaging (BSCI)/ British Society of Cardiovascular CT (BSCCT). Br J Radiol. 2016;89(1061):20150705.
2. Beeres M, Wichmann JL, Frellesen C, et al. ECG-gated versus non-ECG-gated high-pitch dual-source CT for whole body CT angiography (CTA). Acad Radiol. 2016;23(2):163–7.
3. Ippolito D, Talei Franzesi C, Fior D, Bonaffini PA, Minutolo O, Sironi S. Low kV settings CT angiography (CTA) with low dose contrast medium volume protocol in the assessment of thoracic and abdominal aorta disease: a feasibility study. Br J Radiol. 2015;88(1049):20140140.
4. Zhang LJ, Zhao YE, Schoepf UJ, et al. Seventy-peak kilovoltage high-pitch thoracic aortic CT angiography without ECG gating: evaluation of image quality and radiation dose. Acad Radiol. 2015;22(7):890–7.
5. Potthast S, Mitsumori L, Stanescu LA, et al. Measuring aortic diameter with different MR techniques: comparison of three-dimensional (3D) navigated steady-state free-precession (SSFP), 3D contrast-enhanced magnetic resonance angiography (CE-MRA), 2D T2 black blood, and 2D cine SSFP. J Magn Reson Imaging. 2010;31(1):177–84.
6. Bireley WR II, Diniz LO, Groves EM, Dill K, Carroll TJ, Carr JC. Orthogonal measurement of thoracic aorta luminal diameter using ECG-gated high-resolution contrast-enhanced MR angiography. J Magn Reson Imaging. 2007;26(6):1480–5.
7. Groves EM, Bireley W, Dill K, Carroll TJ, Carr JC. Quantitative analysis of ECG-gated high-resolution contrast-enhanced MR angiography of the thoracic aorta. AJR Am J Roentgenol. 2007;188(2):522–8.
8. Abbas A, Brown IW, Peebles CR, Harden SP, Shambrook JS. The role of multidetector-row CT in the diagnosis, classification and management of acute aortic syndrome. Br J Radiol. 2014;87(1042): 20140354.
9. Mussa FF, Horton JD, Moridzadeh R, Nicholson J, Trimarchi S, Eagle KA. Acute aortic dissection and intramural hematoma: a systematic review. JAMA. 2016;316(7):754–63.
10. Nazerian P, Mueller C, Soeiro AM, et al. Diagnostic accuracy of the aortic dissection detection risk score plus D-dimer for acute aortic syndromes: the ADvISED prospective multicenter study. Circulation. 2018;137(3):250–8.
11. Meredith EL, Masani ND. Echocardiography in the emergency assessment of acute aortic syndromes. Eur J Echocardiogr. 2009;10(1):i31–9.
12. Di Marco L, Leone A, Murana G, et al. Acute type A aortic dissection: rationale and outcomes of extensive repair of the arch and distal aorta. Int J Cardiol. 2018;267:145–9.
13. Sailer AM, van Kuijk SM, Nelemans PJ, et al. Computed tomography imaging features in acute uncomplicated stanford type-B aortic dissection predict late adverse events. Circ Cardiovasc Imaging.

2017;10(4):e005709. https://doi.org/10.1161/CIRCIMAGING.116.005709.
14. Williams DM, Joshi A, Dake MD, Deeb GM, Miller DC, Abrams GD. Aortic cobwebs: an anatomic marker identifying the false lumen in aortic dissection–imaging and pathologic correlation. Radiology. 1994;190(1):167–74.
15. Chin AS, Willemink MJ, Kino A, et al. Acute limited intimal tears of the thoracic aorta. J Am Coll Cardiol. 2018;71(24):2773–85.
16. Ueda T, Chin A, Petrovitch I, Fleischmann D. A pictorial review of acute aortic syndrome: discriminating and overlapping features as revealed by ECG-gated multidetector-row CT angiography. Insights Imaging. 2012;3(6):561–71.
17. Hiratzka LF, Bakris GL, Beckman JA, et al. 2010 ACCF/AHA/AATS/ACR/ASA/SCA/SCAI/SIR/STS/SVM Guidelines for the diagnosis and management of patients with thoracic aortic disease. A Report of the American College of Cardiology Foundation/American Heart Association Task Force on Practice Guidelines, American Association for Thoracic Surgery, American College of Radiology,American Stroke Association, Society of Cardiovascular Anesthesiologists, Society for Cardiovascular Angiography and Interventions, Society of Interventional Radiology, Society of Thoracic Surgeons,and Society for Vascular Medicine. J Am Coll Cardiol. 2010;55(14):e27–e129.
18. Ray HM, Durham CA, Ocazionez D, et al. Predictors of intervention and mortality in patients with uncomplicated acute type B aortic dissection. J Vasc Surg. 2016;64(6):1560–8.
19. Ray HM, Besho JM, Au J, et al. The role of ascending aortic size in outcomes of patients with uncomplicated acute type B aortic dissection. J Vasc Surg. 2019;69(4):1011–20.
20. Kubota Y, Yokota H, Mukai H, et al. Low-tube-voltage CT assessment of Adamkiewicz artery: precise comparison between 100-kVp- and 120-kVp protocols. Eur J Radiol. 2019;111:56–61.
21. Clarençon F, Di Maria F, Cormier E, et al. Comparison of intra-aortic computed tomography angiography to conventional angiography in the presurgical visualization of the Adamkiewicz artery: first results in patients with thoracoabdominal aortic aneurysms. Neuroradiology. 2013;55(11):1379–87.
22. Valente T, Rossi G, Lassandro F, et al. MDCT evaluation of acute aortic syndrome (AAS). Br J Radiol. 2016;89(1061):20150825.
23. Gebker R, Gomaa O, Schnackenburg B, Rebakowski J, Fleck E, Nagel E. Comparison of different MRI techniques for the assessment of thoracic aortic pathology: 3D contrast enhanced MR angiography, turbo spin echo and balanced steady state free precession. Int J Cardiovasc Imaging. 2007;23(6):747–56.
24. Oderich GS, Kärkkäinen JM, Reed NR, Tenorio ER, Sandri GA. Penetrating aortic ulcer and intramural hematoma. Cardiovasc Intervent Radiol. 2019;42(3):321–34.
25. Cho KR, Stanson AW, Potter DD, Cherry KJ, Schaff HV, Sundt TM III. Penetrating atherosclerotic ulcer of the descending thoracic aorta and arch. J Thorac Cardiovasc Surg. 2004;127(5):1393–9. discussion 1399-1401
26. Nathan DP, Boonn W, Lai E, et al. Presentation, complications, and natural history of penetrating atherosclerotic ulcer disease. J Vasc Surg. 2012;55(1):10–5.
27. Ganaha F, Miller DC, Sugimoto K, et al. Prognosis of aortic intramural hematoma with and without penetrating atherosclerotic ulcer: a clinical and radiological analysis. Circulation. 2002;106(3):342–8.
28. Maraj R, Rerkpattanapipat P, Jacobs LE, Makornwattana P, Kotler MN. Meta-analysis of 143 reported cases of aortic intramural hematoma. Am J Cardiol. 2000;86(6):664–8.
29. Herrán FL, Bang TJ, Restauri N, et al. CT imaging of complications of aortic intramural hematoma: a pictorial essay. Diagn Interv Radiol. 2018;24(6):342–7.
30. Evangelista A, Mukherjee D, Mehta RH, et al. Acute intramural hematoma of the aorta: a mystery in evolution. Circulation. 2005;111(8):1063–70.
31. Harris KM, Braverman AC, Eagle KA, et al. Acute aortic intramural hematoma: an analysis from the International Registry of Acute Aortic Dissection. Circulation. 2012;126(11 Suppl 1):S91–6.
32. Li Z, Lu B, Chen Y, et al. Acute type B aortic intramural hematoma: the added prognostic value of a follow-up CT. Eur Radiol. 2019;29(12):6571–80.
33. Ko SF, Lu CY, Sheu JJ, Yip HK, Huang CC, Ng SH. Broken-crescent sign at CT indicates impending aortic rupture in patients with acute aortic intramural hematoma. Insights Imaging. 2020;11(1):73.
34. Steverlynck L, Van de Walle S. Mycotic thoracic aortic aneurysm: review of the diagnostic and therapeutic options. Acta Clin Belg. 2013;68(3):193–8.
35. Bendermacher BL, Peppelenbosch AG, Daemen JW, Oude Lashof AM, Jacobs MJ. Q fever (Coxiella burnetii) causing an infected thoracoabdominal aortic aneurysm. J Vasc Surg. 2011;53(5):1402–4.
36. Lopes RJ, Almeida J, Dias PJ, Pinho P, Maciel MJ. Infectious thoracic aortitis: a literature review. Clin Cardiol. 2009;32(9):488–90.
37. Robinson WP, Schuksz M. Surgical and antimicrobial management of a thoracic aortic aneurysm due to Q fever: a case report and brief review. Vasc Endovasc Surg. 2016;50(4):290–4.
38. Narang AT, Rathlev NK. Non-aneurysmal infectious aortitis: a case report. J Emerg Med. 2007;32(4):359–63.
39. Gosavi S, Tyroch AH, Mukherjee D. Cardiac trauma. Angiology. 2016;67(10):896–901.
40. Hogendoorn W, Schlösser FJ, Muhs BE, Popescu WM. Surgical and anesthetic considerations for the endovascular treatment of ruptured descending thoracic aortic aneurysms. Curr Opin Anaesthesiol. 2014;27(1):12–20.
41. Adriaans BP, Wildberger JE, Westenberg JJM, Lamb HJ, Schalla S. Predictive imaging for thoracic aortic

dissection and rupture: moving beyond diameters. Eur Radiol. 2019;29(12):6396–404.
42. Mehard WB, Heiken JP, Sicard GA. High-attenuating crescent in abdominal aortic aneurysm wall at CT: a sign of acute or impending rupture. Radiology. 1994;192(2):359–62.
43. Nguyen VL, Leiner T, Hellenthal FA, et al. Abdominal aortic aneurysms with high thrombus signal intensity on magnetic resonance imaging are associated with high growth rate. Eur J Vasc Endovasc Surg. 2014;48(6):676–84.
44. Kay MD, Davies B, Patel K, Gourevitch D. Aorto-oesophageal fistula following TEVAR: an unusual cause of mediastinal air. BMJ Case Rep. 2013;2013:bcr2013009268.
45. Liu SF, Chen YC, Lin MC, Kao CL. Thoracic aortic aneurysm with aortobronchial fistula: a thirteen-year experience. Heart Lung. 2004;33(2):119–23.
46. Husainy MA, Sayyed F, Puppala S. Acute aortic syndrome-pitfalls on gated and non-gated CT scan. Emerg Radiol. 2016;23(4):397–403.

7 Acute Cardiac Diseases: Evaluation with Computed Tomography and Magnetic Resonance Imaging

7.1 Introduction

Cardiovascular disease can be life threatening, and often necessitates a trip to the emergency department (ED). Coronary CT angiography (CCTA) provides the most reliable and accurate assessment of coronary artery disease. Acute myocardial infarction is also visible, as a low-perfusion area in the left ventricular myocardium, on CT. CT also enables the detection of intracardiac sources of systemic embolization, i.e., cardiac tumors, thrombus, and vegetations. When available, cardiac magnetic resonance imaging (CMR) allows the accurate diagnosis of acute myocardial infarction, acute myocarditis, and pericarditis along with myocardial diseases with heart failure.

7.2 Imaging Techniques

7.2.1 CT Techniques

CT scanners with a 64-slice or higher capacity (detector row) or wide-detector scanners are adequate for cardiac CT. High-temporal-resolution CT scanners are preferred. Calcium scoring CT is first performed without contrast injection.

Drugs may be administered to patients with heart rates ≥65 beats per minute (bpm) before CCTA. Intravenous injection of a beta-blocker is preferred to oral medication. Contraindications to the use of beta-blockers, calcium channel blockers, and nitroglycerin should be considered before drug administration. Beta-blockers should not be given to patients with asthma or chronic obstructive pulmonary disease on a beta-2-agonist inhaler, or those with heart failure [1].

Regarding scan coverage, areas from the thoracic inlet to the diaphragm level are generally included and the whole aorta is covered in cases suspected of aortic dissection or aneurysm.

Contrast material is injected as a bolus at a rate of 3–7 mL/s (40–120 mL in total, 300–400 mg I/kg) followed by a 30–50 mL saline chaser or a mixture of contrast material and saline in a ratio of 2:8 or 3:7. The amount of iodine that is delivered should be designed to achieve optimal cardiovascular contrast enhancement. For example, the iodine flux (iodine delivery rate, IDR) of 4 mL/s contrast material is 1.48 g I/s for iopromide 370 mg I/mL, while it is 1.60 g I/s for iomeprol 400 mg I/mL. A lower tube voltage of 70, 80, 90, or 100 kVp may result in greater relative vascular enhancement compared to a tube voltage of 120 or 140 kVp. Therefore, iodine delivery rates differ according to the tube voltage (1.6–2.0 g I/s at 120 kVp and 1.3–1.5 g I/s at 70 kVp) [2]. Biphasic or triphasic contrast injection should be considered to reduce contrast dose, achieve uniform contrast enhancement of the right- and left-side chambers, and eliminate streak artifacts from the superior vena cava [2].

Electrocardiography (ECG) gating is applied in helical (retrospective reconstruction), axial (step-and-shoot; prospective recon-

T. J. Kim et al., *Emergency Chest Radiology*, https://doi.org/10.1007/978-981-33-4396-2_7

struction), or high-pitch modes (pitch factor, 3.2). Variable helical pitch (VHP) mode scanning refers to CT scanning using two pitch changes (Fig. 7.1). These scan techniques have led to simultaneous acquisition of images of the aorta and heart during single contrast injection with a reduction in radiation and contrast doses [3]. In VHP scanning, prospective/retrospective ECG-gated scanning (cardiac pitch, 0.15) proceeds from the carina to the base of the heart. Non-ECG-gated scanning (vascular pitch, 0.81) is used for the upper chest and abdominal/pelvic areas.

Arterial phase imaging is usually sufficient for the assessment of cardiac and coronary structures. Delayed-phase imaging is optionally adopted to diagnose intracardiac thrombus, tumor, abscess, chest wall bleeding, or myocardial diseases. Stress perfusion CT is not indicated in an acute setting.

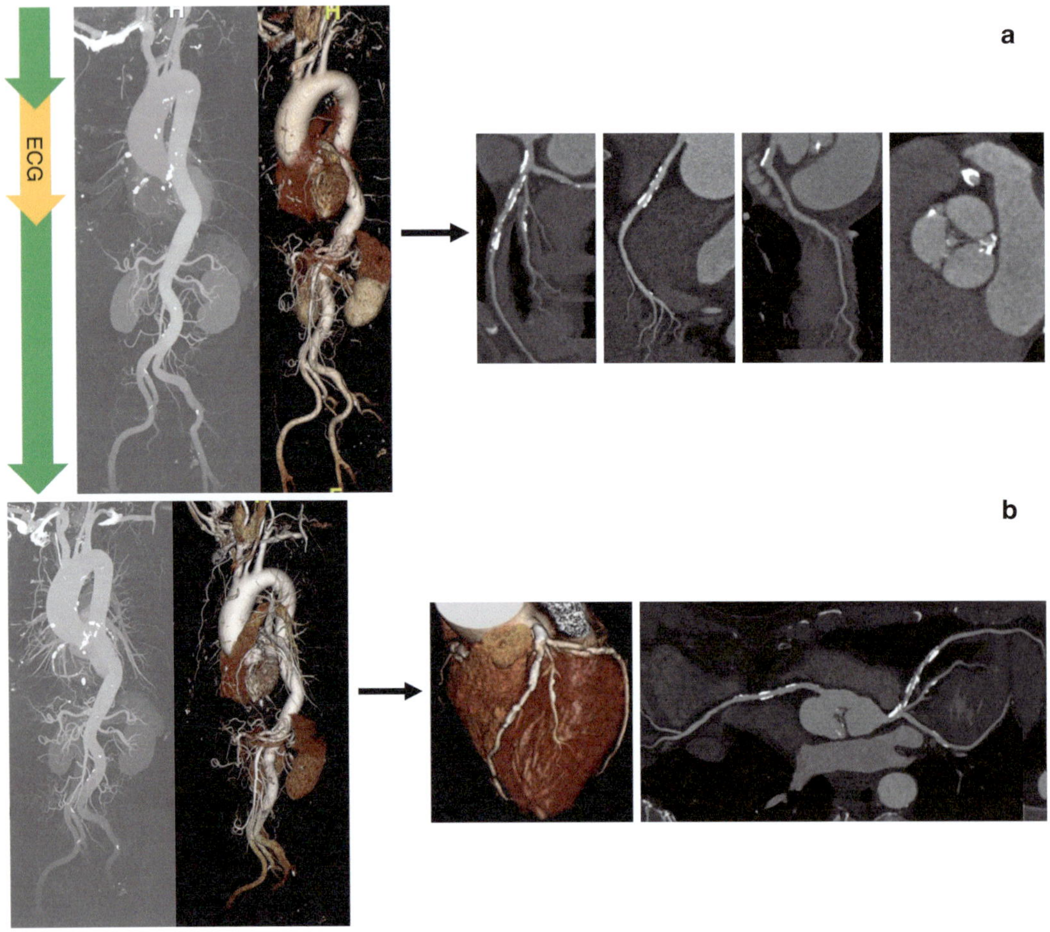

Fig. 7.1 Comparison of variable helical-pitch mode with an area-detector CT and high-pitch mode scanning with a dual-source CT for simultaneous evaluation of the coronary arteries and aorta. The patient was a 74-year-old male with an aneurysmal ascending aorta and mild aortic valvular stenosis. A single injection of contrast material was given and one scan was performed. (**a**) In variable helical-pitch mode scanning, electrocardiography (ECG)-gated CT angiography was performed in the cardiac area with a heart-dedicated pitch (0.15). Non-ECG-gated scanning was performed in the upper chest and abdominopelvic area with a medium pitch (0.81). The total dose–length product was 576 mGy·cm at 100 kVp. (**b**) In high-pitch mode scanning, the whole aorta and coronary artery system were scanned with a pitch factor of 3.2. The image of the coronary arteries is of diagnostic quality on this follow-up scan, taken 2 years after the initial scan in **A**. Calcific lesions can be seen in the left anterior descending and right coronary arteries. The total dose–length product was 170 mGy·cm at 90 kVp

7.2.2 Cardiac MRI Techniques

Typical imaging sequences for CMR include cine MRI, T2-weighted imaging, and late Gd-enhanced imaging. Cine MRI is performed in 4-, 2-, 3-chamber, and short-axial views in balanced steady-state free precession (SSFP) sequence using a 1.5T or 3T scanner. T2-weighted short-axial images are acquired before contrast injection. Late Gd-enhanced (LGE) images are taken in short-axial planes 5 to 20 min after Gd-based contrast material injection (0.1–0.2 mmol/kg; macrocyclic Gd contrast agents preferred) with inversion times according to the manufacturer's recommendations and field strength. T1, T2, and T2* mapping and coronary MR angiography can also be performed. Velocity-encoded cine MRI may be performed in cases with valvular stenosis or regurgitation.

7.3 Acute Coronary Syndrome

Many patients who seek care for acute chest pain are diagnosed with acute myocardial infarction. Approximately 0.4 million patients in the United States alone have acute coronary syndrome (ACS) [4]. CCTA is an attractive noninvasive imaging modality for use in the emergency department (ED) for the evaluation of acute chest pain due to its high negative predictive value. Recent studies have demonstrated that CCTA can be used for safe, rapid, and efficient triage of ED patients. High heart rates (>65 bpm) in patients with acute chest pain may cause blurring of the coronary arteries and stairstep artifacts on imaging. Therefore, CT techniques should be optimized and tailored for each patient.

Along with the recently introduced high-resolution troponin assay, acute myocardial infarction, or severe coronary stenosis causing myocardial ischemia can be reliably diagnosed with CCTA. Recently introduced guidelines encourage the use of CCTA in appropriate clinical cases. The role of CCTA is mainly to exclude patients without CAD and discharge patients from the ED, thus avoiding unnecessary hospitalization. CCTA helps to detect CAD causing myocardial ischemia or infarction by allowing visualization of significant coronary stenosis (> 50% luminal narrowing) and/or low myocardial perfusion even without pharmacological stress in cases of acute myocardial infarction (Fig. 7.2).

7.3.1 CCTA for Diagnosis of Acute Coronary Syndrome

CCTA has a high diagnostic accuracy to rule out clinically significant CAD in patients with non-ST-segment elevation acute coronary syndrome (NSTEACS) by invasive coronary angiography (ICA), as in the VERDICT (Very Early Versus Deferred Invasive Evaluation Using Computerized Tomography in Patients With Acute Coronary Syndromes) trial ($n = 1023$). The per-patient diagnostic accuracy of CCTA for detection of coronary stenosis ≥50% by ICA was 88.7% and the area under the curve was 0.84, with a negative predictive value (NPV), positive predictive value (PPV), sensitivity, and specificity of 90.9%, 87.9%, 96.5%, and 72.4%, respectively [5].

Interpretation of CCTA in patients with acute chest pain should be prompt. When a cardiac radiologist is not available, automatic CAD detection algorithms with or without deep-learning seem promising. According to one article, a CAD detection algorithm enabled detection of CAD in the ED with high sensitivity and NPV for the detection of stenosis of at least 50% on CCTA. As a second "reader," the CAD algorithm may help to exclude significant coronary stenosis in patients with acute chest pain. Min et al. investigated 128 consecutive patients who presented with acute chest pain and underwent 128-slice dual-source CCTA and ICA in an ED. The CCTA data were analyzed using customized software for the detection of coronary artery stenosis, without any human interaction. On a per-vessel basis, the CAD algorithm yielded 90.0% sensitivity, 62.4% specificity, 40.1% PPV, and 95.7% NPV (Fig. 7.3). Human interpretation of CCTA data yielded 96.7% sensitivity, 95.0% specificity, 84.5% PPV, and 99.0% NPV for

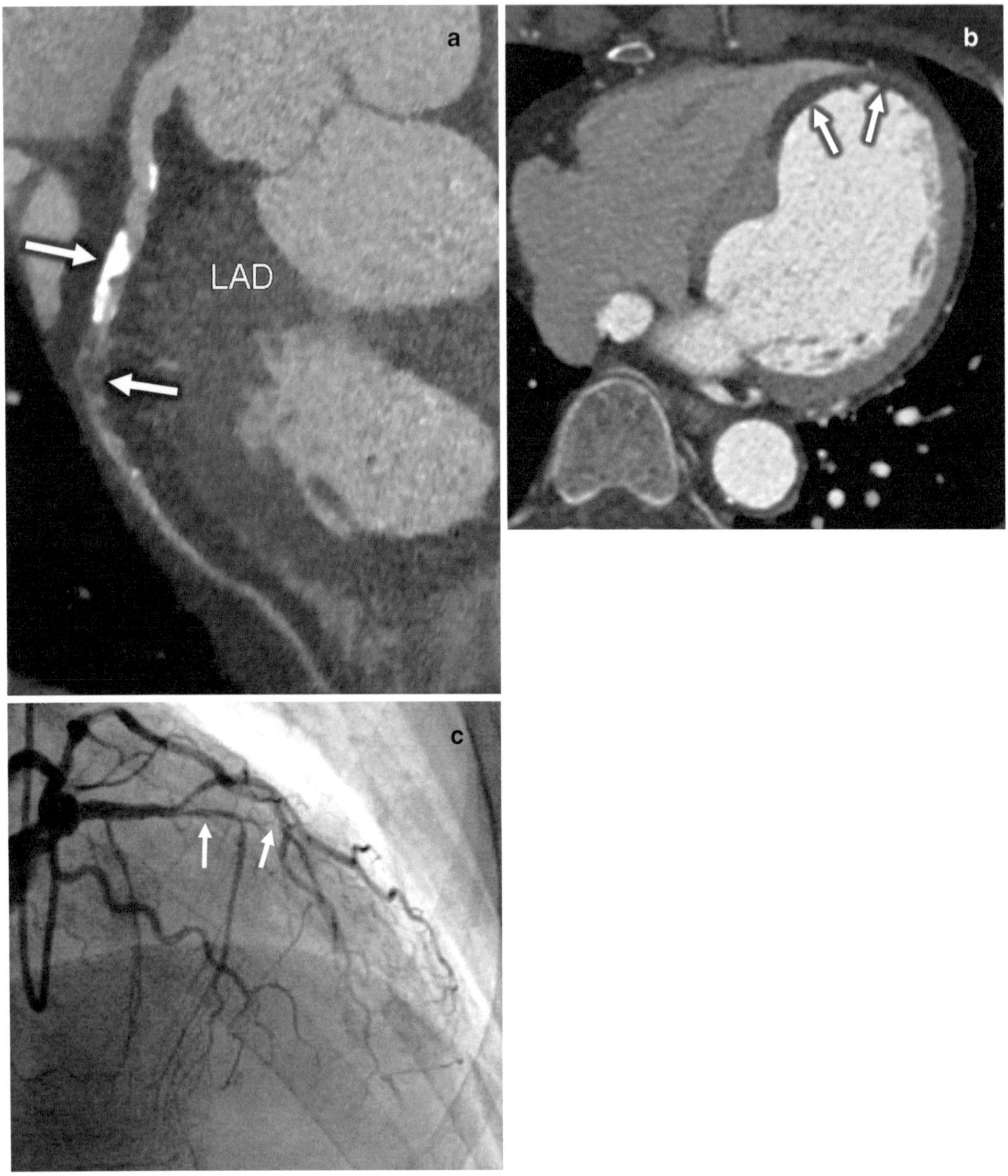

Fig. 7.2 Non-ST-elevation acute myocardial infarction in a 69-year-old female. (**a**) Coronary CT angiography (CCTA) shows severe stenosis (arrows) in the proximal to middle left anterior descending artery (LAD). (**b**) Transverse CCTA image shows a low-perfusion area (arrows), indicating myocardial infarction in the apical interventricular septum. (**c**) Invasive angiography shows severe stenosis (arrows) in the LAD. The patient had a 3-vessel disease and stenting was performed in the LAD

diagnosing significant stenosis, respectively, on a per-vessel basis [6].

In acute, low-risk chest pain patients in the ED, CCTA leads to more rapid and cost-efficient diagnosis than rest-stress nuclear myocardial perfusion imaging (MPI) [7]. CCTA has higher diagnostic performance than dobutamine-stress echocardiography for evaluation of patients with recent chest pain, normal ECG findings, and negative troponine to exclude CAD [8].

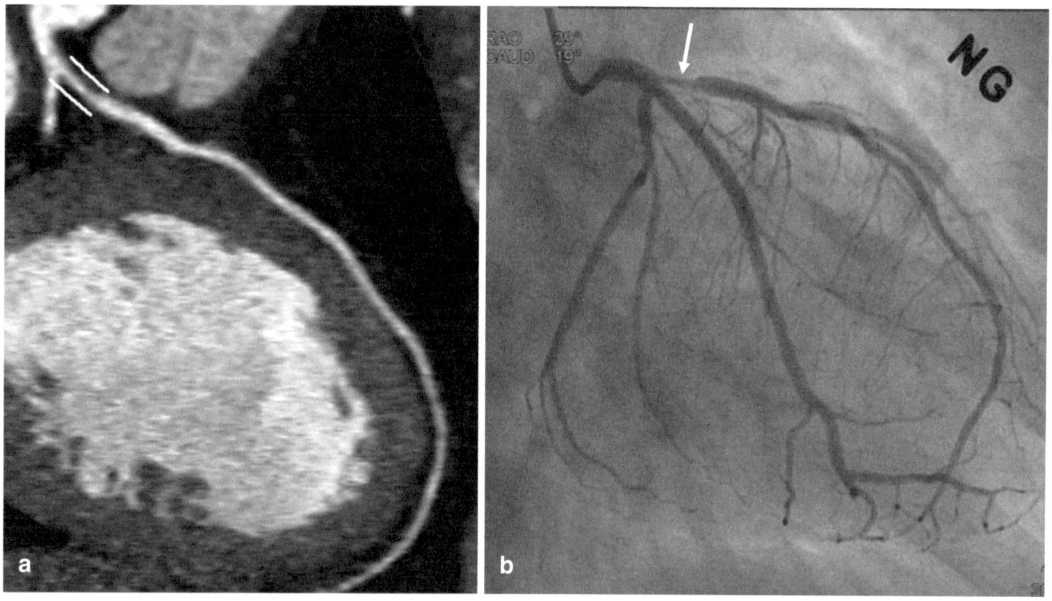

Fig. 7.3 Algorithm-based detection of coronary stenosis in a 52-year-old male. (**a**) A coronary artery disease (CAD) detection algorithm identified a stenotic lesion in the proximal LAD. (**b**) Confirmation of a severely stenotic lesion (arrow) in the LAD with invasive coronary angiography

7.3.2 Clinical Studies of Patient Triage in the Emergency Department

A CCTA-based strategy for low-to-intermediate-risk patients presenting with possible ACS appears to allow the safe, expedited discharge of many patients from the ED. In a study by Litt et al., patients in the CCTA group had a higher rate of discharge from the ED (49.6% vs. 22.7%), a shorter length of stay (median, 18.0 h vs. 24.8 h; $P < 0.001$), and a higher rate of detection of CAD (9.0% vs. 3.5%) compared to patients receiving traditional care [9]. No patients with a negative CCTA examination died or had a myocardial infarction within 30 days after presentation.

According to Hoffmann et al., in a multicenter trial in 1000 patients, the rate of ACS was 8% [10]. After early CCTA, as compared with a standard evaluation, the mean length of stay in the hospital was reduced by 7.6 h ($P < 0.001$) and more patients were discharged directly from the ED (47% vs. 12%, $P < 0.001$). There were no cases of undetected ACS and no significant differences in major adverse cardiovascular events at 28 days. After CCTA, there was more downstream testing and higher total radiation exposure.

In the CATCH trial (299 patients treated with a CCTA-guided strategy and 301 given standard care), major adverse cardiovascular events (MACE: cardiac death, myocardial infarction, hospitalization for unstable angina pectoris, and late symptom-driven revascularization) were observed in a smaller number of patients in the CCTA-guided group ($n = 5$) than the standard care group ($n = 14$) ($P = 0.04$; hazard ratio: 0.36) [11].

An early CCTA-based strategy can benefit women with symptoms suggestive of ACS by excluding CAD. In the ROMICAT-II (Rule Out Myocardial Infarction/Ischemia Using Computer Assisted Tomography) trial, women in the CCTA arm had a greater reduction in length of stay, lower hospital admission rates, and a lesser increase in cumulative radiation dose than men [12]. In comparison to men, women had lower ACS rates (3% vs. 12%; $P < 0.0001$) and more normal CCTA examinations (58% vs. 37%; $P < 0.0001$). Women were also less likely to be diagnosed with obstructive CAD by CCTA (5%

versus 17%; P = 0.0001). Notably, diabetic patients had fewer normal CCTA examinations than nondiabetic patients (32% vs. 50%, P = 0.003). Diabetic patients with >50% stenosis had a high prevalence of ACS, ICA, and revascularization [13].

In a pooled analysis of data from the ACRIN-PA (American College of Radiology Imaging Network-Pennsylvania) 4005 and ROMICAT-II studies, which compared an initial CCTA strategy to standard of care (SOC) in patients with acute chest pain, of 1234 patients, the prevalence of obstructive CAD (1–64%), ACS (1–44%), downstream testing (4–72%), and total and diagnostic cost increased across coronary artery calcium (CAC) strata (P < 0.001) [14]. A study of 204 patients found that a CAC score of zero had a 97% NPV for excluding ACS, and that a positive CAC score was a significant, independent predictor of ACS [15].

A recent study concluded that CCTA may not identify more patients with significant CAD requiring coronary revascularization, shorten hospital stay, or allow for more direct discharge from the ED compared to standard care including high-sensitivity (hs)-troponins (hsTnI) testing. In a study (n = 500) by Dedic et al. which compared CCTA and SOC encompassing high-sensitivity troponin assays, there was no difference in the primary endpoint and incidence of undetected ACS [16]. Twenty-two (9%) patients underwent coronary revascularization within 30 days in the CCTA group, compared to 17 (7%) in the SOC group (P = 0.40). Discharge from the ED was not more frequent after CCTA (65% vs. 59%, P = 0.16), and length of stay was similar (6.3 h in both groups; P = 0.80). However, there have been reports that hsTnI at the time of presentation followed by early advanced CCTA assessment improves the risk stratification and diagnostic accuracy for ACS as compared to conventional troponin and traditional CCTA assessment [17]. Inclusion of high-sensitivity troponin testing increases sensitivity for the detection of myocardial infarction; however, it may decrease specificity and increase clinical uncertainty.

7.3.3 CCTA Findings of Acute Coronary Syndrome

The presence of high-risk plaques (plaques with lipid-rich components, positive remodeling, scattered microcalcifications, napkin-ring sign; minimum lumen area <4 mm^2, plaque burden ≥70%) on CCTA increases the likelihood of ACS independent of clinical risk assessment and significant CAD [18]. Although it is generally believed that most acute coronary events result from the rupture of nonobstructive plaques, progression of early, uncomplicated atherosclerosis may be necessary before plaque rupture (Figs. 7.4 and 7.5). Serial studies have clarified that nonobstructive lesions progressively enlarge relatively rapidly before an acute event occurs, while CCTA data have shown that lesions without voluminous progression over time rarely lead to events, regardless of baseline high-risk plaque morphology or the extent of luminal stenosis [19].

Perivascular fat stranding may indicate an increased risk of ACS in patients with significant stenosis or spontaneous coronary artery dissection. In a study by Sandeep et al., perivascular fat stranding was seen in 11 of 1403 patients, nine with atherosclerotic lesions and two with spontaneous coronary artery dissections, with a mean fat stranding length of 19.2 mm and an average circumferential extent of 2.9 quadrants [20]. The mean attenuation of perivascular fat stranding was 17 HU. The prevalence of ACS was 45.4% in cases and 3.8% in control subjects (P = 0.001).

Coronary artery spasm is also considered important in the pathogenesis of ACS. Detection of coronary spasm is not easy with CCTA. However, coronary spasm may accompany coronary artery lesions (Fig. 7.6). In one study, spasm-induced ACS was diagnosed in 20% of 1601 patients with non-ST-segment elevation acute coronary syndrome (NSTE ACS) [21]. A double-acquisition CCTA protocol in the presence and absence of intravenous vasodilator infusion for detecting vasospastic angina showed a sensitivity, specificity, PPV, and NPV for CCTA on a per-patient basis of 73%, 100%, 100%, and 56%, respectively [22]. Microvascular coronary

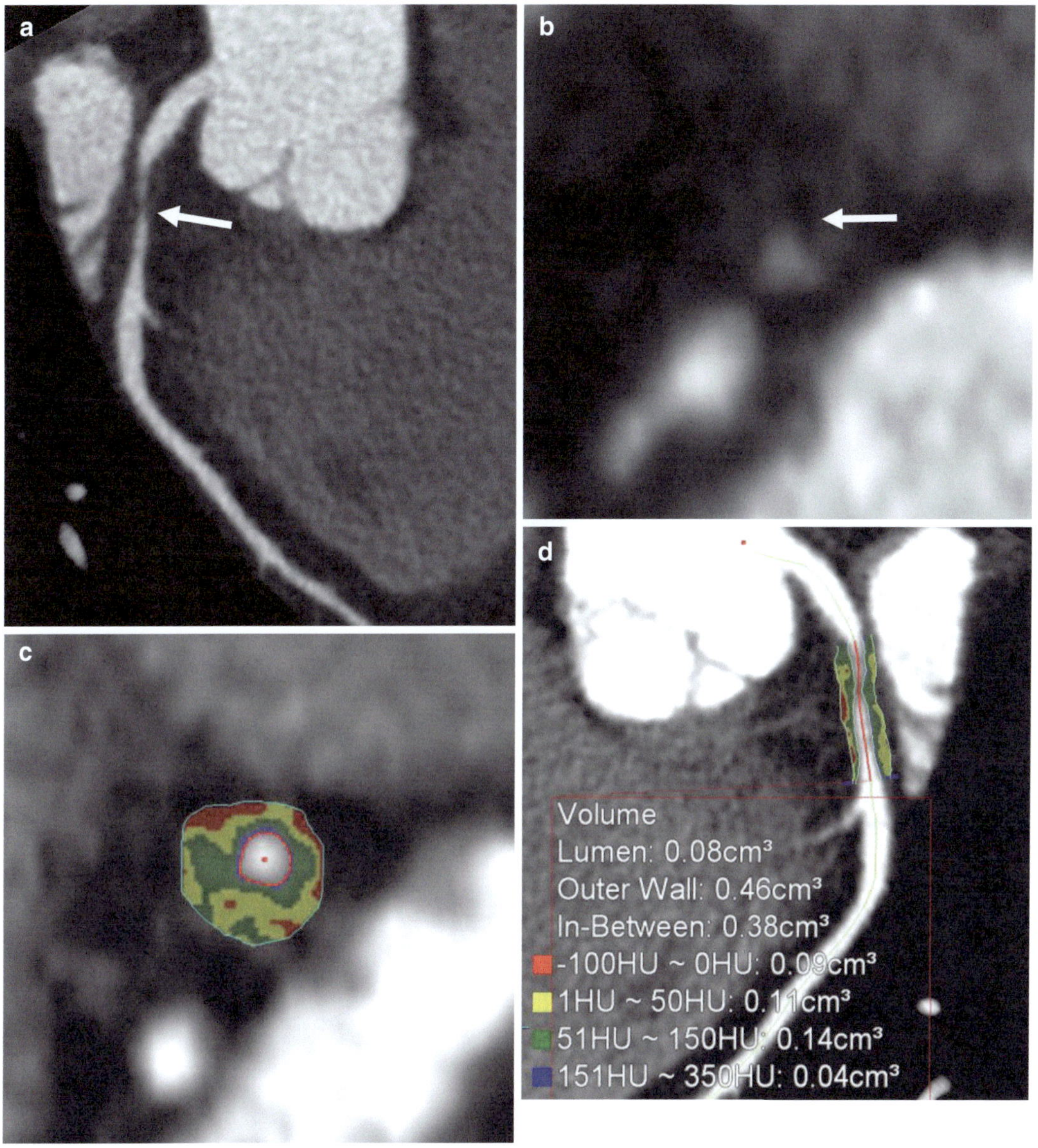

Fig. 7.4 Acute coronary syndrome in a 55-year-old male. (**a**) CCTA shows severe stenosis (arrow) in the proximal LAD. (**b**) Cross-sectional image of the LAD shows a noncalcific plaque with a focal lipid-rich component (arrow). (**c**, **d**) Plaque analysis shows that most of the plaque consisted of a fibrous component

artery spasm with endothelial dysfunction can be the cause of nonobstructive CAD [23]. Ohyama posited that coronary spasm is associated with inflammation of the coronary adventitia and perivascular adipose tissue, and that F-18 fluorodeoxy-glucose (FDG) positron emission tomography (^{18}F-FDG PET)/CT can be useful for assessment of disease activity [24].

Isolated pulmonary thromboembolism (PTE) and aortic dissection (AD) outside of the CCTA display field of view (DFOV) rarely occur (Fig. 7.7). Therefore, a modified triple-rule-out (TRO) CT protocol using cardiac scan coverage was adopted to detect PTE (1.9%) and AD (0.8%) in 1224 patients with reduced radiation dose [25]. In another study, of a total of 309 cases, 6 (1.9%)

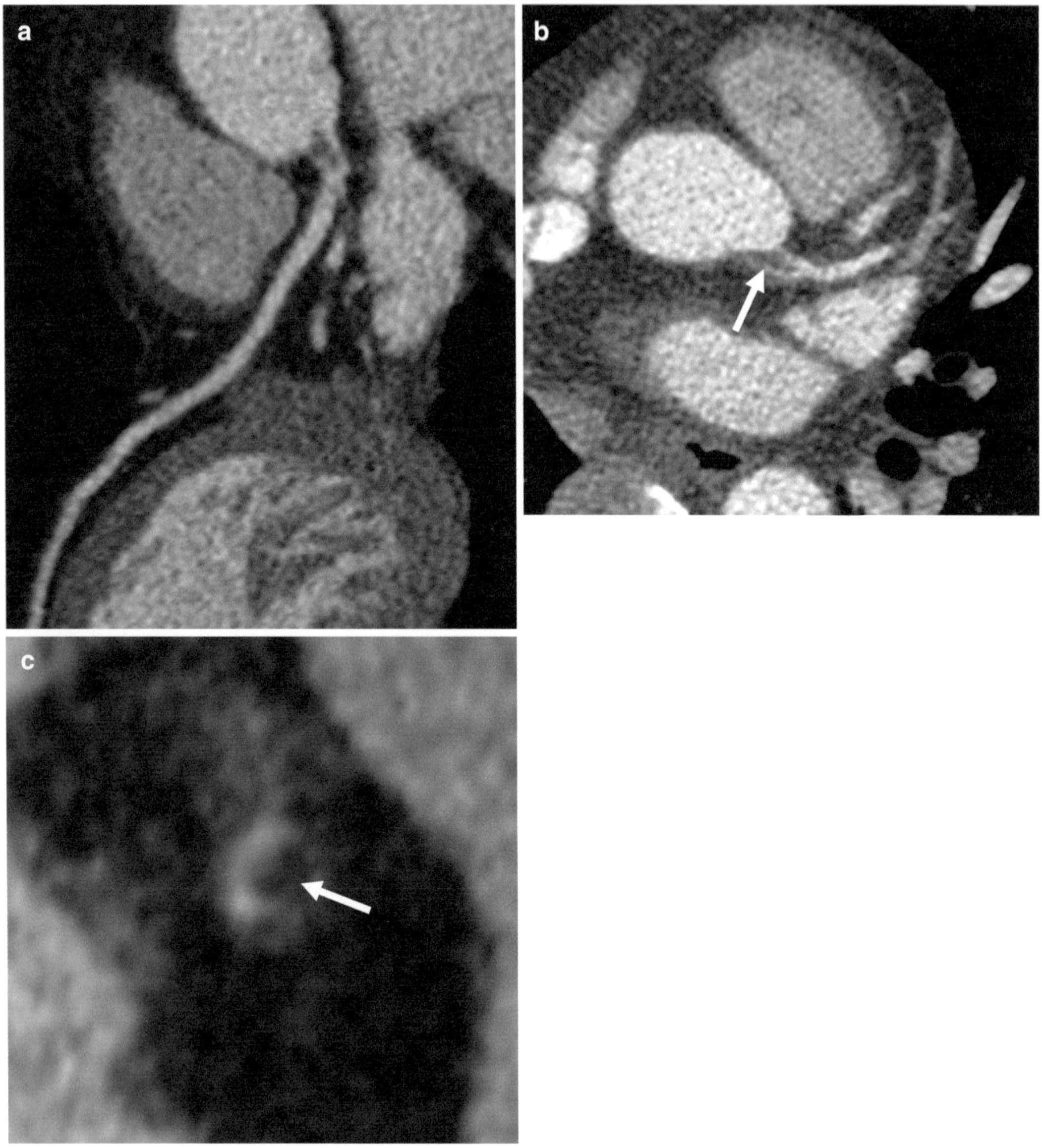

Fig. 7.5 Acute coronary artery thrombosis with possible plaque rupture in a 47-year-old male. (**a, b**) Curved-planar reformatted image (**a**) and transverse image (**b**) (both on CCTA) show a filling defect (arrow) in the left main coronary artery. (**c**) Cross-sectional image shows the lesion (arrow) obstructing the left main coronary artery. It measured 8 HU. A red thrombus was extracted during a thrombo-aspiration procedure

patients had aortic lesions outside of the cardiac scan range [26].

Adenosine-stress CT perfusion may not be feasible for detection of physiologically significant CAD in ED patients because it cannot be done with sufficient urgency. Rest-only CT perfusion may aid the risk stratification of patients presenting to the ED with nontraumatic acute chest pain [27]. Color-coded myocardial perfusion may also enable easier detection of myocardial infarction, even on arterial-phase images (Fig. 7.8).

Spontaneous coronary artery dissection (SCAD) has emerged as an important cause of ACS, myocardial infarction, and sudden death, particularly in young women and patients with

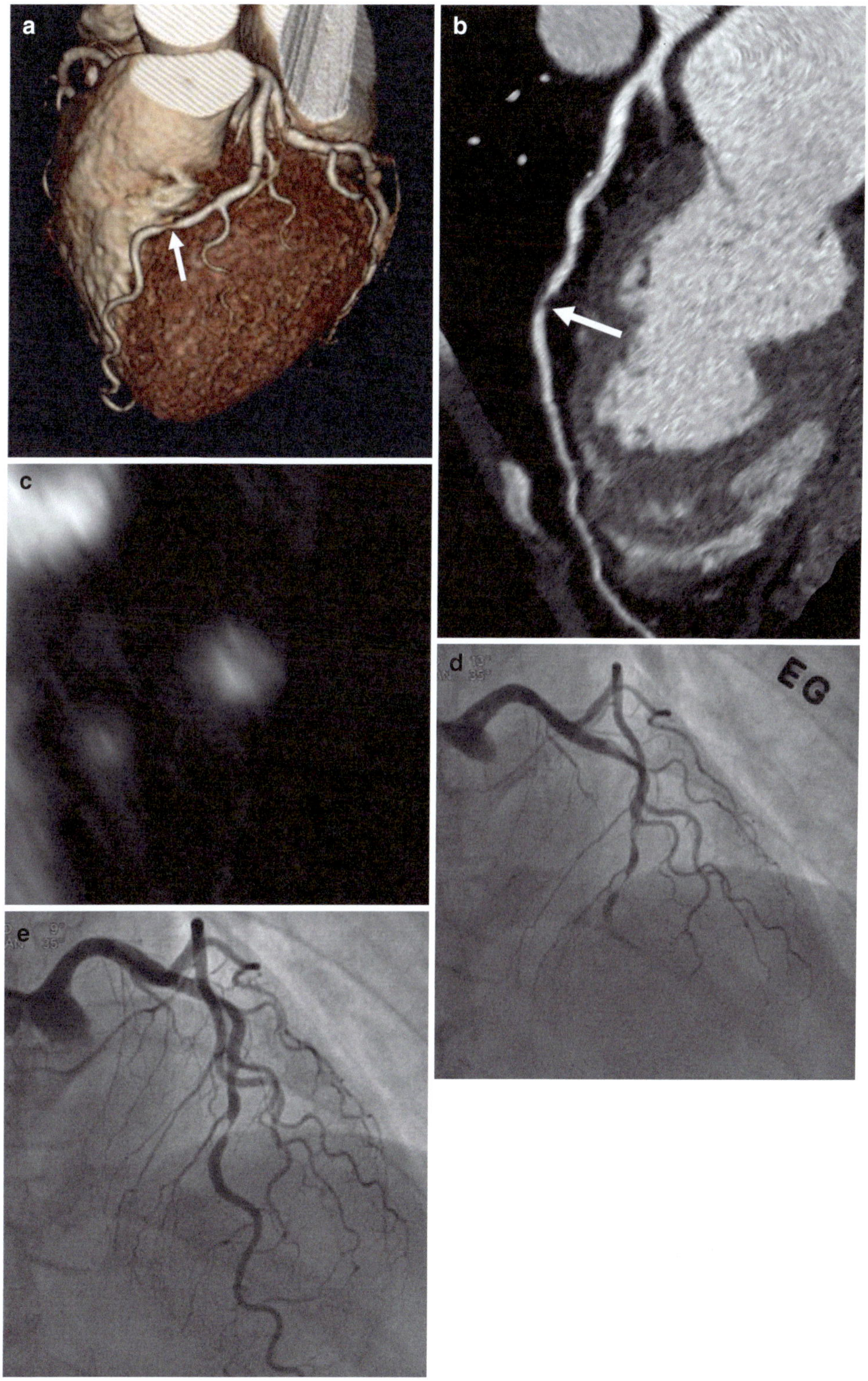

Fig. 7.6 Coronary artery spasm in a 57-year-old female. (**a–c**) A focal severe stenosis (arrow) with noncalcific plaque found in the middle of the LAD on CCTA. (**d**, **e**) A spasm was evoked in the LAD by ergonovine (**d**) and relieved by nitroglycerin injection (**e**)

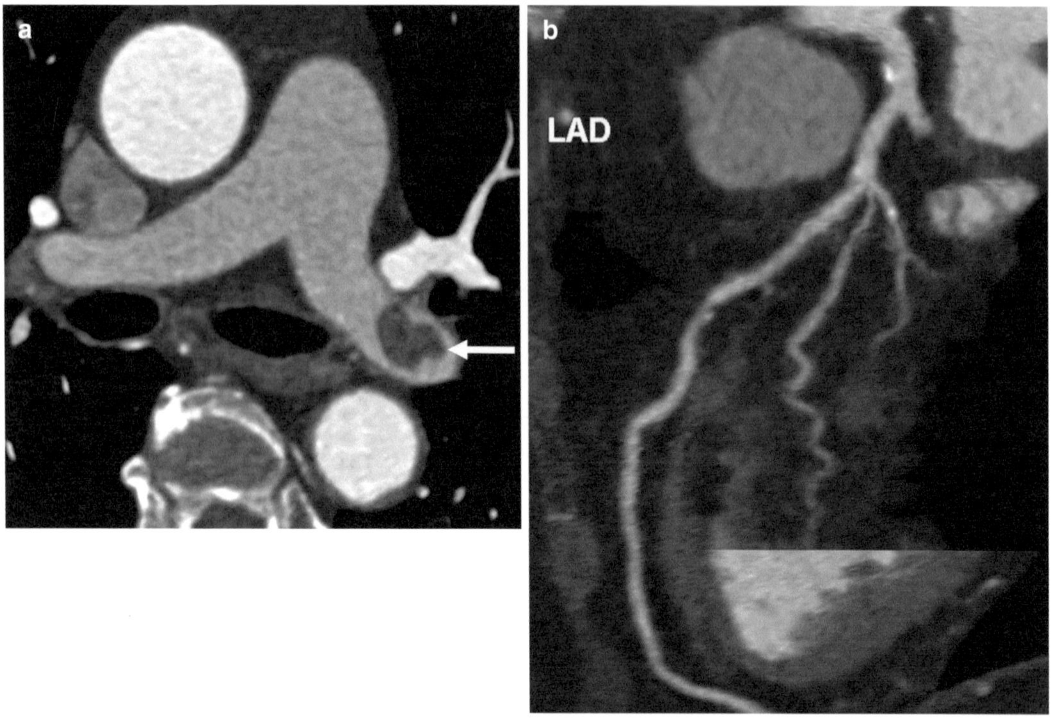

Fig. 7.7 Pulmonary artery embolism in a 71-year-old female. (**a**) A filling defect (arrow) can be seen in the left pulmonary artery, which was included in the CCTA display field of view. (**b**) Curved-planar reformatted image shows coronary calcifications in the left coronary artery

few conventional atherosclerotic risk factors [28]. CT may show a "classical" dual lumen or compression of the true lumen by a hematoma, without contrast penetration (Fig. 7.9) [29]. The sensitivity and specificity of CCTA as a primary diagnostic tool for SCAD are not known and CCTA is expected to play a role in the follow-up of patients with SCAD.

A CCTA-guided diagnostic algorithm may incorporate CT-fractional flow reserve (CT-FFR). After CCTA, patients may be triaged to CT-FFR if the CCTA findings reflect 30% to 90% diameter stenosis. Patients with CT-FFR > 0.84 should be referred for medical treatment. Those with CT-FFR of 0.75 to 0.84 (gray zone) are likely to undergo invasive FFR for definitive evaluation. Patients with CT-FFR of <0.75 will undergo angiography with or without invasive FFR, while invasive FFR may be reserved for cases with diffuse disease, which requires further localization of ischemia [30].

7.3.4 Cardiac MRI in Acute Coronary Syndrome

CMR imaging is increasingly used for initial work-up of chest pain and evaluation of acute myocardial infarction early after coronary intervention [31–35]. CMR can be used to evaluate regional ventricular wall motion, infarct distribution, depth, size, myocardium at risk, microvascular obstruction, and intramyocardial hemorrhage (Fig. 7.10). CMR can be used as a one-stop imaging modality to identify the cause of chest pain, which may include aortic dissection, pulmonary embolism, acute myocardial infarction, acute myocarditis, Takotsubo syndrome, and hypertrophic cardiomyopathy, especially in patients with ACS and unobstructed coronary arteries [31, 32].

According to Kwong et al., CMR accurately detected a high fraction of patients with ACS, including patients with enzyme-negative unstable angina. For detecting ACS, the respective

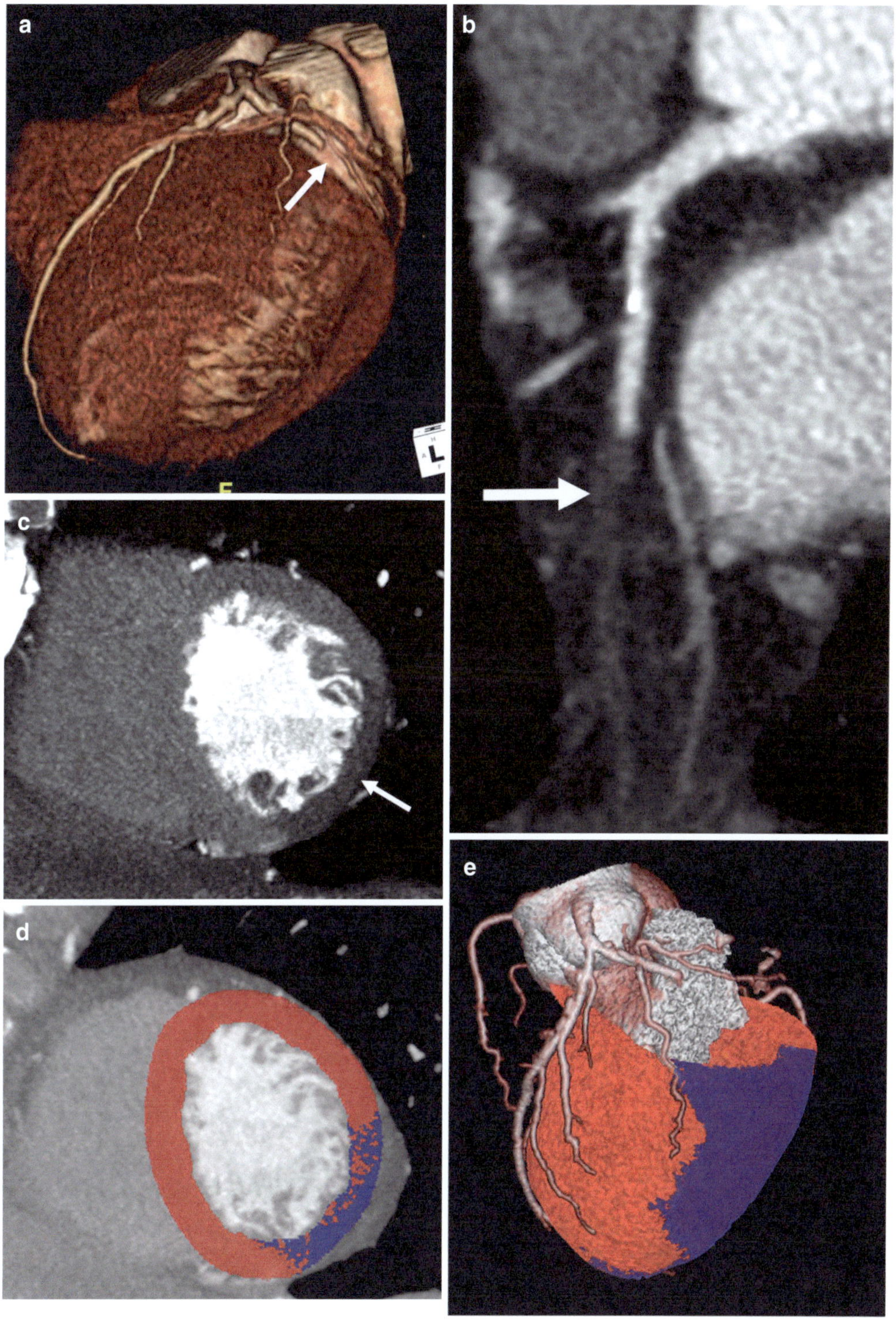

Fig. 7.8 Acute myocardial infarction in a 55-year-old male. (**a**, **b**) On CCTA, occlusion (arrows) of the left circumflex artery is noted on a volume-rendered (**a**) and curved planar reformatted image (**b**). (**c**) Reformatted short-axial image shows a subtle low-attenuation area (arrow) in the middle inferolateral wall. (**d**, **e**) On color-coded short-axial and 3-dimensional volume-rendered images, a large area of decreased myocardial enhancement (purple) due to thrombotic occlusion of the left circumflex artery is more easily seen than on conventional reformatted images

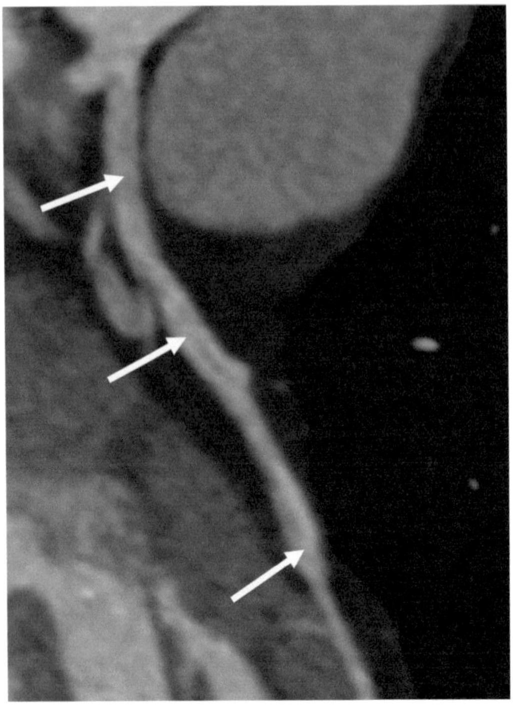

Fig. 7.9 Spontaneous coronary dissection in a 50-year-old male. Curved reformatted CCTA image shows a dissecting flap (arrows) in the proximal to middle LAD. Invasive coronary angiography confirmed the presence of coronary dissection (not shown)

sensitivity and specificity were 84% and 85% for CMR, 16% and 95% for strict ECG criteria for ischemia (ST depression or T-wave inversion), 40% and 97% for peak troponin-I, and 48% and 85% for TIMI risk score ≥ 3. Multivariate logistic regression analysis revealed that CMR was the strongest predictor of ACS, with additional diagnostic value over clinical parameters ($P < 0.001$).

Stress-induced cardiomyopathy or Takotsubo syndrome (TTS) mimics acute myocardial infarction in the absence of culprit CAD (Fig. 7.11). SCAD shows left ventricular wall motion abnormalities similar to those seen in TTS, and the two conditions share a predilection for women.

7.4 Acute Pericardial Disease

More than 85% of patients with acute pericarditis present with chest pain [36]. In patients with acute pericarditis, CT and CMR show pericardial effusion and thickened pericardium. CMR is the preferred imaging modality for assessment of pericardial disease with regard to pericardial tissue characterization and assessment of cardiac

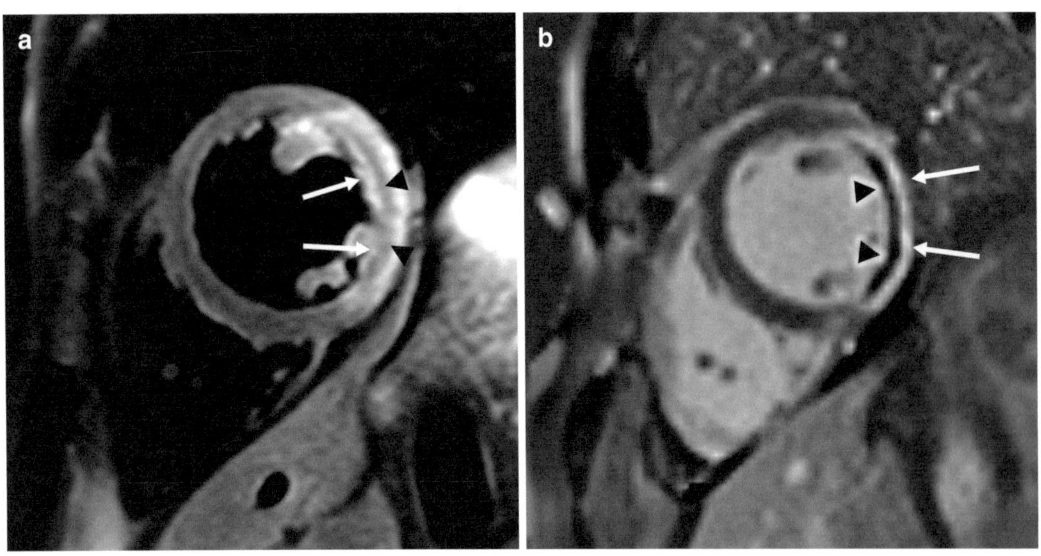

Fig. 7.10 Acute myocardial infarction in a 52-year-old male. (**a**) T2-weighted MR image shows myocardial edema with bright signal intensity (arrows). A thin band of low signal intensity (arrowheads) represents intramyocardial hemorrhage. (**b**) Late gadolinium-enhanced (LGE) image shows full-thickness myocardial infarction (arrows) with microvascular occlusion (arrowheads). (**c**) T2-star map shows intramyocardial hemorrhage (arrow) with short $T2^*$ relaxation time

Fig. 7.10 (continued)

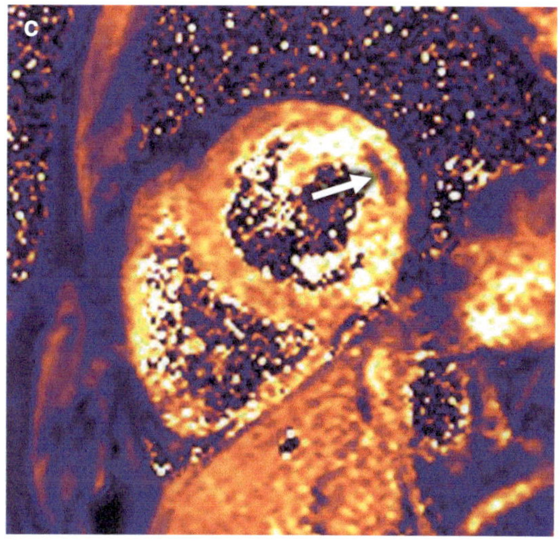

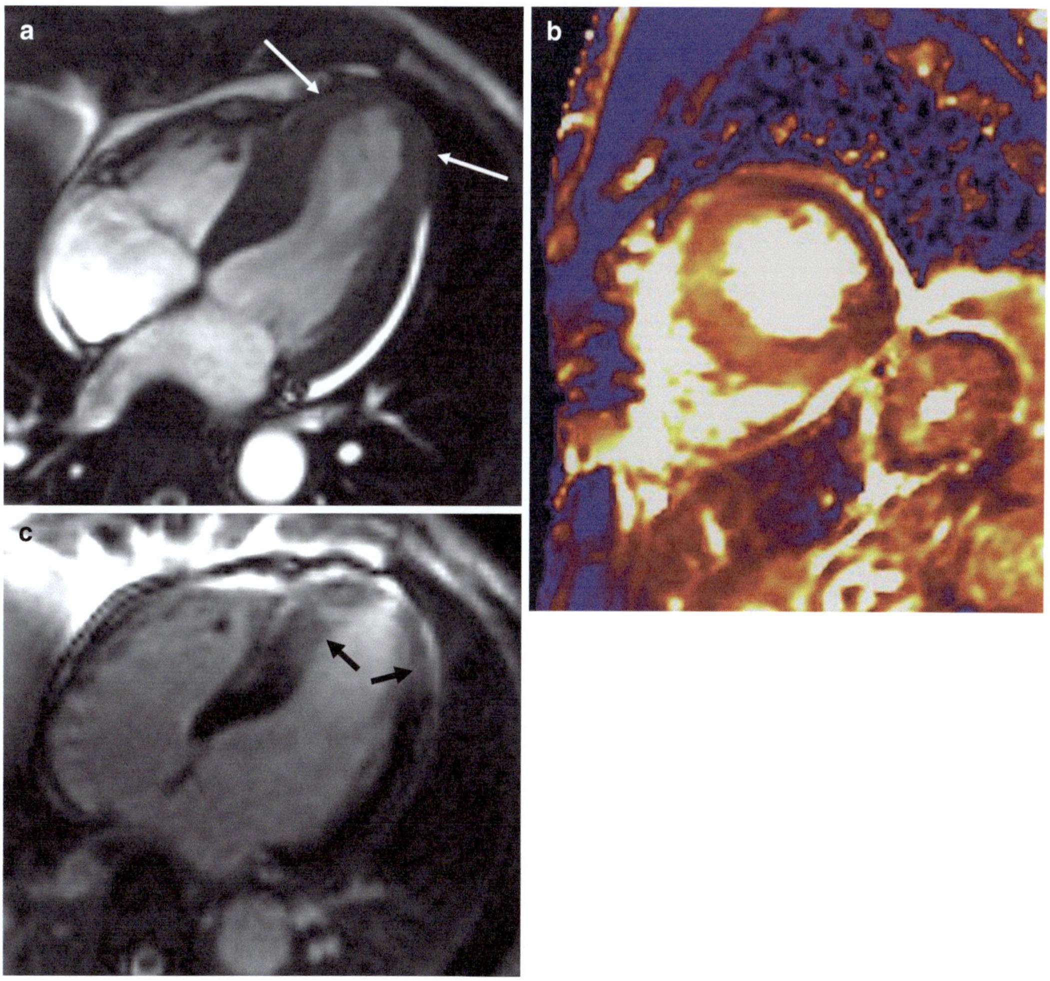

Fig. 7.11 Stress-induced cardiomyopathy in a 58-year-old male. (**a**) Systolic-phase cine MR image shows left ventricular apical ballooning (arrows). (**b**) T2 mapping reveals a longer T2 relaxation time (100 ms) in the apical septum compared with that seen in remote areas (55 ms). (**c**) A mild degree of hyperenhancement (arrows) is seen in the mid-to-apical segments of the left ventricle on an LGE image. Coronary angiography revealed normal coronary arteries (not shown)

function and filling patterns [36]. Pericardial thickening and enhancement are the main CT findings in acute pericarditis (Fig. 7.12) [37]. LGE MRI may show hyperenhancement in the thickened pericardium (Fig. 7.13).

Cardiac tamponade may occur in cases with rapid accumulation of pericardial fluid, regardless of the amount of fluid. CT findings associated with cardiac tamponade include pericardial effusion (usually a large amount) with distention

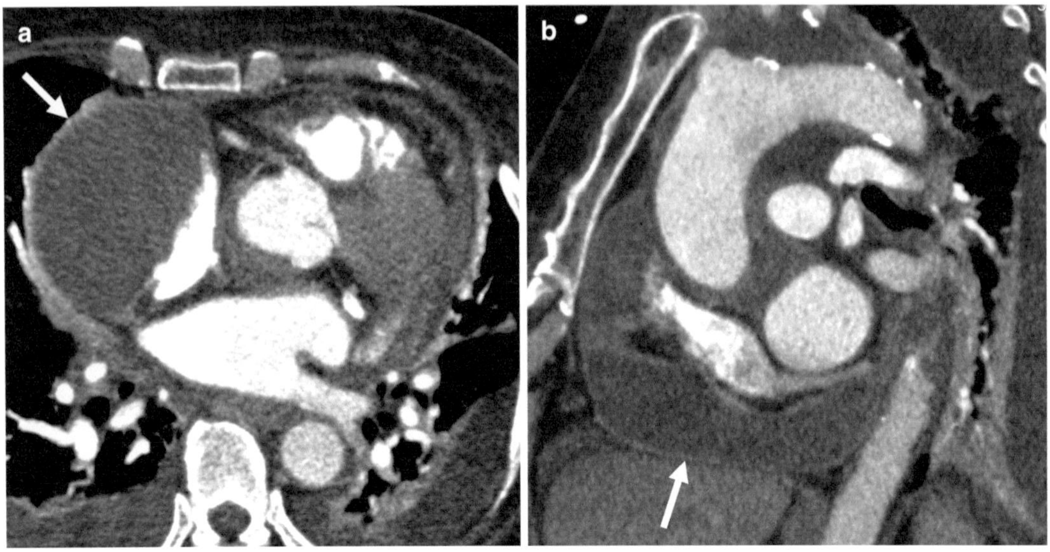

Fig. 7.12 Pyogenic pericarditis with *Salmonella* infection. (**a**, **b**) Contrast-enhanced CT (**a** transverse image; **b** oblique sagittal image) shows a large amount of pericardial effusion and diffusely thickened pericardium. The right atrium is markedly compressed by loculated pericardial effusion (arrows)

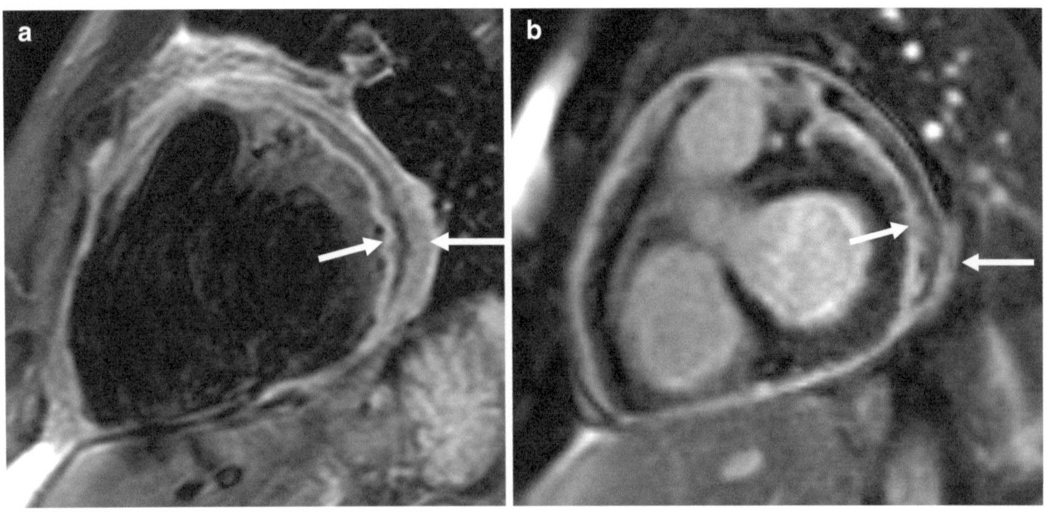

Fig. 7.13 Tuberculous pericarditis in a 40-year-old male. (**a**) Short-axial T2-weighted image shows thickened visceral and parietal pericardium (arrows) with increased signal intensity. (**b**) LGE image shows hyperenhancement of the thickened pericardium (arrows), suggesting active pericardial inflammation. (**c**) F-18 fluoro-deoxy-glucose (FDG) positron emission tomography shows increased FDG uptake (arrows)

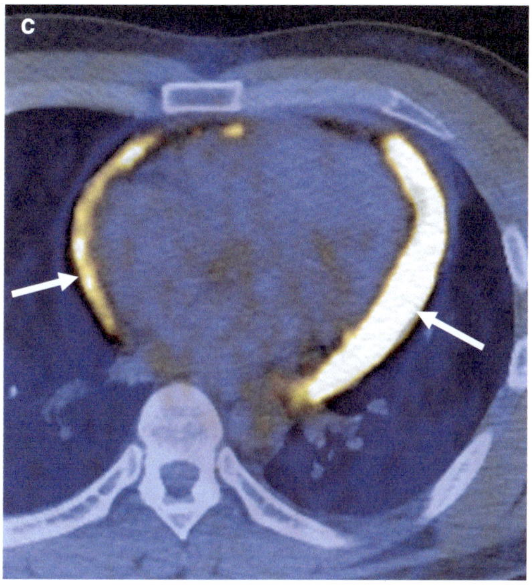

Fig. 7.13 (continued)

of the superior and inferior caval veins; deformity and compression of the cardiac chambers and other intrapericardial structures; bowing of the interventricular septum, and reflux of contrast material into the azygos vein and inferior vena cava [38].

7.5 Acute Myocarditis

CMR is the most comprehensive and accurate diagnostic tool for evaluation of patients with acute myocarditis. It can be used to assess the activity and severity of myocarditis and determine the necessity of endomyocardial biopsy [39]. CMR has a sensitivity of 67% and a specificity of 91% for acute myocarditis [40]. Detection of tissue edema, hyperemia, and necrosis in both the acute and the chronic stages of myocarditis provide the foundation of the Lake Louise Criteria (CLL) [41]. CMR features of myocarditis include myocardial edema on T2-weighted images and contrast enhancement on LGE images (Fig. 7.14). T1 and T2 quantifications are now recommended over T1- and T2-weighted imaging (Fig. 7.15). Late Gd enhancement remains in the updated criteria, whereas early Gd enhancement has been replaced by T1 quantification [42]. Texture analysis applied to CMR T1 and T2 mapping delivers quantitative imaging parameters for the diagnosis of acute or chronic myocarditis and may be superior to the Lake Louise criteria or averaged myocardial T1 or T2 values [43].

FDG PET/CT provides metabolic information on inflammation in the form of increased myocardial FDG uptake in the lesions of myocarditis. PET/MR may detect more cases of myocarditis than FDG PET/CT due to the delayed PET acquisition time on PET/MR [40]. CT may demonstrate myocardial edema and contrast enhancement in patients with acute myocarditis, but with low sensitivity and specificity.

LGE is associated with future cardiovascular death and ventricular arrhythmia among patients referred for MRI for known or suspected cardiac sarcoidosis [44].

7.6 Cardiogenic Sources of Systemic Embolism

Approximately 20%–40% of all stroke cases are associated with embolism from the heart or aorta [45]. Cardiogenic thromboembolism is associated with thrombus formation in the left atrial appendage (LAA) in patients with atrial fibrillation (AF) and can also occur in the absence of clinical AF as a result of various pathological conditions [46]. Left atrial thrombus occurs in 8% of patients with AF [47]. Cardiac CT is a reliable alternative imaging modality to transesophageal echocardiography (TEE) for the evaluation of cardioembolic sources in patients with ischemic stroke [48].

Poor enhancement in the LAA on CT suggests a high risk of stroke [49]. Delayed CT after 1–2 min after contrast injection may exclude slow flow in the atrial appendages and left atrial cavity (Fig. 7.16) [50]. The protocol can adopt dual-phase CT, double-bolus single-phase, or prone-position CT (Fig. 7.17) [51, 52]. Dual-energy CT may show decreased iodine content in the thrombi. With TEE as the reference standard,

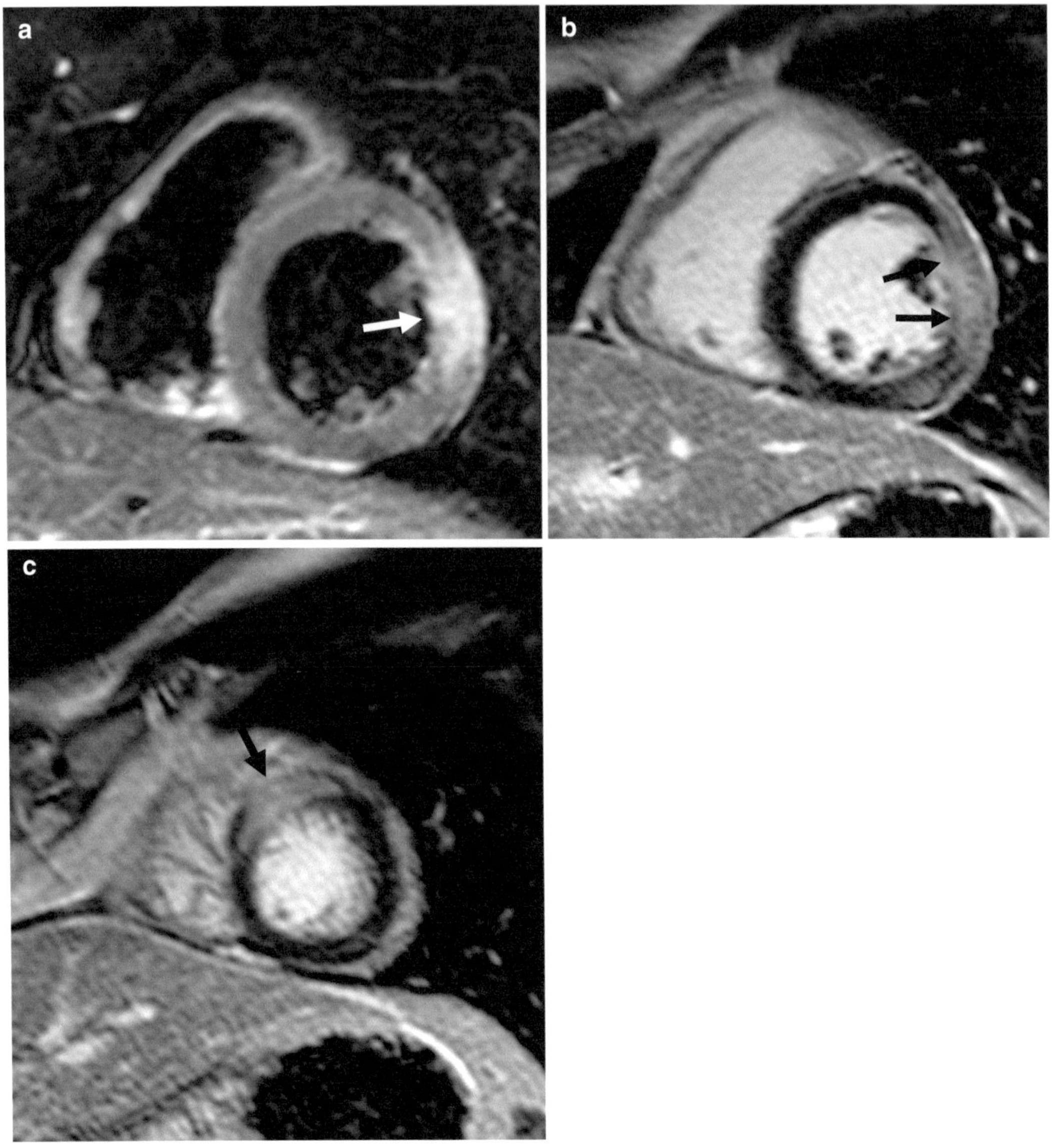

Fig. 7.14 Acute myocarditis of presumed viral origin in a 34-year-old male. (**a**) T2-weighted MRI shows high signal intensity (arrow) in the middle lateral wall of the left ventricle. (**b**, **c**) LGE images taken 15 min after contrast injection show hyperenhancement (arrows) in the middle lateral and apical septal segments of the left ventricle. Coronary angiography showed no stenotic lesions (not shown)

the overall sensitivity, specificity, PPV, and NPV of dual-energy cardiac CT for the detection of thrombi and spontaneous echo contrast (SEC) in the LAA were 97%, 100%, 100%, and 97%, respectively [53].

Other cardiac lesions, such as aortic valve fibroelastoma, myxoma, and valvular vegetation may develop systemic embolization [54]. In patients with infective endocarditis, CT may reveal perivalvular abscess or pseudoaneurysms, vegetation, valvular thrombi, and foci of endocarditis (Fig. 7.18). Delayed CT or LGE CMR may reveal foci of enhancement as the consequence of inflammation, while PET-CT plays an important role in the detection of inflammation. Cardiac CT can accurately demonstrate infective

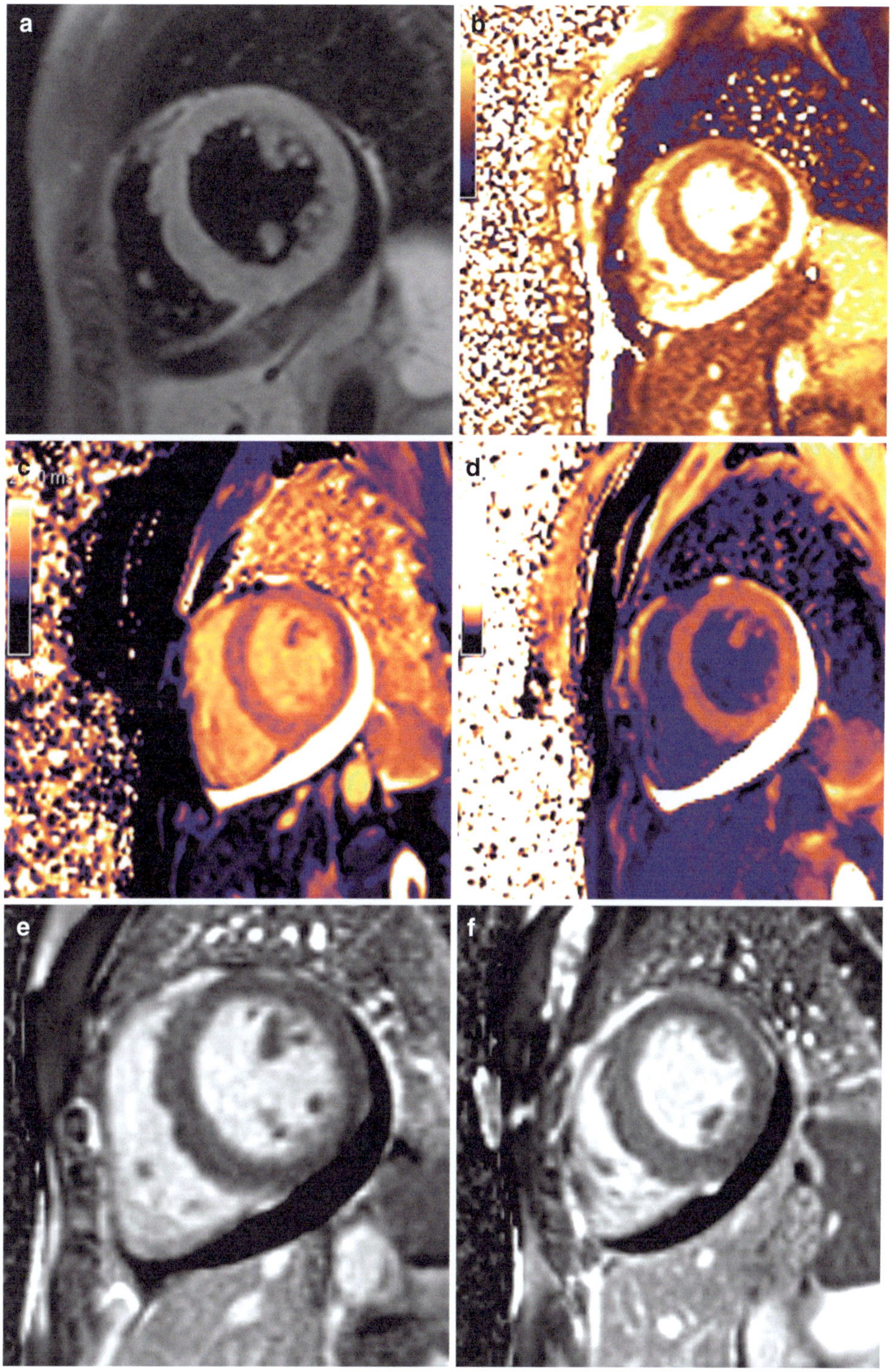

Fig. 7.15 Acute eosinophilic myocarditis in a 28-year-old female. (**a**) T2-weighted image shows no significant myocardial abnormalities, except a small amount of pericardial effusion. (**b**) T2 mapping reveals an increased left ventricular myocardial T2 relaxation time of 65 ms. (**c**, **d**) Pre-contrast (**c**) and post-contrast (15 min after contrast injection) T1 mapping resulted in an increased left ventricular myocardial extracellular volume fraction of 0.37. (**e**, **f**) LGE images in contiguous sections show no remarkable abnormalities. In this case, T1 and T2 mapping helped to establish a diagnosis of acute myocarditis

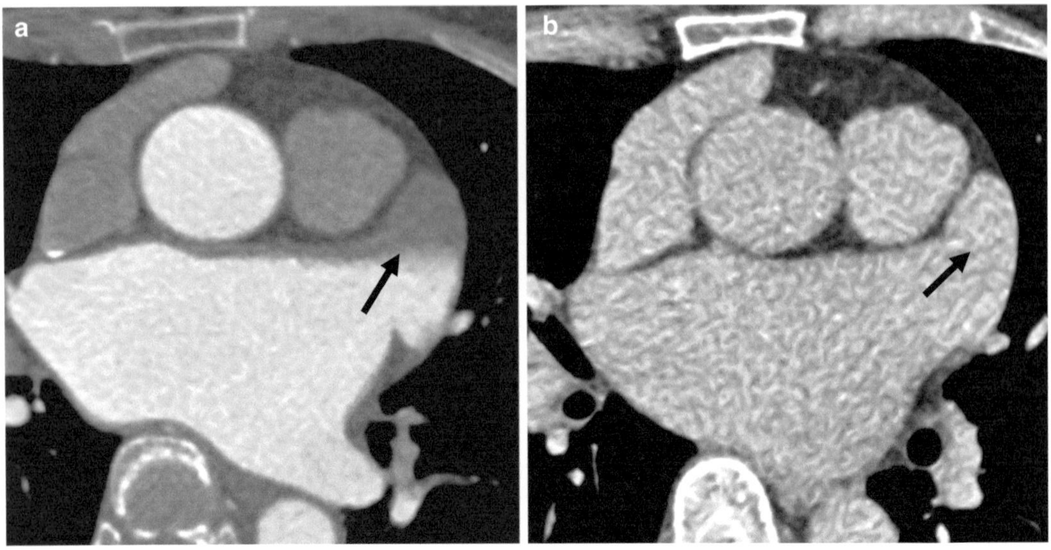

Fig. 7.16 Slow flow with poor enhancement of the atrial appendage in a patient with atrial fibrillation. (**a**) Early (arterial)-phase CT shows poor contrast enhancement (arrow) in the atrial appendage. (**b**) Delayed-phase CT (1-minute delay) shows no filling defect (arrow) in the atrial appendage

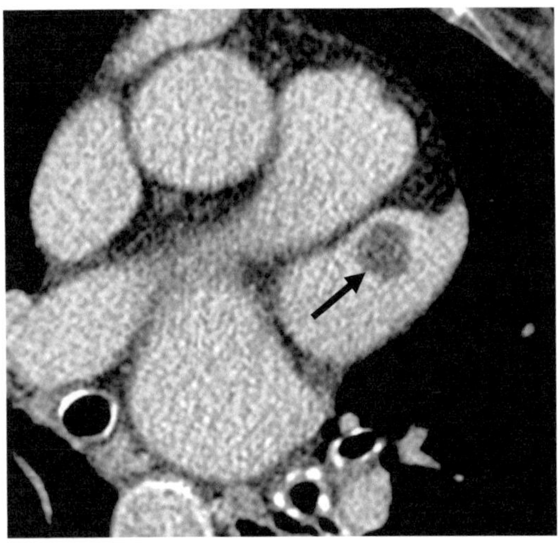

Fig. 7.17 Thrombus in the left atrial appendage in a 69-year-old female with mitral valve disease. Delayed-phase CT shows a round filling defect (arrow) in the left atrial appendage

endocarditis in preoperative patients, with a similar diagnostic accuracy to TEE [55]. In a study by Koo et al., the rates of detection of infective endocarditis per patient with CT and TEE were 93.9% (46/49) and 95.9% (47/49), respectively. In per-imaging analysis, the sensitivities of CT and TEE did not significantly differ for both native and prosthetic valve infective endocarditis (sensitivity: vegetation, 100% in TEE and 90.9% on CT; leaflet perforation, 87.5% on TEE and 50.0% on CT; abscess/pseudoaneurysm, 40.0% on TEE and 60.0% on CT; paravalvular leakage, 100% on TEE and 50.0% on CT).

Paradoxical embolism is an important clinical entity among patients with venous thromboembolism in the presence of intracardiac or pulmonary shunts [56]. The main risk factors of patent foramen ovale (PFO)-attributable strokes are young age, large PFO size, right-to-left shunt degree, PFO morphology, presence of atrial septal aneurysm, intrinsic imbalance of coagulation–anticoagulation systems, and co-existence of other atrial abnormalities, such as right atrial septal pouch, Eustachian valve and Chiari's network (Fig. 7.19) [57]. The TEE bubble study is considered the gold standard for diagnosing PFO. A meta-analysis of studies assessing the accuracy of TEE for detection of PFO (with confirmation by autopsy, cardiac surgery, and/or catheterization as the reference) found that some PFOs may still be missed or misdiagnosed on TEE bubble study, which had a sensitivity of 89.2% and a

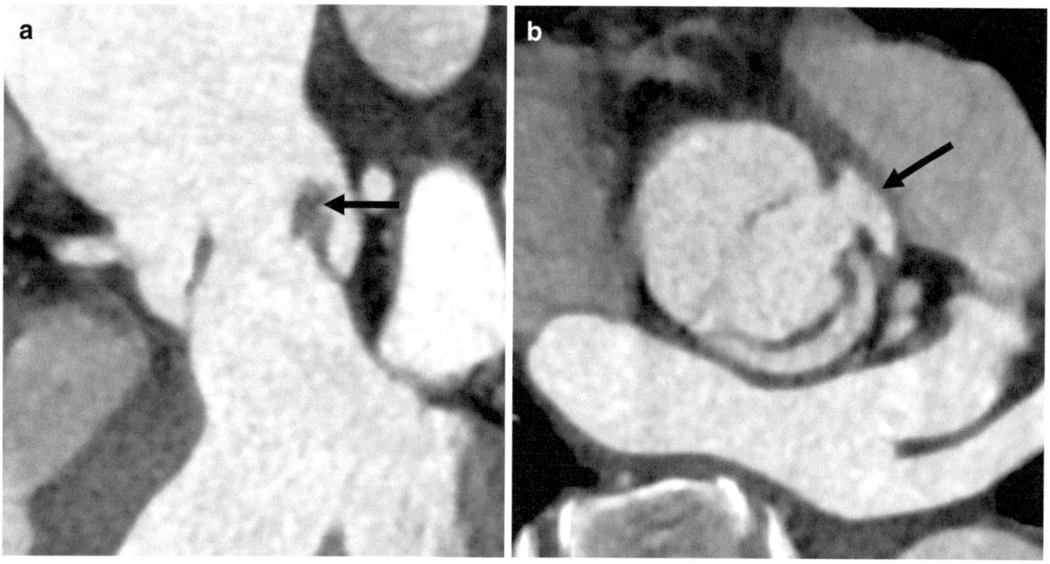

Fig. 7.18 Acute infective endocarditis in a 59-year-old male with a bicuspid aortic valve. (**a**, **b**) Reformatted CT images show a vegetation (arrow, **a**) and perivalvular pseudoaneurysm (arrow, **b**) in the aortic valve

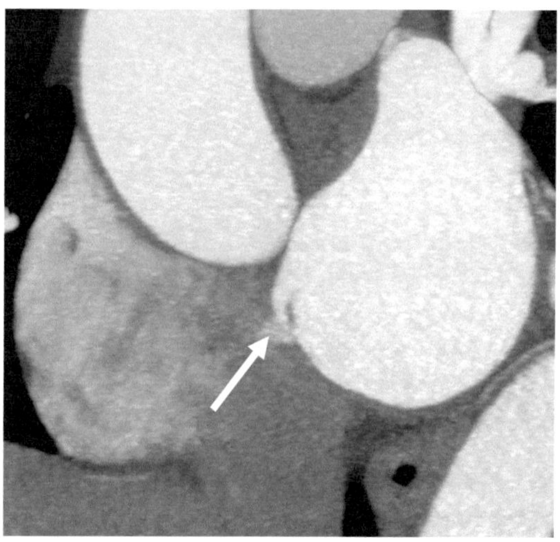

Fig. 7.19 Wide patent foramen ovale in a 68-year-old male. CT depicts a contrast jet (arrow) from the left atrium to the right atrium

specificity of 91.4% [58]. Cardiac CT demonstrates a contrast agent jet from the left to the right atrium toward the inferior vena cava along with a channel-like appearance of the interatrial septum. CT showed a sensitivity of 73.1% and a specificity of 98.4% for detection of PFO in 152 stroke patients, as compared with TEE [59].

Cardiac CT can be used to simultaneously diagnose CAD in stroke patients (Fig. 7.20). Stroke is associated with CAD (≥50% stenosis on CCTA) in 20%–48% of patients [60]. Currently, after ischemic stroke/transient ischemic attack the risk of myocardial infarction is less than 2% per year [61]. Asymptomatic CAD detected on CCTA is associated with increased risks of vascular events or death in acute stroke patients [62]. According to a study by Yoo et al., 654 of 1893 patients (34.5%) with acute stroke had significant (≥50%) CAD on CCTA and MACE occurred in 230 patients (12.2%) during follow-up (median, 4.4 years) [62]. The event rates of MACE increased with increasing extent of CAD. In a study by Yoon et al., the prevalence of CAD (stenosis ≥50%) was 30.2% among 1418 patients with acute stroke who had no previous cardiac disease and underwent CCTA [63]. Increasing Framingham risk score (FRS), CAC score, and stenosis degree were positively associated with MACE (all $p < 0.05$). Patients with high-risk plaques showed the highest incidence of MACE, followed by non-calcified, mixed, and calcified plaque, respectively (log-rank $P < 0.001$).

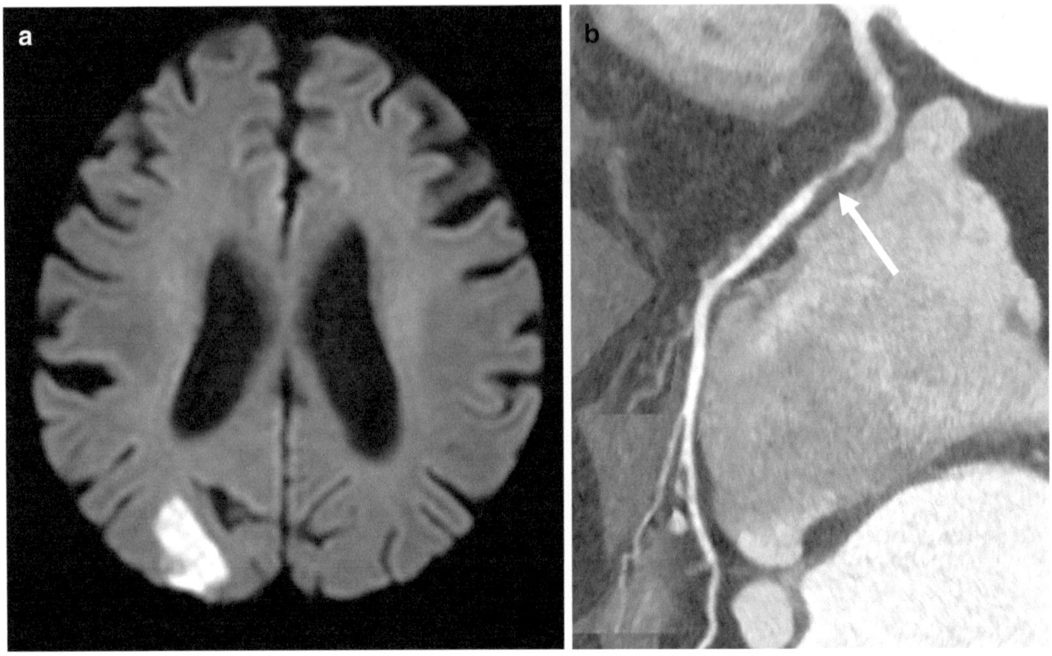

Fig. 7.20 Coronary artery disease in an 82-year-old female with stroke. (**a**) Diffusion-weighted brain MRI shows an acute right cerebral infarct. (**b**) CCTA shows severe focal stenosis (arrow) in the right coronary artery

7.7 Cardiac Trauma

CT signs of severe thoracic trauma should be regarded as indirect evidence of potential blunt cardiac injury. Myocardial hypo-enhancement on CT has poor sensitivity as the evidence of myocardial contusion. Patients with myocardial hypo-attenuation on contrast-enhanced CT could undergo echocardiography or CMR to evaluate wall motion abnormalities [64]. The right ventricle is the most common site of entry in penetrating cardiac injuries due to its anterior location, at 62% of cases. Although the left ventricle is less often affected in cases with penetrating injuries, the mortality rate is quite high at 98% [65].

7.8 Complications of Cardiac Surgery and Transcatheter Aortic Valve Implantation

Mechanical complications of cardiac surgery include spasm or occlusion of a coronary artery graft, prosthetic valve paravalvular regurgitation, cardiac tamponade, and hematoma. CT may demonstrate immediate or early postoperative complications after aortic valve replacement, such as paravalvular dehiscence, abscess, thrombus, pseudoaneurysm around prosthetic aortic valves, and coronary artery occlusion [66, 67].

Acute valvular thrombus and coronary artery occlusion may occur after transcatheter aortic valve implantation (TAVI) [68–70]. Recently, subclinical leaflet thrombosis was described as a commonly observed imaging finding seen in all transcatheter and surgical bioprostheses. Subclinical leaflet thrombosis is readily detectable on CT with a high degree of concordance with transthoracic echocardiography (TTE) findings. The CT hallmarks of the condition are hypoattenuated leaflet thickening associated with reduced leaflet motion [71].

Contained rupture of the aortic root in balloon-expandable TAVI is associated with severe prosthesis oversizing (Fig. 7.21). In a study of 72 patients undergoing balloon-expandable TAVI

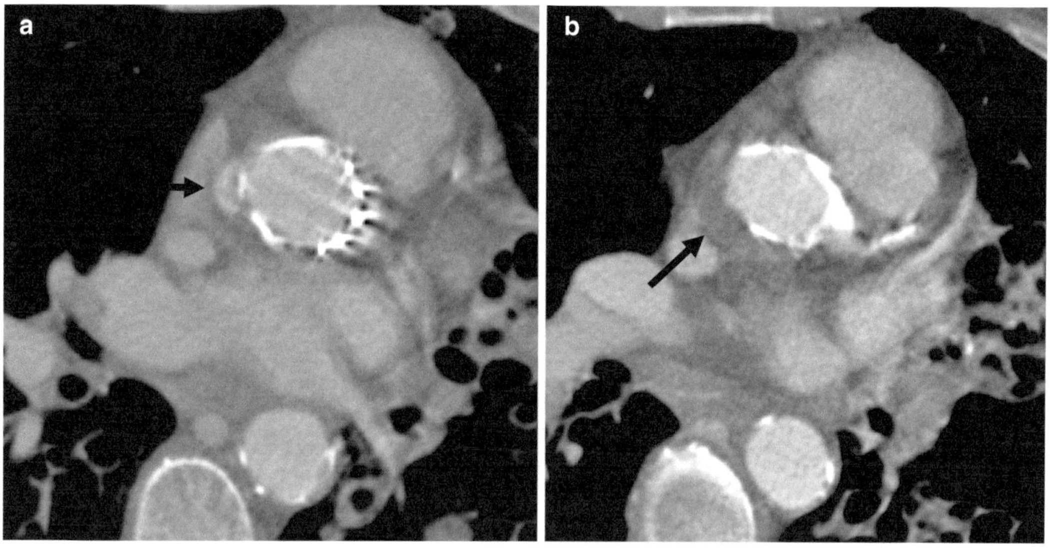

Fig. 7.21 Aortic root rupture after TAVI in a 62-year-old female. (**a**, **b**) CCTA shows a focal pseudoaneurysm (arrow, **a**) and hematoma (arrow, **b**) around the aortic root, 2 days after TAVI. Pre-interventional CT showed severe calcifications in the aortic root (not shown)

using the Edwards SAPIEN Transcatheter Heart Valve, contained aortic root rupture was diagnosed in 3 patients [72]. Relative oversizing was significantly higher in patients with contained rupture compared with patients without contained rupture (24.6% versus 9.1%, $P < 0.001$). CT-based assessment of the dimensions of the aortic annulus may reduce the incidence of aortic rupture.

CMR is considered a reproducible, accurate, and reliable method of assessing the severity of paravalvular aortic regurgitation (PAR) after TAVI with quantification of AR. In a study by Salaun et al., regurgitation volume (RV) and regurgitation fraction (RF) on CMR were significantly correlated with AR severity at TTE ($P < 0.001$), with mean RF values of 9.2 ± 7.6% in mild ($n = 22$), 20.3 ± 4.2% in moderate ($n = 3$), and 46.8 ± 10.8% in severe PAR patients ($n = 5$) [73]. A cut-off value of RF < 14% on CMR accurately differentiated mild from moderate/severe PAR (sensitivity, 100%; specificity, 82%).

7.9 Coronary Vasculitis

Patients with Takayasu's arteritis display thickening, stenosis, and aneurysmal changes of the aorta, neck vessels, abdominal visceral arteries, and lower extremity arteries. Edema and vasculitis activity can be evaluated with T2-weighted and LGE MRI or contrast-enhanced delayed CT [74, 75]. CCTA may reveal accelerated atherosclerosis, coronary ostial stenosis or occlusion, and coronary aneurysm (Fig. 7.22) [74]. A study of 111 patients by Kang et al. identified three main radiologic features: coronary ostial stenosis (28.0%), nonostial coronary arterial stenosis (36.9%), and coronary aneurysm (8.1%) [74].

ACS may occur in adults long after confirmed or missed Kawasaki disease (KD) (Fig. 7.23). A Japanese nationwide questionnaire demonstrated nationwide emergence of initial ACS in young adults at low coronary risks who were followed up or lost to follow-up after initial coronary aneurysms ≥6 mm and confirmation of KD [76]. CMR can be per-

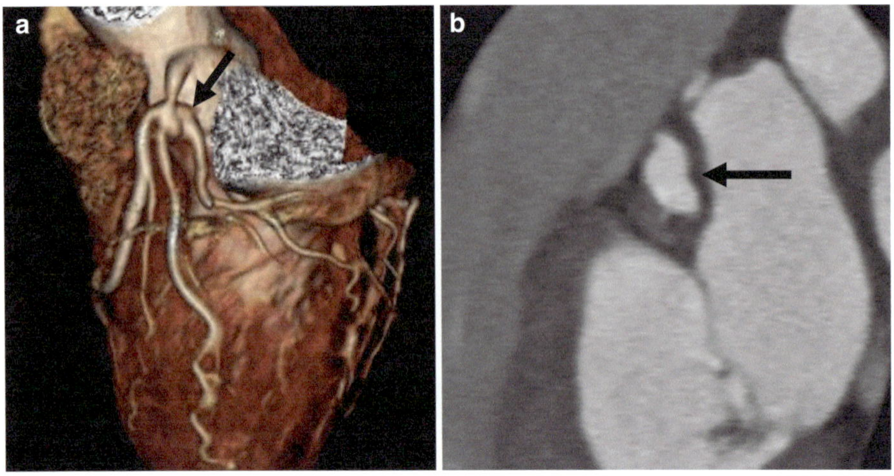

Fig. 7.22 Coronary artery aneurysm in a 20-year-old female with Takayasu's arteritis. (**a**, **b**) Volume-rendered (**a**) and reformatted CT images show a 10-mm aneurysm (arrow) involving the left coronary artery

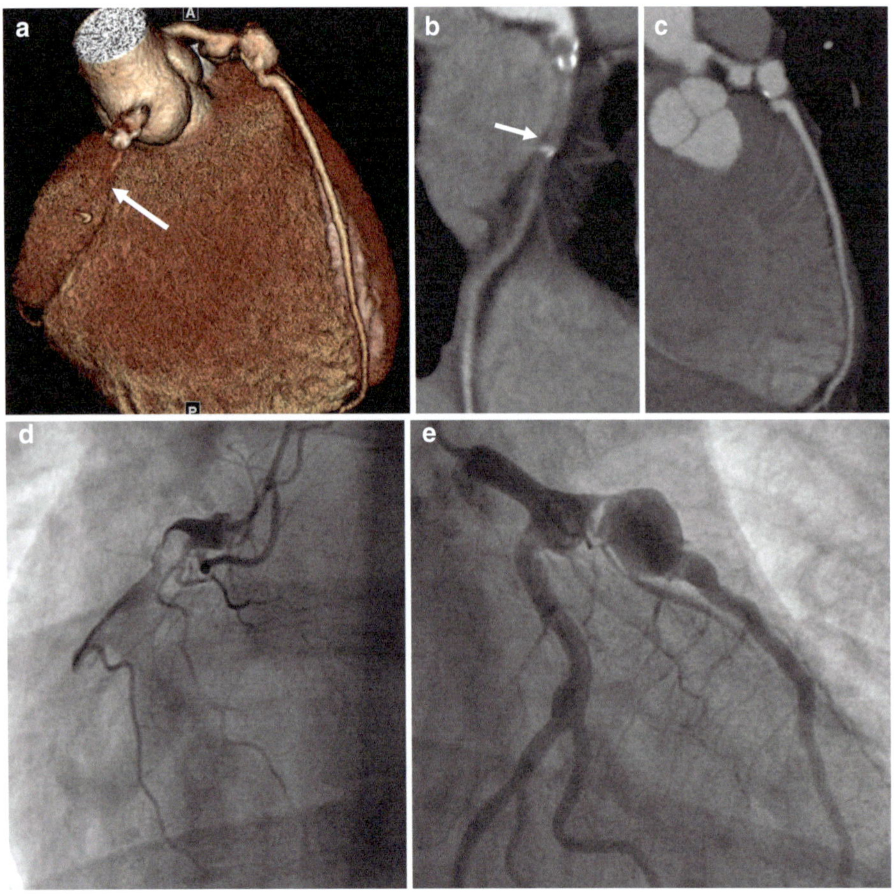

Fig. 7.23 Coronary artery aneurysms in a 28-year-old male with Kawasaki disease and acute myocardial infarction. (**a**) Volume-rendered CT images show aneurysms in the proximal LAD and RCA. There is occlusion of the RCA (arrow) distal to the aneurysm. (**b–e**) Curved planar reformatted CT images (**b**, **c**) and invasive angiograms (**d**, **e**) show aneurysms in the coronary arteries, occlusion of the RCA (arrow), and severe stenosis in the proximal LAD

formed to identify coronary artery aneurysm (CAA), left ventricular functional abnormalities, myocardial ischemia, and myocardial infarction. Low-dose CCTA can be performed in children and young adults when CMR is not feasible [77]. Although CCTA and MR coronary angiography (MRCA) show comparable performance in per-patient analysis, CCTA shows higher diagnostic performance than MRCA for evaluating coronary artery abnormalities in patients with KD [78].

Churg-Strauss syndrome is an autoimmune vasculitis seen in patients with a history of atopy or late-onset asthma that can lead to myocardial injury mimicking ACS with or without coronary artery aneurysms [79].

7.10 Coronary Artery Anomalies

Coronary artery anomalies are an uncommon but important cause of chest pain. Potentially hazardous coronary anomalies include ectopic origin from the pulmonary artery, ectopic origin from the opposite aortic sinus, single coronary artery, and large coronary fistulae [80–83]. CCTA allows accurate depiction of the origin, course, and termination of anomalous coronary arteries. CCTA is superior to ICA in delineating the ostial origin and proximal path of an anomalous coronary artery [80, 83].

Anomalous aortic origin of a coronary artery (AAOCA) from the inappropriate sinus of Valsalva is increasingly recognized by CCTA (Fig. 7.24). Although most AAOCA subtypes are

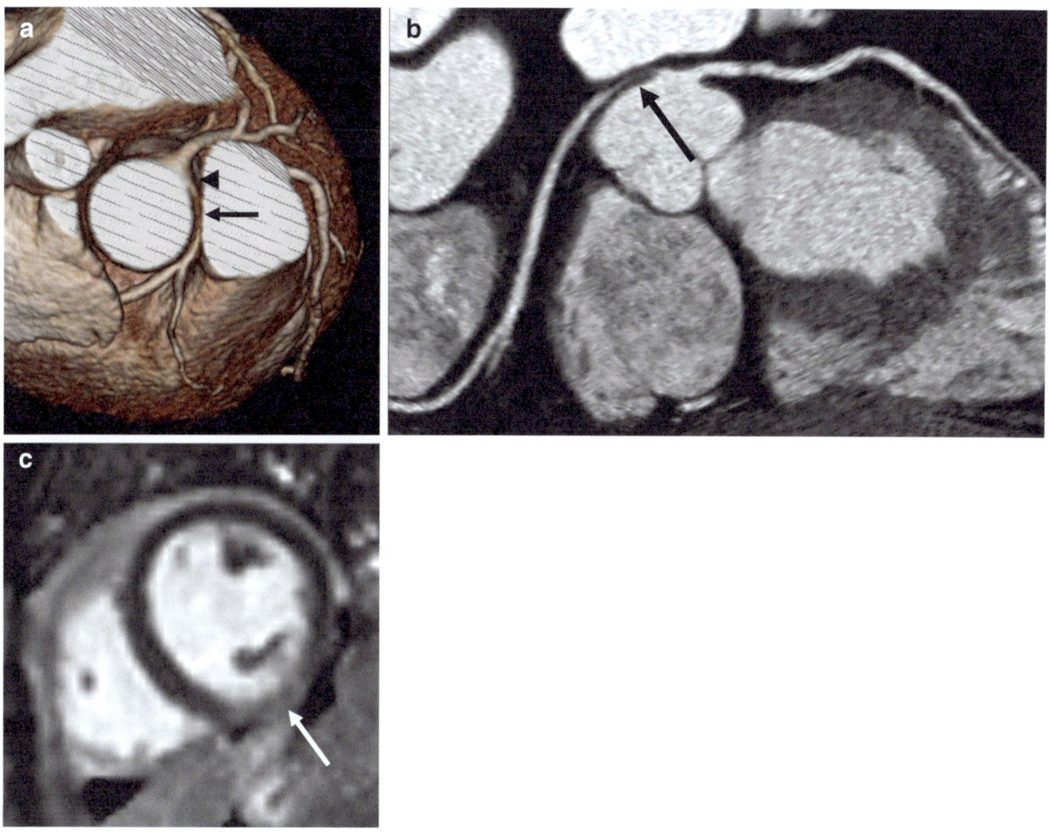

Fig. 7.24 Anomalous right coronary artery arising from just above the left coronary sinus in a 60-year-old female. (**a**) Volume-rendered CT image shows anomalous origin (arrowhead) of the RCA and interatrial course (arrow) of the RCA. (**b**) Curved planar reformatted image shows severe compression of the proximal segment (arrow) of the RCA. (**c**) LGE image shows acute myocardial infarction in the middle inferior wall of the left ventricle with areas of high signal intensity (arrow)

benign, autopsy studies report an increased risk of sudden death associated with interarterial anomalous left coronary artery (ALCA) and anomalous right coronary artery (ARCA). Cheezum et al. comprehensively reviewed 77 studies on the prevalence of AAOCA among >1 million patients and 20 studies examining outcomes in interarterial ALCA/ARCA patients [84]. Observational data suggests that interarterial ALCA is rare (weighted prevalence = 0.03%) compared with interarterial ARCA (weighted prevalence = 0.23%). CCTA can shed light on otial type (shared or separate ostia), percentage luminal diameter and area stenosis, length of the narrowed segments, ostial shape (oval or slit-like), presence of intramural location, and takeoff angles on multiplanar reconstruction.

Anomalous origin of the left coronary artery from the pulmonary artery (ALCAPA) syndrome is a rare coronary artery anomaly that affects 1/300,000 live births and represents 0.25%–0.5% of all congenital heart defects [83]. It is characterized by an anomalous origin of the left coronary artery from the pulmonary trunk or from a pulmonary artery. In the absence of collateral supply, myocardial infarction, secondary mitral regurgitation, and ischemic cardiomyopathy occur in the first weeks to months of life. This anomaly is rarely encountered in adults with well-developed collateral circulation and may cause mitral regurgitation and heart failure (Fig. 7.25) [85].

The coronary angiographic incidence of coronary artery fistula (CAF) is 0.1%–0.2%, representing 0.13% of all congenital heart defects. The right coronary artery is the most commonly affected vessel (60%, vs. 40% in the left coronary artery). CAF primarily drains into the right ventricle (45%), followed by communication with the right atrium (25%) or a pulmonary artery (15%) [83]. Coronary-to-pulmonary artery fistula (CPAF) is the most common type of CAF found incidentally on CCTA, with a prevalence ranging from 0.17% to 0.68% [81]. According to a study by Kim et al., the most common origin of CPAF is both coronary arteries, in 58.0% of cases.

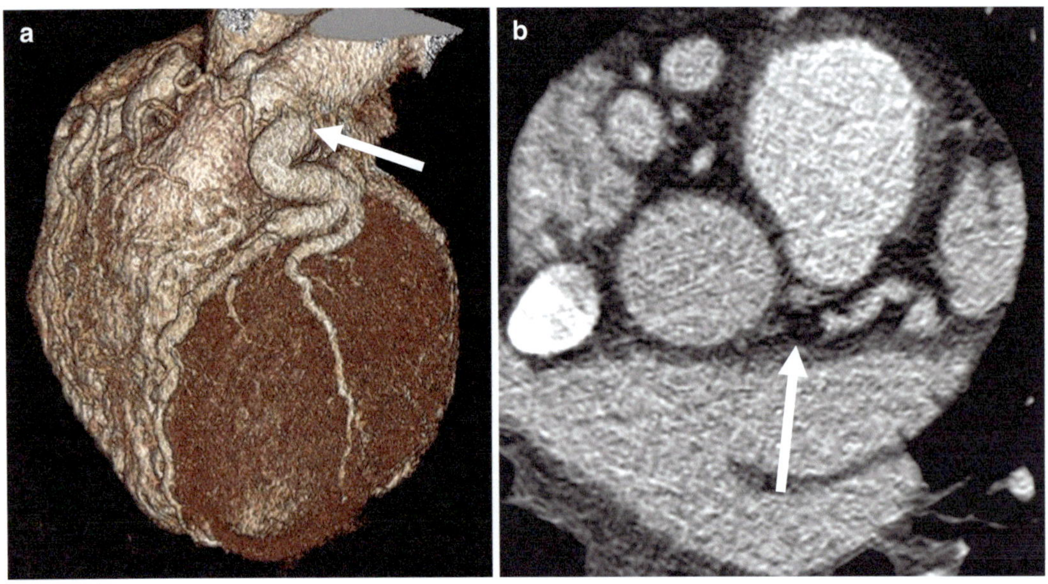

Fig. 7.25 Anomalous left coronary artery arising from the pulmonary artery in a 40-year-old female. (**a**) Volume-rendered CT image shows anomalous origin (arrow) of the left coronary artery (LCA) from the main pulmonary artery. (**b**) Transverse CT image shows the absence (arrow) of the normal LCA connection with the aortic sinus of Valsalva. (**c**) Right coronary angiography shows opacification of the LCA via collateral circulation draining into the main pulmonary artery (arrow)

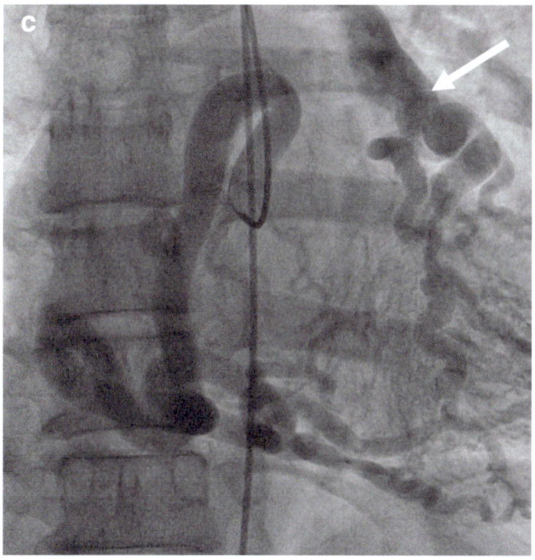

Fig. 7.25 (continued)

Aneurysms of anomalous coronary arteries are present in 31.3% of cases [81].

7.11 Hypertrophic Cardiomyopathy

The causes of chest pain in patients with hypertrophic cardiomyopathy (HCM) include myocardial ischemia due to microvascular dysfunction, increased left ventricular wall stress, and left ventricle outflow tract obstruction (Fig. 7.26). Deep myocardial bridging of the left anterior descending artery or atherosclerotic CAD may also account for chest pain. Invasive angiography or CCTA should be considered before septal reduction therapy in all patients aged 40 years or more

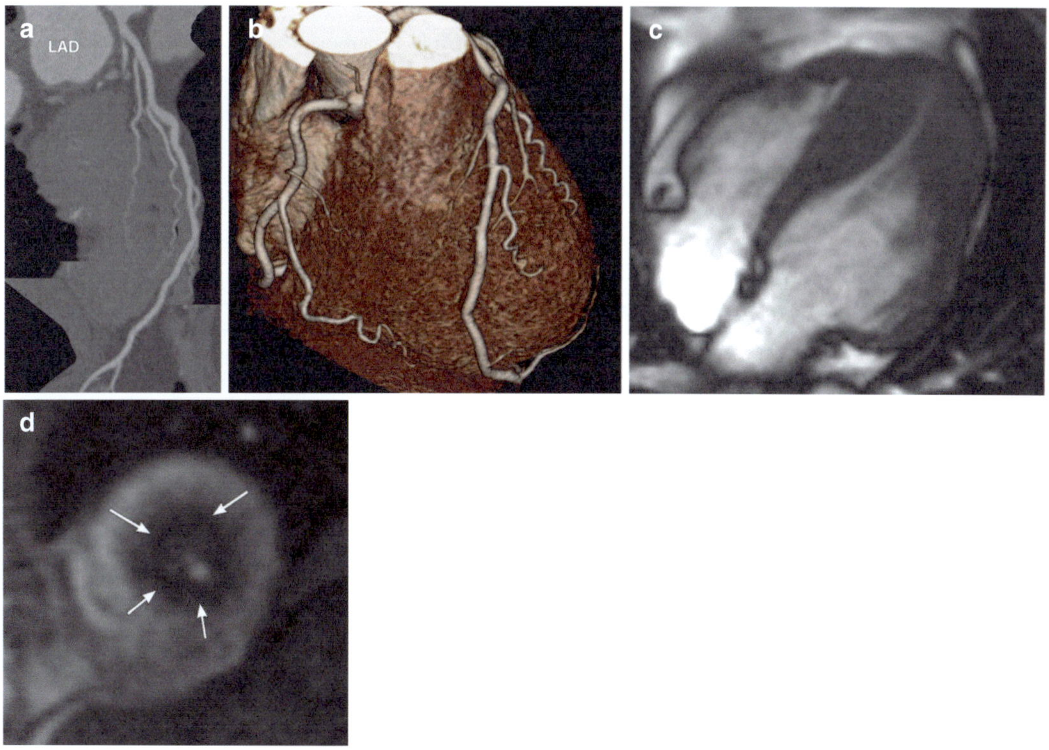

Fig. 7.26 Hypertrophic cardiomyopathy with chest pain in a 55-year-old male. (**a**, **b**) CCTA shows no significant stenosis in the epicardial coronary arteries. (**c**) Cine MRI in 4-chamber view shows apical hypertrophy. (**d**) Adenosine-stress perfusion imaging reveals perfusion defects (arrows) in the hypertrophied apical segments, probably due to microvascular ischemia

[86]. CCTA allows for visualization of the coronary arteries and valves and can guide catheter ablation of supraventricular arrhythmia. Cardiac CT should be considered in patients with inadequate echocardiographic imaging and contraindications for CMR. CMR shows gadolinium hyperenhancement in 65% of patients (range, 33–84%) with HCM in a patchy mid-wall pattern in the areas of hypertrophy [87].

7.12 New-Onset Heart Failure

CCTA can be performed to exclude CAD as the cause of new-onset heart failure (HF). CCTA enables assessment of CAD and CMR can show the severity and etiology of myocardial damage and the presence of myocardial ischemia [88]. CMR plays a role in differentiation between HF with reduced ejection fraction (EF) (HFrEF) versus preserved EF (HFpEF). CMR-based distinction between ischemic and nonischemic etiologies facilitates further planning [89].

7.13 Summary

CCTA has a high diagnostic accuracy for ruling out clinically significant CAD in patients with ACS; a CCTA-based strategy may allow safe and fast discharge of many patients at low-to-intermediate risk from the ED. Adoption of hs-Tn followed by early CCTA assessment improves risk stratification and diagnostic accuracy for ACS. High-risk plaques, which increase the likelihood of ACS, can be identified on CCTA. CMR accurately detects patients with ACS and helps to assess myocardial diseases mimicking ACS as well as acute myopericarditis. CCTA enables evaluation of cardiogenic sources of systemic embolism and CAD in stroke patients. CT shows acute complications of cardiovascular surgery and TAVI, such as valvular thrombosis, perivalvular pseudoaneurysms, and coronary artery occlusion. In cases with vasculitis, CCTA plays a role in the detection of coronary artery stenosis and aneurysms and CMR enables the evaluation of myocardial inflammation or infarction associated with vasculitis. CCTA allows accurate depiction of anomalous coronary arteries in ED patients.

Key Points
- CCTA and hs-Tn (especially in those with intermediate results) can contribute equally to ED patient management.
- CMR can be used as a one-stop imaging modality to identify causes of acute chest pain, such as acute myocardial infarction, acute myocarditis, Takotsubo syndrome, and hypertrophic cardiomyopathy, especially in patients with unobstructed coronary arteries.
- Asymptomatic CAD detected on CCTA is associated with increased risk of cardiovascular events or death in acute stroke patients.
- ACS may occur in patients with vasculitis, such as Takayasu's arteritis and Kawasaki disease.
- CCTA is superior to ICA in delineating the ostial origin and proximal path of an anomalous coronary artery.

References

1. Pannu HK, Alvarez W Jr, Fishman EK. Beta-blockers for cardiac CT: a primer for the radiologist. AJR Am J Roentgenol. 2006;186(6 Suppl 2):S341–5.
2. Vardhanabhuti V, Nicol E, Morgan-Hughes G, et al. Recommendations for accurate CT diagnosis of suspected acute aortic syndrome (AAS): on behalf of the British Society of Cardiovascular Imaging (BSCI)/British Society of Cardiovascular CT (BSCCT). Br J Radiol. 2016;89(1061):20150705.
3. Shin N, Kim SM, Choe YH. Protocol using wide-detector CT with single contrast injection for the aorta and coronary artery: variable helical pitch versus volume scan following helical scan. Int J Cardiovasc Imaging. 2019;35(10):1935–42.
4. Raff GL, Hoffmann U, Udelson JE. Trials of imaging use in the Emergency Department for acute chest pain. JACC Cardiovasc Imaging. 2017;10(3):338–49.
5. Linde JJ, Kelbæk H, Hansen TF, et al. Coronary CT angiography in patients with non-ST-segment elevation acute coronary syndrome. J Am Coll Cardiol. 2020;75(5):453–63.
6. Min JH, Kim SM, Lee S, Choi JH, Chang SA, Choe YH. Diagnostic performance of algorithm for computer-assisted detection of significant coronary artery disease in patients with acute chest pain: com-

parison with invasive coronary angiography. AJR Am J Roentgenol. 2014;202(4):730–7.
7. Goldstein JA, Chinnaiyan KM, Abidov A, et al. The CT-STAT (coronary computed tomographic angiography for systematic triage of acute chest pain patients to treatment) trial. J Am Coll Cardiol. 2011;58(14):1414–22.
8. Durand E, Bauer F, Mansencal N, et al. Head-to-head comparison of the diagnostic performance of coronary computed tomography angiography and dobutamine-stress echocardiography in the evaluation of acute chest pain with normal ECG findings and negative troponin tests: a prospective multicenter study. Int J Cardiol. 2017;241:463–9.
9. Litt HI, Gatsonis C, Snyder B, et al. CT angiography for safe discharge of patients with possible acute coronary syndromes. N Engl J Med. 2012;366(15):1393–403.
10. Hoffmann U, Truong QA, Schoenfeld DA, et al. Coronary CT angiography versus standard evaluation in acute chest pain. N Engl J Med. 2012;367(4):299–308.
11. Linde JJ, Hove JD, Sorgaard M, et al. Long-term clinical impact of coronary CT angiography in patients with recent acute-onset chest pain: the randomized controlled CATCH trial. JACC Cardiovasc Imaging. 2015;8(12):1404–13.
12. Truong QA, Hayden D, Woodard PK, et al. Sex differences in the effectiveness of early coronary computed tomographic angiography compared with standard emergency department evaluation for acute chest pain: the rule-out myocardial infarction with computer-assisted tomography (ROMICAT)-II trial. Circulation. 2013;127(25):2494–502.
13. Truong QA, Schulman-Marcus J, Zakroysky P, et al. Coronary CT angiography versus standard emergency department evaluation for acute chest pain and diabetic patients: is there benefit with early coronary CT angiography? Results of the randomized comparative effectiveness ROMICAT II trial. J Am Heart Assoc. 2016;5(3):e003137.
14. Bittner DO, Mayrhofer T, Bamberg F, et al. Impact of coronary calcification on clinical management in patients with acute chest pain. Circ Cardiovasc Imaging. 2017;10(5):e005893.
15. Hinzpeter R, Higashigaito K, Morsbach F, et al. Coronary artery calcium scoring for ruling-out acute coronary syndrome in chest pain CT. Am J Emerg Med. 2017;35(10):1565–7.
16. Dedic A, Lubbers MM, Schaap J, et al. Coronary CT angiography for suspected ACS in the era of high-sensitivity troponins: randomized multicenter study. J Am Coll Cardiol. 2016;67(1):16–26.
17. Ferencik M, Liu T, Mayrhofer T, et al. hs-Troponin I followed by CT angiography improves acute coronary syndrome risk stratification accuracy and work-up in acute chest pain patients: results from ROMICAT II trial. JACC Cardiovasc Imaging. 2015;8(11):1272–81.
18. Puchner SB, Liu T, Mayrhofer T, et al. High-risk plaque detected on coronary CT angiography predicts acute coronary syndromes independent of significant stenosis in acute chest pain: results from the ROMICAT-II trial. J Am Coll Cardiol. 2014;64(7):684–92.
19. Ahmadi A, Argulian E, Leipsic J, Newby DE, Narula J. From subclinical atherosclerosis to plaque progression and acute coronary events: JACC state-of-the-art review. J Am Coll Cardiol. 2019;74(12):1608–17.
20. Hedgire S, Baliyan V, Zucker EJ, et al. Perivascular epicardial fat stranding at coronary CT angiography: a marker of acute plaque rupture and spontaneous coronary artery dissection. Radiology. 2018;287(3):808–15.
21. Nakayama N, Kaikita K, Fukunaga T, et al. Clinical features and prognosis of patients with coronary spasm-induced non-ST-segment elevation acute coronary syndrome. J Am Heart Assoc. 2014;3(3):e000795.
22. Kang EJ, Kim MH, De Jin C, et al. Noninvasive detection of coronary vasospastic angina using a double-acquisition coronary CT angiography protocol in the presence and absence of an intravenous nitrate: a pilot study. Eur Radiol. 2017;27(3):1136–47.
23. Ohba K, Sugiyama S, Sumida H, et al. Microvascular coronary artery spasm presents distinctive clinical features with endothelial dysfunction as nonobstructive coronary artery disease. J Am Heart Assoc. 2012;1(5):e002485.
24. Ohyama K, Matsumoto Y, Takanami K, et al. Coronary adventitial and perivascular adipose tissue inflammation in patients with vasospastic angina. J Am Coll Cardiol. 2018;71(4):414–25.
25. Kim HS, Kim SM, Cha MJ, et al. Triple rule-out CT angiography protocol with restricting field of view for detection of pulmonary thromboembolism and aortic dissection in emergency department patients: simulation of modified CT protocol for reducing radiation dose. Acta Radiol. 2017;58(5):521–7.
26. Park J, Kim J, Kim K. Limiting scan range of cardiac CT and the chance of missed acute aortic syndrome. Am J Emerg Med. 2016;34(10):2007–10.
27. Thomas DM, Larson CW, Cheezum MK, et al. Rest-only myocardial CT perfusion in acute chest pain. South Med J. 2015;108(11):688–94.
28. Hayes SN, Kim ESH, Saw J, et al. Spontaneous coronary artery dissection: current state of the science: a scientific statement from the American Heart Association. Circulation. 2018;137(19):e523–57.
29. Adlam D, Alfonso F, Maas A, Vrints C. European Society of Cardiology, acute cardiovascular care association, SCAD study group: a position paper on spontaneous coronary artery dissection. Eur Heart J. 2018;39(36):3353–68.
30. Hecht HS, Narula J, Fearon WF. Fractional flow reserve and coronary computed tomographic angiography: a review and critical analysis. Circ Res. 2016;119(2):300–16.
31. Abanador-Kamper N, Kamper L, Castello-Boerrigter L, Haage P, Seyfarth M. MRI findings in patients with acute coronary syndrome and unobstructed coronary arteries. Diagn Interv Radiol. 2019;25(1):28–34.

32. Chu G, Zhang G, Zhu M, Zhang Z, Wu Y, Zhang H. Acute one-stop cardiovascular magnetic resonance imaging for differential diagnosis in patients with acute coronary syndrome and unobstructed coronary arteries. Med Princ Pract. 2015;24(4):325–31.
33. De Filippo M, Capasso R. Coronary computed tomography angiography (CCTA) and cardiac magnetic resonance (CMR) imaging in the assessment of patients presenting with chest pain suspected for acute coronary syndrome. Ann Transl Med. 2016;4(13):255.
34. Kwong RY, Schussheim AE, Rekhraj S, et al. Detecting acute coronary syndrome in the emergency department with cardiac magnetic resonance imaging. Circulation. 2003;107(4):531–7.
35. Saremi F. Cardiac MR imaging in acute coronary syndrome: application and image interpretation. Radiology. 2017;282(1):17–32.
36. Adler Y, Charron P, Imazio M, et al. ESC Guidelines for the diagnosis and management of pericardial diseases: the task force for the diagnosis and management of pericardial diseases of the European Society of Cardiology (ESC)Endorsed by: The European Association for Cardio-Thoracic Surgery (EACTS). Eur Heart J. 2015;36(42):2921–64.
37. Fadl SA, Nasrullah A, Harris A, Edwards R, Kicska G. Comprehensive review of pericardial diseases using different imaging modalities. Int J Cardiovasc Imaging. 2020;36(5):947–69.
38. Restrepo CS, Lemos DF, Lemos JA, et al. Imaging findings in cardiac tamponade with emphasis on CT. Radiographics. 2007;27(6):1595–610.
39. Friedrich MG, Marcotte F. Cardiac magnetic resonance assessment of myocarditis. Circ Cardiovasc Imaging. 2013;6(5):833–9.
40. Chen W, Jeudy J. Assessment of myocarditis: cardiac MR, PET/CT, or PET/MR? Curr Cardiol Rep. 2019;21(8):76.
41. Gannon MP, Schaub E, Grines CL, Saba SG. State of the art: evaluation and prognostication of myocarditis using cardiac MRI. J Magn Reson Imaging. 2019;49(7):e122–31.
42. Wheen P, Armstrong R, Daly CA. Recent advances in T1 and T2 mapping in the assessment of fulminant myocarditis by cardiac magnetic resonance. Curr Cardiol Rep. 2020;22(7):47.
43. Baessler B, Luecke C, Lurz J, et al. Cardiac MRI and texture analysis of myocardial T1 and T2 maps in myocarditis with acute versus chronic symptoms of heart failure. Radiology. 2019;292(3):608–17.
44. Hulten E, Agarwal V, Cahill M, et al. Presence of late gadolinium enhancement by cardiac magnetic resonance among patients with suspected cardiac sarcoidosis is associated with adverse cardiovascular prognosis: a systematic review and meta-analysis. Circ Cardiovasc Imaging. 2016;9(9):e005001.
45. Hur J, Choi BW. Cardiac CT imaging for ischemic stroke: current and evolving clinical applications. Radiology. 2017;283(1):14–28.
46. Smietana J, Plitt A, Halperin JL. Thromboembolism in the absence of atrial fibrillation. Am J Cardiol. 2019;124(2):303–11.
47. Niku AD, Shiota T, Siegel RJ, Rader F. Prevalence and resolution of left atrial thrombus in patients with nonvalvular atrial fibrillation and flutter with oral anticoagulation. Am J Cardiol. 2019;123(1):63–8.
48. Pathan F, Hecht H, Narula J, Marwick TH. Roles of transesophageal echocardiography and cardiac computed tomography for evaluation of left atrial thrombus and associated pathology: a review and critical analysis. JACC Cardiovasc Imaging. 2018;11(4):616–27.
49. Inoue T, Suematsu Y. Poor enhancement pattern of left atrial appendage in cardiac computed tomography is associated with stroke in persistent atrial fibrillation patients. J Thorac Dis. 2019;11(8):3315–24.
50. Bilchick KC, Mealor A, Gonzalez J, et al. Effectiveness of integrating delayed computed tomography angiography imaging for left atrial appendage thrombus exclusion into the care of patients undergoing ablation of atrial fibrillation. Heart Rhythm. 2016;13(1):12–9.
51. Crimm HA, Taylor JR, Fogarty BT, Villines TC. Prone patient positioning to exclude left atrial appendage thrombus using cardiac CT. J Cardiovasc Comput Tomogr. 2018;12(2):176–8.
52. Teunissen C, Habets J, Velthuis BK, Cramer MJ, Loh P. Double-contrast, single-phase computed tomography angiography for ruling out left atrial appendage thrombus prior to atrial fibrillation ablation. Int J Cardiovasc Imaging. 2017;33(1):121–8.
53. Hur J, Kim YJ, Lee HJ, et al. Cardioembolic stroke: dual-energy cardiac CT for differentiation of left atrial appendage thrombus and circulatory stasis. Radiology. 2012;263(3):688–95.
54. Kim EY, Choe YH, Sung K, Park SW, Kim JH, Ko YH. Multidetector CT and MR imaging of cardiac tumors. Korean J Radiol. 2009;10(2):164–75.
55. Koo HJ, Yang DH, Kang JW, et al. Demonstration of infective endocarditis by cardiac CT and transoesophageal echocardiography: comparison with intraoperative findings. Eur Heart J Cardiovasc Imaging. 2018;19(2):199–207.
56. Windecker S, Stortecky S, Meier B. Paradoxical embolism. J Am Coll Cardiol. 2014;64(4):403–15.
57. Ioannidis SG, Mitsias PD. Patent foramen ovale in cryptogenic ischemic stroke: direct cause, risk factor, or incidental finding? Front Neurol. 2020;11:567.
58. Mojadidi MK, Bogush N, Caceres JD, Msaouel P, Tobis JM. Diagnostic accuracy of transesophageal echocardiogram for the detection of patent foramen ovale: a meta-analysis. Echocardiography. 2014;31(6):752–8.
59. Kim YJ, Hur J, Shim CY, et al. Patent foramen ovale: diagnosis with multidetector CT-comparison with transesophageal echocardiography. Radiology. 2009;250(1):61–7.
60. Auer J. Coronary evaluation in patients with stroke: recognizing the risk. Atherosclerosis. 2015;238(2):427–9.
61. Boulanger M, Béjot Y, Rothwell PM, Touzé E. Long-term risk of myocardial infarction compared to recurrent stroke after transient ischemic attack and ischemic stroke: systematic review and meta-analysis. J Am Heart Assoc. 2018;7(2):e007267.

62. Yoo J, Song D, Baek JH, et al. Poor long-term outcomes in stroke patients with asymptomatic coronary artery disease in heart CT. Atherosclerosis. 2017;265:7–13.
63. Yoon SH, Kim E, Jeon Y, et al. Prognostic value of coronary CT angiography for predicting poor cardiac outcome in stroke patients without known cardiac disease or chest pain: the assessment of coronary artery disease in stroke patients study. Korean J Radiol. 2020;21(9):1055–64.
64. Hammer MM, Raptis DA, Cummings KW, et al. Imaging in blunt cardiac injury: computed tomographic findings in cardiac contusion and associated injuries. Injury. 2016;47(5):1025–30.
65. Gosavi S, Tyroch AH, Mukherjee D. Cardiac trauma. Angiology. 2016;67(10):896–901.
66. Koo HJ, Lee HN, Anh TT, et al. Postoperative complications after surgical aortic valve replacement. Cardiovasc Imaging Asia. 2017;1(4):222–30.
67. Sanchez-Recalde A, Gonzalez-Obeso E, Oliver JM. Bilateral coronary artery occlusion after aortic valve replacement in a patient with porcelain ascending aorta. Eur Heart J. 2007;28(13):1553.
68. Soschynski M, Capilli F, Ruile P, Neumann FJ, Langer M, Krauss T. Post-TAVI follow-up with MDCT of the valve prosthesis: technical application, regular findings and typical local post-interventional complications. Rofo. 2018;190(6):521–30.
69. Ribeiro HB, Nombela-Franco L, Urena M, et al. Coronary obstruction following transcatheter aortic valve implantation: a systematic review. JACC Cardiovasc Interv. 2013;6(5):452–61.
70. Barbanti M, Petronio AS, Ettori F, et al. 5-year outcomes after transcatheter aortic valve implantation with CoreValve prosthesis. JACC Cardiovasc Interv. 2015;8(8):1084–91.
71. Jilaihawi H, Asch FM, Manasse E, et al. Systematic CT methodology for the evaluation of subclinical leaflet thrombosis. JACC Cardiovasc Imaging. 2017;10(4):461–70.
72. Blanke P, Reinöhl J, Schlensak C, et al. Prosthesis oversizing in balloon-expandable transcatheter aortic valve implantation is associated with contained rupture of the aortic root. Circ Cardiovasc Interv. 2012;5(4):540–8.
73. Salaun E, Jacquier A, Theron A, et al. Value of CMR in quantification of paravalvular aortic regurgitation after TAVI. Eur Heart J Cardiovasc Imaging. 2016;17(1):41–50.
74. Kang EJ, Kim SM, Choe YH, Lee GY, Lee KN, Kim DK. Takayasu arteritis: assessment of coronary arterial abnormalities with 128-section dual-source CT angiography of the coronary arteries and aorta. Radiology. 2014;270(1):74–81.
75. Choe YH, Han BK, Koh EM, Kim DK, Do YS, Lee WR. Takayasu's arteritis: assessment of disease activity with contrast-enhanced MR imaging. AJR Am J Roentgenol. 2000;175(2):505–11.
76. Mitani Y, Tsuda E, Kato H, et al. Emergence and characterization of acute coronary syndrome in adults after confirmed or missed history of Kawasaki disease in Japan: a Japanese Nationwide survey. Front Pediatr. 2019;7:275.
77. Dietz SM, Tacke CE, Kuipers IM, et al. Cardiovascular imaging in children and adults following Kawasaki disease. Insights Imaging. 2015;6(6):697–705.
78. Kim JW, Goo HW. Coronary artery abnormalities in Kawasaki disease: comparison between CT and MR coronary angiography. Acta Radiol. 2013;54(2):156–63.
79. Gue YX, Prasad S, Isenberg D, Gorog DA. A case of repetitive myocardial infarction with unobstructed coronaries due to Churg-Strauss syndrome. Eur Heart J Case Rep. 2019;3(2):ytz041.
80. Kim SY, Seo JB, Do KH, et al. Coronary artery anomalies: classification and ECG-gated multi-detector row CT findings with angiographic correlation. Radiographics. 2006;26(2):317–33.
81. Kim H, Beck KS, Choe YH, Jung JI. Coronary-to-pulmonary artery fistula in adults: natural history and management strategies. Korean J Radiol. 2019;20(11):1491–7.
82. Lee BY. Anomalous right coronary artery from the left coronary sinus with an interarterial course: is it really dangerous? Korean Circ J. 2009;39(5):175–9.
83. Heermann P, Heindel W, Schülke C. Coronary artery anomalies: diagnosis and classification based on cardiac CT and MRI (CMR) - from ALCAPA to anomalies of termination. Rofo. 2017;189(1):29–38.
84. Cheezum MK, Liberthson RR, Shah NR, et al. Anomalous aortic origin of a coronary artery from the inappropriate sinus of Valsalva. J Am Coll Cardiol. 2017;69(12):1592–608.
85. Boutsikou M, Shore D, Li W, et al. Anomalous left coronary artery from the pulmonary artery (ALCAPA) diagnosed in adulthood: varied clinical presentation, therapeutic approach and outcome. Int J Cardiol. 2018;261:49–53.
86. Elliott PM, Anastasakis A, Borger MA, et al. ESC guidelines on diagnosis and management of hypertrophic cardiomyopathy: the task force for the diagnosis and management of hypertrophic cardiomyopathy of the European Society of Cardiology (ESC). Eur Heart J. 2014;35(39):2733–79.
87. Rudolph A, Abdel-Aty H, Bohl S, et al. Noninvasive detection of fibrosis applying contrast-enhanced cardiac magnetic resonance in different forms of left ventricular hypertrophy relation to remodeling. J Am Coll Cardiol. 2009;53(3):284–91.
88. Hamilton-Craig C, Strugnell WE, Raffel OC, Porto I, Walters DL, Slaughter RE. CT angiography with cardiac MRI: non-invasive functional and anatomical assessment for the etiology in newly diagnosed heart failure. Int J Cardiovasc Imaging. 2012;28(5):1111–22.
89. White RD, Kirsch J, Bolen MA, et al. ACR appropriateness criteria(®) suspected new-onset and known nonacute heart failure. J Am Coll Radiol. 2018;15(11):S418–31.

8 Pulmonary Infection (Pneumonia)

8.1 Introduction

Pneumonia is a common condition seen in the emergency department (ED); it is the leading cause of death owing to infectious disease. In the United States, there are an estimated 1.1 million cases of community-acquired pneumonia (CAP) requiring hospitalization each year [1]. Pneumonia is responsible for >50 million days of restricted activity from work and is the sixth leading cause of death in the United States, with a mortality rate of 13.4 per 100,000 patients [2].

More structured approaches have been evolving for the treatment of pneumonia. The diagnosis of pneumonia requires clinical acumen, appropriate microbiologic testing, and imaging. In the ED, accurate diagnosis of pneumonia and grading of pneumonia severity is important because clinicians must determine whether to manage pneumonia on an outpatient basis, in a hospital ward, or in the intensive care unit. US national guidelines suggest that local pneumonia protocols be established at each hospital. The use of local protocols should facilitate improved patient care [3].

Imaging studies should always be interpreted with full awareness of the clinical features of the disease, such as symptom duration, presence of fever, cough, and dyspnea, and the presence or absence of leukocytosis. Knowledge of a patient's exposure status (community-acquired pneumonia, CAP, or healthcare-associated pneumonia, HCAP) and immune status are important for differential diagnosis and determination of the most likely causative organisms [4].

The pneumonia severity index (PSI) is a clinical prediction tool that medical practitioners can use to calculate the probability of morbidity and mortality among patients with CAP [5]. The PSI is often used to predict the need for hospitalization in people with pneumonia, helping physicians make more rational decisions. Mortality prediction is similar to that done using CURB-65 [6]. The CURB-65, curb criterion, is a clinical prediction rule that has been validated for predicting mortality in CAP and infection of any site. The CURB-65 is based on the early CURB score and is recommended by the British Thoracic Society for the assessment of the severity of pneumonia [7]. It was developed in 2002 at the University of Nottingham by Lim WS et al. [8]. In 2018 a new toolkit was presented on the basis of CURB-65. The score is an acronym for each of the risk factors measured. Each risk factor scores one point if relevant (zero if not relevant), for a maximum score of 5: Confusion of new onset, Blood urea nitrogen >7 mmol/l (19 mg/dL), Respiratory rate of ≥30 breaths per minute or greater, Blood pressure <90 mmHg, systolic or diastolic blood pressure <60 mmHg, and age ≥65.

T. J. Kim et al., *Emergency Chest Radiology*, https://doi.org/10.1007/978-981-33-4396-2_8

8.2 Morphologic Classification of Pneumonia

Pulmonary infection can be classified into several radiologic and pathologic patterns according to its morphologic features. The three most common patterns are lobar pneumonia, bronchopneumonia, and interstitial pneumonia. Less common forms of infection include cellular (inflammatory) bronchiolitis, septic embolism, miliary infection, and lung abscess. In this section, we describe the three most common patterns of pneumonia.

8.2.1 Lobar Pneumonia

Lobar pneumonia is characterized histopathologically by filling of alveolar airspaces with an exudate of edema fluid and neutrophils. This filling is usually uniform within the affected lung and typically extends across pulmonary segments. Consolidation usually begins in the periphery of the lung adjacent to the visceral pleura and spreads centripetally via interalveolar pores and small airways, sometimes to involve the entire lobe. Bronchi that remain filled with gas and become surrounded by the expanding inflammatory exudate are often seen as air-bronchograms on CT scans. The most common causative organisms in lobar pneumonia are *Streptococcus pneumoniae* (*S. pneumoniae*), *Klebsiella pneumoniae* (*K. pneumoniae*) (Fig. 8.1), and *Legionella pneumophila* (*L. pneumophila*) (Fig. 8.2).

On CT scans, homogeneous airspace consolidation involving adjacent segments of a lobe (in a unilateral lung) is the predominant finding. On thin-section CT (TSCT), areas of ground-glass opacities (GGOs) denoting incomplete filling of alveoli can be seen adjacent to the areas of airspace consolidation (Figs. 8.1 and 8.2) [9]. The consolidation typically extends across lobular and segmental boundaries. A segmental or lobar form of tuberculous pneumonia may occur in adults, particularly acquired immune deficiency syndrome (AIDS) patients and non-AIDS immunocompromised patients including pregnant women, the elderly, diabetes, alcoholics, and transplant patients. Multiple small cavities may be shown within the consolidative lesion in tuberculous pneumonia [10, 11].

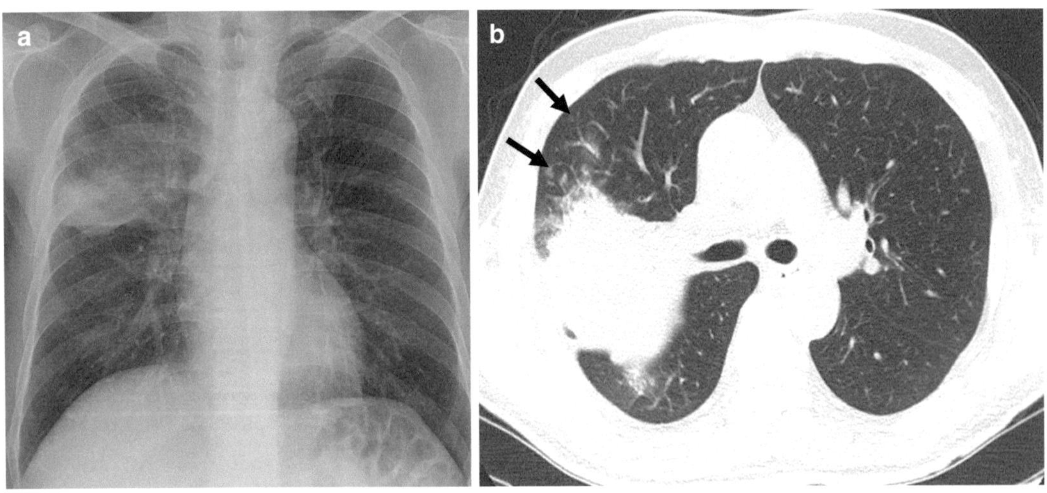

Fig. 8.1 *Klebsiella* pneumonia manifesting as a segmental consolidative lesion in a 64-year-old man. (**a**) Chest radiograph demonstrates a mass-like lesion in the right upper lung zone. (**b**) Lung window image of a CT scan obtained at the level of the main bronchi shows mass-like consolidation occupying the posterior segment of the right upper lobe. Also note the small centrilobular nodules (arrows) with fluffy margin representing cellular bronchiolitis. (**c**) Mediastinal window image of an enhanced CT scan depicts necrotic consolidation showing internal CT-angiogram sign (arrows: enhancing vascular structures within consolidation)

Fig. 8.1 (continued)

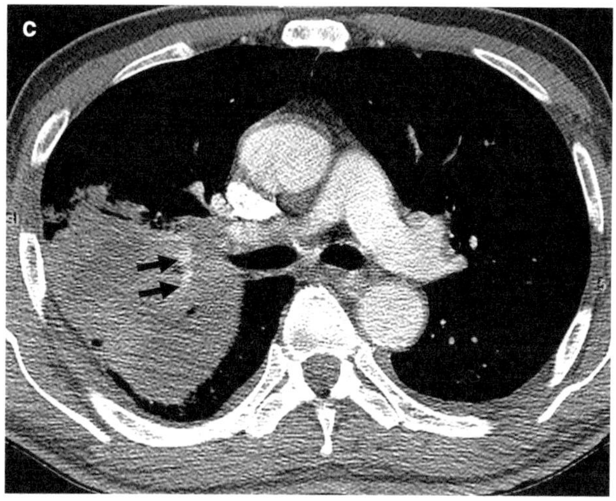

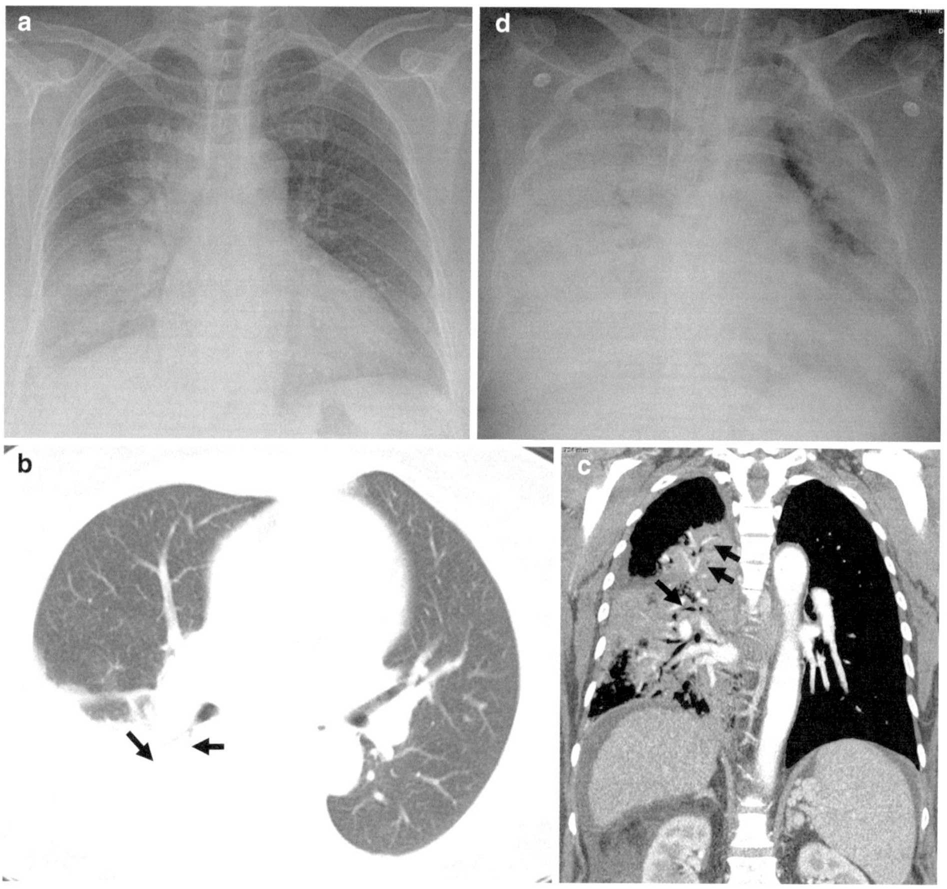

Fig. 8.2 Legionella pneumonia in a 61-year-old woman. (**a**) Chest radiograph shows lobar consolidation in the right lower lobe territory. (**b**) Lung window image of a CT scan obtained at the level of the distal bronchus intermedius demonstrates lobar consolidation in the right lower lobe. CT air-bronchogram signs (arrows: aerated bronchi within consolidation) are also seen. (**c**) Mediastinal window image of an enhanced CT scan depicts extensive lobar pneumonia in the right lower lobe. Also note CT angiogram signs (arrows). (**d**) Follow-up radiograph obtained 10 days after **a** discloses extensive parenchymal consolidation occupying both lungs. An endotracheal intubation tube, central line, and L-tube are in situ

8.2.2 Bronchopneumonia

Bronchopneumonia is characterized histopathologically by patchy, predominantly peribronchiolar inflammation. It is not clear why this localization is different from that seen in lobar pneumonia, but the difference may be related to relatively less abundant edema formation (associated with more difficult spread of infection within the lung) and an increased presence of virulent organisms (resulting in greater tissue destruction in bronchopneumonia). Although initially patchy, progression of the disease may result in lobular and segmental consolidation. The main causative organisms are *Staphylococcus aureus* (*S. aureus*), *Hemophilus influenzae* (*H. influenzae*), *Pseudomonas aeruginosa* (*P. aeruginosa*), and anaerobic bacteria.

Characteristic findings on HRCT include centrilobular small nodules (airspace nodules), branching nodular structures with fluffy margins, acinus-sized nodules, and multi-focal lobular consolidation or GGO (Figs. 8.3 and 8.4) [9]. The small nodules and branching nodular opacities result in an appearance that resembles a budding tree; they are related to the presence of the inflammatory exudate in the lumen and walls of membranous and respiratory bronchioles as well as within alveolar spaces adjacent to the involved respiratory bronchioles (Fig. 8.2). Inflammatory exudate is present within alveoli, airway lumens, and walls, so the nodules are usually fluffy in CAP. By contrast, with much less inflammatory exudate in the alveolar spaces and with inflammatory cells mainly located in the airway walls and lumens, the tree-in-bud signs are sharp in margin and clearly branching in tuberculosis (Fig. 8.5).

This small centrilobular nodular appearance is similar in cellular (inflammatory) bronchiolitis caused by viruses, *Mycoplasma pneumonia* (*M. pneumonia*) (Figs. 8.3 and 8.4), and *Chlamydia* [9, 12]. Unlike the latter (atypical pneumonias), however, the tree-in-bud pattern usually comprises only a small proportion of the TSCT abnormalities in bacterial bronchopneumonia, where additional acinar or lobular nodule or consolidation features are predominant. Moreover, in atypical pneumonia, thickening of bronchovascular bundles is more frequently observed, and individual opacity tends to be distributed at the inner zone in addition to the middle and outer zones and tends to be smaller than that seen in bacterial pneumonias [9]. Lesions in bacterial bronchopneumonia may involve the unilateral lobe or lung. However, in viral pneumonia, particularly in influenza pneumonia (H1N1) in immunocompetent hosts, the lung lesions may manifest as bilateral lung abnormalities in up to 82% of patients. In this particular condition, the lesions on TSCT may simulate interstitial lung disease [13, 14].

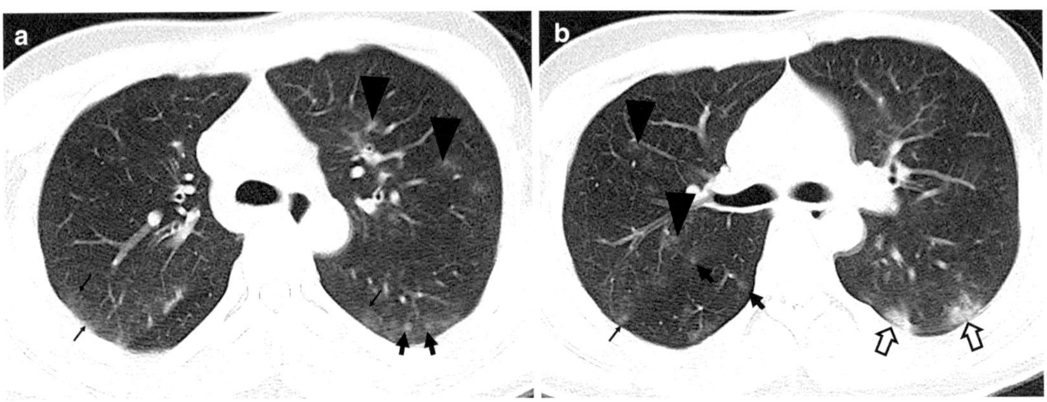

Fig. 8.3 Metapneumovirus pneumonia in a 20-year-old man. (**a**, **b**) Lung window images of CT scans obtained at the levels of the azygos arch (**a**) and main bronchi (**b**) show ground-glass opacity nodules (arrows) with fluffy margin in the centrilobular areas or along bronchovascular bundles (arrowheads). Also note subtle acinus-sized ground-glass nodules (small arrows) and lobular areas of consolidation (open arrows) in both lungs

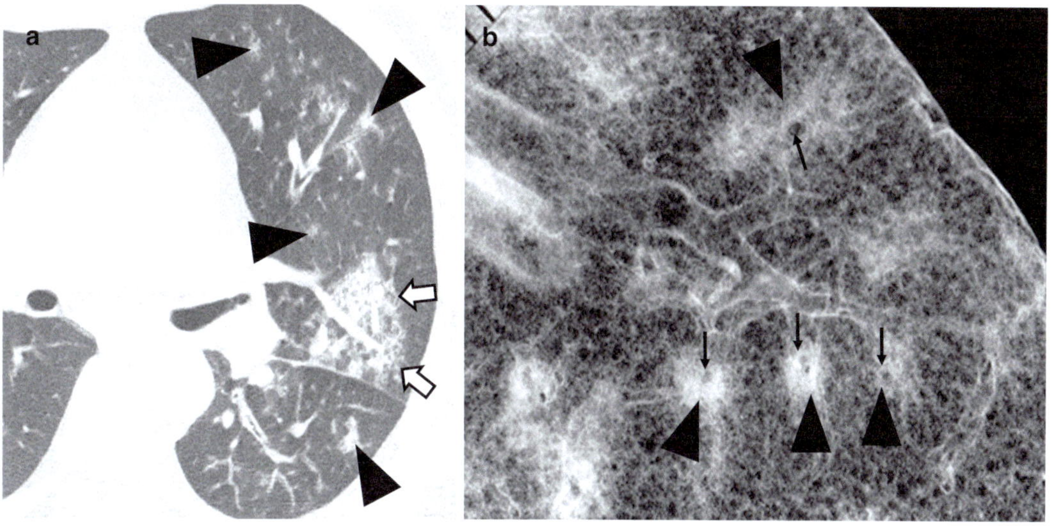

Fig. 8.4 Community-acquired pneumonia showing morphologic bronchopneumonia in a 56-year-old woman (organisms not identified). (**a**) Lung window image of a CT scan obtained at the level of the bronchus intermedius shows fluffy nodules (arrowheads) along the bronchovascular bundles. Also note subsegmental opacity (open arrows) in the superior lingular segment of the left upper lobe. (**b**) Contact radiograph of a pathologic specimen from a different patient suffering from symptoms of pneumonia demonstrates fluffy nodules (arrowheads) along the bronchovascular bundles; fluffy margin is caused by inflammatory cell extension from respiratory bronchioles (small arrows) into alveolar spaces. Case courtesy of Dr. Kiyoshi Murata, Department of Radiology, Shiga University of Medical Science, Otsu, Japan

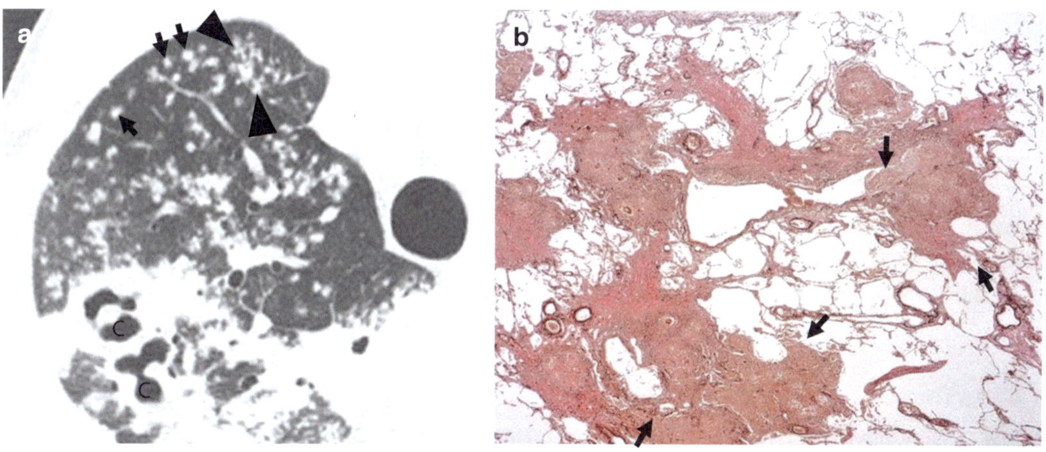

Fig. 8.5 Bronchopneumonia of pulmonary tuberculosis in a 47-year-old man. (**a**) Lung window image of a CT scan obtained at the level of the great vessels in the thoracic inlet shows typical dense centrilobular nodules (arrows), branching nodular lesions appearing as tree-in-bud signs (arrowheads), and cavities (C) within consolidative lesions in the right upper lobe. (**b**) Low-magnification pathologic specimen obtained from a different patient demonstrates inflammatory lesions and granulomas, mainly in the walls and lumens (arrows) of the respiratory bronchioles. Also note the paucity of inflammatory cells or granulomas in alveolar spaces. The combination of these features (bronchiolar or airway luminal location and paucity of alveolar space involvement) on histopathology results in centrilobular small nodules or branching nodular lesions with dense margin and without fluffy nodules on CT scans

8.2.3 Interstitial Pneumonia

Interstitial pneumonia is characterized histologically by a mononuclear inflammatory cell infiltrate in the alveolar walls and interstitial tissue surrounding small parenchymal vessels and airways (bronchioles). The most common causative organisms are *Mycoplasma pneumoniae (M. pneumoniae)*, viruses, and *Pneumocystis jirovecii* (*P. jirovecii*).

Viral pneumonia is associated with several pathologic forms of low respiratory tract infection, including tracheobronchitis, cellular bronchiolitis, and pneumonia. Because viral organisms replicate within cells, the most prominent histologic changes are observed in the epithelium and in the adjacent interstitium. In tracheobronchitis, the airway walls are congested and the lumen contains mononuclear cell infiltrates. Cellular (inflammatory) bronchiolitis, which is particularly important in children, appears with epithelial necrosis, neutrophilic exudate in the airway lumen, and predominantly mononuclear cell infiltrates in the airway walls. Parenchymal involvement begins with the involvement of the lung adjacent to the terminal and respiratory bronchioles; however, extension throughout the lobule may occur. Pneumonia may progress rapidly, particularly in the elderly and in immunocompromised patients; in such cases, the histological findings include diffuse alveolar damage comprising interstitial lymphocyte infiltration, airspace hemorrhage, edema, and fibrin, type 2 cell hyperplasia, and hyaline membrane formation [15].

Viral pneumonias manifest radiologically as poorly defined fluffy nodules (airspace nodules 4–10 mm in diameter) and patchy areas of peribronchial GGO and airspace consolidation. Because of the associated cellular bronchiolitis, hyperinflation is commonly present [15–17]. Progressive pneumonia involves the rapid confluence of consolidation leading to diffuse alveolar damage, consisting of homogeneous or patchy unilateral or bilateral airspace consolidation and GGO or poorly defined small centrilobular nodules (Table 8.1 and Fig. 8.6) [15].

At the time of writing, COVID-19 (coronavirus disease-19; the respiratory disease caused by severe acute respiratory syndrome coronavirus 2 [SARS-CoV-2]) is pandemic throughout the globe. SARS-CoV-2 appeared in Wuhan, China in late December 2019 and rapidly spread around the world. During the first two decades of the twenty-first century, there have been three coronavirus-related outbreaks, one of SARS-CoV, one of Middle East respiratory syndrome coronavirus (MERS-CoV), and one of SARS-CoV-2. Although the mortality rate of SARS-CoV-2 infection is the lowest among the three, the number of confirmed cases of SARS-CoV-2 infection worldwide exceed 10,580,000 on July 01, 2020, which is about 4230 times larger than the number of people ever infected with MERS-CoV (2500), and the outbreak is ongoing. Males are more susceptible to MERS-CoV and SARS-

Table 8.1 Summary of CT findings in viral pneumonias

	Centrilobular nodules	GGO with lobular distribution	Segmental consolidation	Thickened interlobular septae	Diffuse GGO
Influenza	+++	+++			+
Measles	++	+	+	+	+
Hantavirus			++	+	+++
Adenovirus	++	+	+++		
HSV	+	+++	+++		+
VZV	+++	+			
CMV	++	++	+	+	++
EBV	+	+	+		+

HSV herpes simplex virus; *VZV* varicella-zoster virus; *CMV* cytomegalovirus; *EBV* Epstein–Bar virus; *GGO* ground-glass opacity

Reprinted from reference 15 (Kim EA et al. *Radiographics* 2002; 22:S137–S149) with permission

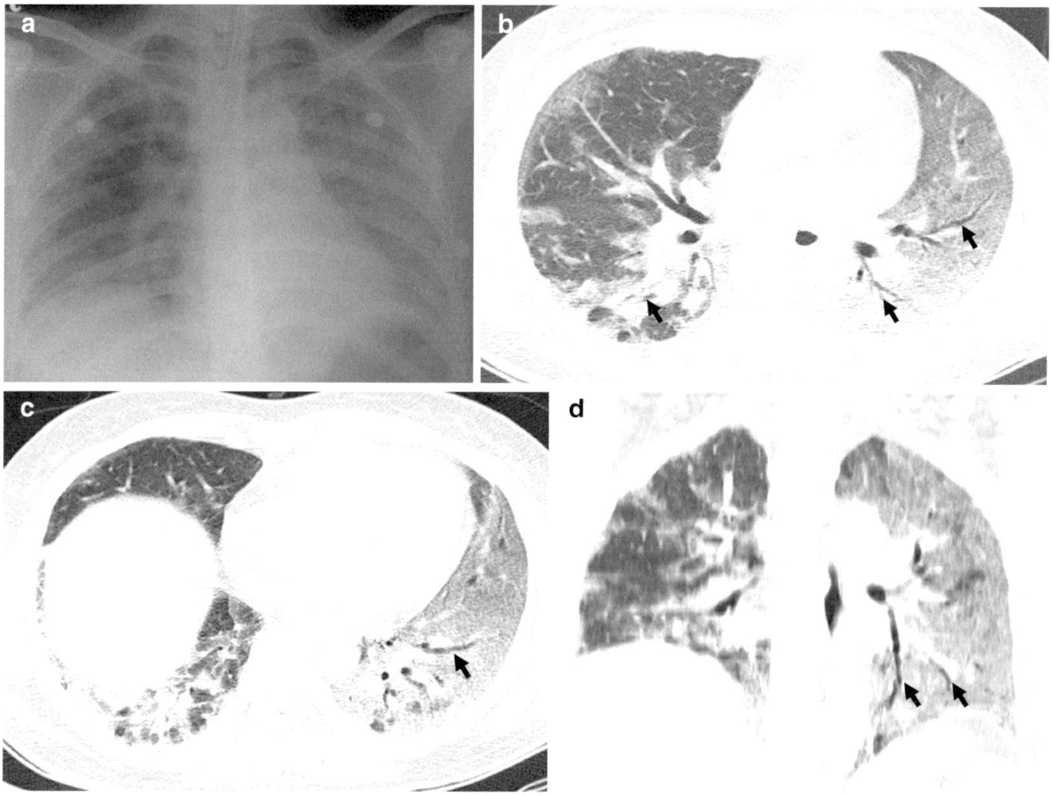

Fig. 8.6 Adenovirus pneumonia in a 44-year-old immunocompetent woman. (**a**) Chest radiograph shows diffuse ground-glass opacity in both lungs. An endotracheal tube and L-tube have been inserted. (**b**, **c**) Lung window images obtained at the levels of the beginning of the right middle bronchus (**b**) and liver dome (**c**) demonstrate patchy and wide areas of parenchymal opacity in both lungs. Also note CT air-bronchogram signs (arrows). (**d**) Coronal reformation image depicts opacity lesions in both lungs with CT air-bronchogram signs (arrows)

CoV-2 infections than females. Chronic underlying diseases, such as diabetes, hypertension, and cardiovascular disease, may increase the risk of coronavirus infection and older age has been reported as an important predictor of increased mortality in coronavirus infection [18–20].

Approximately 15%–20% of patients with coronavirus infection have normal initial CXR findings at the time of diagnosis (usually done with reverse transcription–polymerase chain reaction [RT-PCR]) [21–23]. The most common initial CXR findings in coronavirus infection are peripheral focal or multifocal airspace consolidation, ground-glass opacity (GGO), or both [21–24] (Figs. 8.7, 8.8, and 8.9). However, initial radiographs in SARS-CoV and MERS-CoV infection usually show unilateral and middle-to-lower lung zone involvement of lung parenchymal lesions, whereas bilateral lung involvement with lower lung zone or no zonal predominance is more common in SARS-CoV-2 infection [21–23]. Cavity and nodular opacity are rare in coronavirus infection. Pleural effusion is rare in SARS-CoV-2 infection, but it occurs in approximately 15% and 30% of SARS-CoV and MERS-CoV infections, respectively, during the first week of infection [21–23] (Fig. 8.8). As the disease progresses, parenchymal abnormalities eventually spread to both lungs in coronavirus infection (Figs. 8.8 and 8.9).

CT findings include GGO with or without interlobular septal thickening, consolidation, or a combination of both; these are the most common findings during the first 2 weeks of corona-

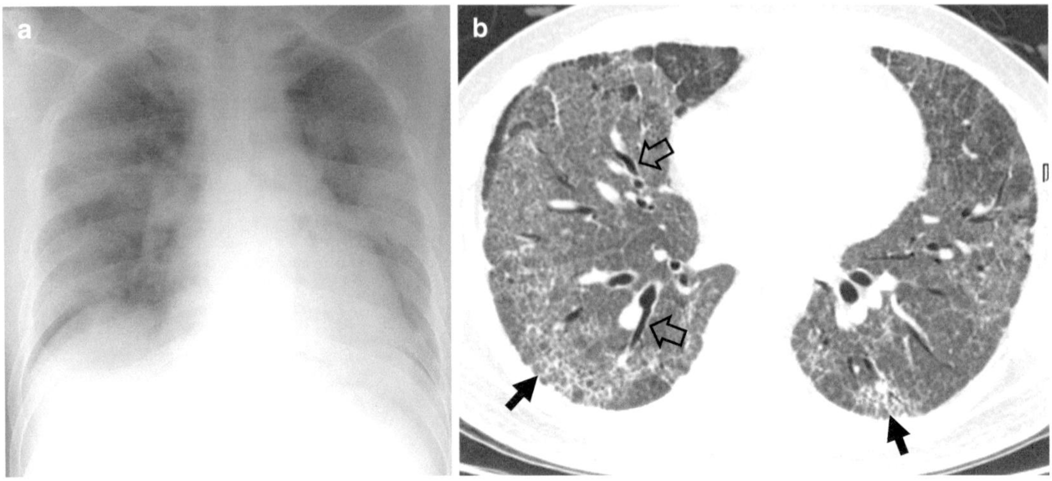

Fig. 8.7 Severe Acute Respiratory Syndrome-coronavirus (SARS-CoV) pneumonia in a 31-year-old man. (**a**) Chest radiograph obtained 4 days after admission shows rapidly progressive bilateral diffuse opacity lesions comprised of ground-glass opacity and consolidation. (**b**) Lung window image of a CT scan obtained at the level of the right inferior pulmonary vein 1 month after **a** demonstrates bilateral diffuse ground-glass opacity with superimposed areas of intralobular interstitial thickening and reticulation (arrows) and bronchial dilatation (open arrows), features suggestive of ongoing pulmonary fibrosis. Case courtesy of Franquet T et al. *British J Radiol* 2020 Jun 25;20200515. doi: https://doi.org/10.1259/bjr.20200515

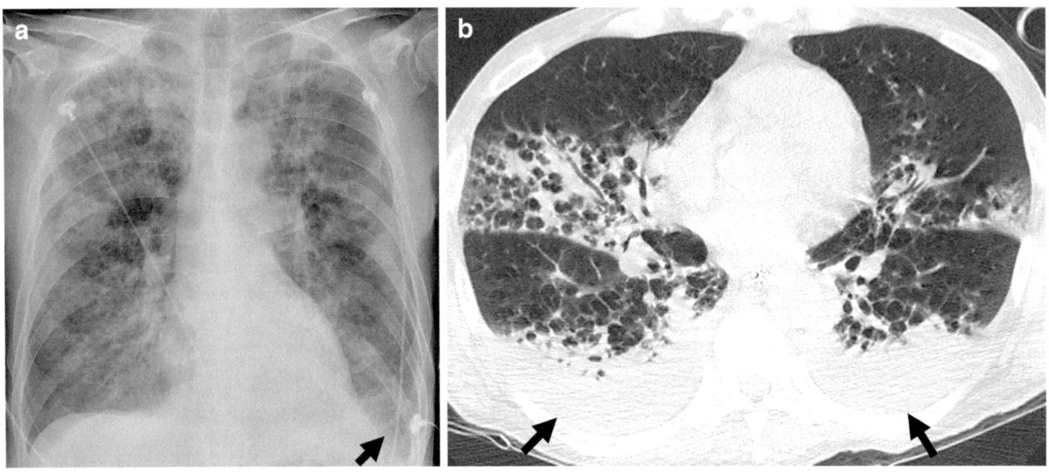

Fig. 8.8 Middle East Respiratory Syndrome-coronavirus (MERS-CoV) pneumonia in a 68-year-old man. (**a**) Chest radiograph obtained 2 weeks after symptom onset shows rapidly progressive parenchymal opacity composed of ground-glass opacity and consolidation in both lungs. Also note obliteration (arrow) of the left costophrenic angle, suggesting the presence of left pleural effusion. (**b**) Lung window image of a CT scan obtained at the level of the basal trunks 4 days after **a** demonstrates bilateral patchy areas of consolidation and ground-glass opacity and bilateral pleural effusions (arrows). This patient died of respiratory failure. Case courtesy of Franquet T et al. *British J Radiol* 2020 Jun 25;20200515. doi: https://doi.org/10.1259/bjr.20200515

virus infection [25–27] (Fig. 8.9). In SARS-CoV infection, reticulation is evident after the second week of infection and persists in half of all patients after 4 weeks [25] (Fig. 8.7). In MERS-CoV infection, crazy-paving signs and organizing pneumonia (OP) pattern are seen during the second and third weeks of infection [26]. In SARS-CoV-2 infection, GGO and consolida-

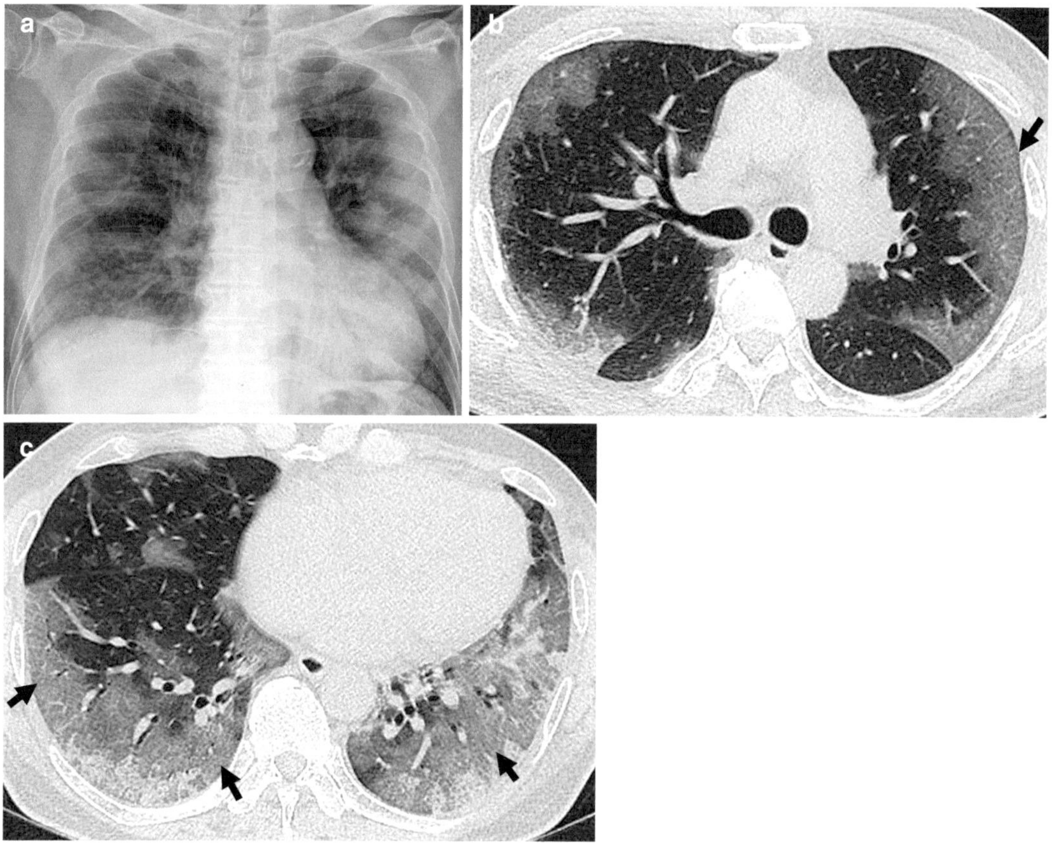

Fig. 8.9 Severe Acute Respiratory Syndrome-coronavirus-2 (SARS-CoV-2) pneumonia in a 64-year-old man. (**a**) Chest radiograph obtained 7 days after symptom onset shows bilateral multi-focal and patchy opacity with peripheral lung-predominant distribution. (**b**, **c**) Lung window images of CT scans obtained at the levels of the main bronchi (**b**) and cardiac ventricle (**c**) demonstrate parenchymal opacity comprised of both ground-glass opacity and consolidation with subpleural and lower lung zone predominance. Also note the large area of crazy-paving signs (arrows: ground-glass opacity and internal linear networks). Case courtesy of Franquet T et al. *British J Radiol* 2020 Jun 25;20200515. doi: https://doi.org/10.1259/bjr.20200515

tion are decreased in extent, whereas the mixed pattern of GGO and consolidation demonstrates an increase after the second week of infection [27]. Cavity, centrilobular nodules, and mediastinal or hilar lymph node enlargement are rarely seen in coronavirus infection. During the early stage of the disease, parenchymal abnormalities are usually located in the peripheral lung; from there, they eventually spread to the entire bilateral lungs when the disease progresses. Parenchymal abnormalities usually have a peripheral and basilar predilection in MERS-CoV infection [26], whereas bilateral multilobar lesions are seen in SARS-CoV-2 infection with peripheral or both peripheral and central predilection [27, 28] (Fig. 8.9). In the chronic stage of coronavirus infection, variable-sized GGO with interlobular septal and intralobular reticular lesions are the most common findings. Signs of fibrosis such as parenchymal bands, reticulation, traction bronchiectasis, and irregular interface signs are also seen [25–27] (Figs. 8.7 and 8.9). In SARS-CoV infection, GGO and interstitial opacity in the convalescent stage usually resolve over time but air trapping may persist [29].

8.3 Pneumonia in Immunocompetent Subjects

8.3.1 Community-Acquired Pneumonia

In one study [8] (Lim WS et al.) of 309 patients admitted with CAP, 267 fulfilled the study criteria; 135 (50.6%) were men and the mean (SD) age was 65.4 (19.6) years. Etiological agents were identified from 199 (75%) patients (one pathogen in 124 [46%], two in 53 [20%], and three or more in 22 [8%]): *Streptococcus pneumoniae* 129 (48%), influenza A virus 50 (19%), *Chlamydia pneumoniae* 35 (13%), *Hemophilus influenzae* 20 (7%), *Mycoplasma pneumoniae* 9 (3%), *Legionella pneumophilia* 9 (3%) (Fig. 8.2), other Chlamydia spp. 7 (2%), *Moraxella catarrhalis* 5 (2%), *Coxiella burnetii* 2 (0.7%), and others 8 (3%). Atypical pathogens were less common in patients aged 75 years and over than in younger patients (16% v 27%; OR 0.5, 95% CI 0.3 to 0.9). The 30-day mortality was 14.9%. Mortality risk could be stratified by the presence of four "core" adverse features (CURB-65). Three of 60 patients (5%) infected with an atypical pathogen died.

CAP in patients <60 years of age without comorbidities is usually caused by *Streptococcus pneumoniae* (*St. pneumoniae*), *Mycoplasma pneumonia pneumoniae* (*M. pneumonia pneumoniae*), respiratory viruses, *Hemophilus influenzae*, *Chlamydia pneumoniae*, and *Legionella* (Fig. 8.2). On the other hand, CAP in patients >60 years of age and those with comorbidities is usually caused by *S. pneumoniae*, respiratory viruses, *H. influenzae*, anaerobic Gram-negative bacteria, and *Staphylococcus aureus* (*S. aureus*) (Fig. 8.10). According to one study [30, 31], among 2259 patients with CAP who had radiographic evidence of pneumonia and specimens available for both bacterial and viral testing, a pathogen was detected in only 853 (38%): one or more viruses in 530 (23%), bacteria in 247 (11%), bacterial and viral pathogens in 59 (3%), and a fungal or mycobacterial pathogen in 17 (1%). The most common pathogens were human rhinovirus (in 9% of patients), influenza virus (in 6%), and *S. pneumoniae* (in 5%). The incidence of CAP requiring hospitalization was highest among older adults. Despite current diagnostic tests, no pathogen was detected in the majority of patients. Respiratory viruses were detected more frequently than bacteria.

It seems that patients with CAP requiring hospitalization suffer from more extensive pneumonia with bilateral lung abnormalities and with symptoms and signs of infection which lead them to visit an ED. Furthermore, patients with pneumonia associated with adult respiratory syndrome (ARDS) or those who are immunocompromised would also be more likely to visit the ED. Thus, in this chapter, we introduce types of pneumonia that are frequently seen in the ED, describe their imaging features, and elaborate on differential diagnostic features of pneumonia vs. conditions that can simulate pneumonia (drug-induced lung disease, acute eosinophilic pneumonia, organizing pneumonia or acute fibrinous organizing pneumonia [AFOP], and pulmonary vasculitis). Please also refer to the non-infectious pulmonary emergency chapter (Chap. 11).

8.3.2 Healthcare-Associated Pneumonia (HCAP)

Healthcare-associated pneumonia (HCAP) refers to adult pneumonia contracted in a clinical setting such as an acute care hospital or chronic care center. HCAP is usually caused by multidrug resistant bacteria, namely Methicillin-resistant *S. aureus* and Gram-negative bacteria (*Pseudomonas aeruginosa*, extended-spectrum beta-lactamase-producing *Klebsiella pneumoniae*, and *Acinetobacter* species) [32].

Hospital-acquired pneumonia (HAP) is defined as pneumonia that occurs after admission to a hospital which was neither present nor in a period of incubation at the time of admission [33]. HAP includes healthcare-associated pneumonia (HCAP) and ventilator-associated pneumonia. HAP is the leading cause of death from hospital-acquired infections and an important public health problem. HAP most commonly occurs in intensive care unit (ICU)

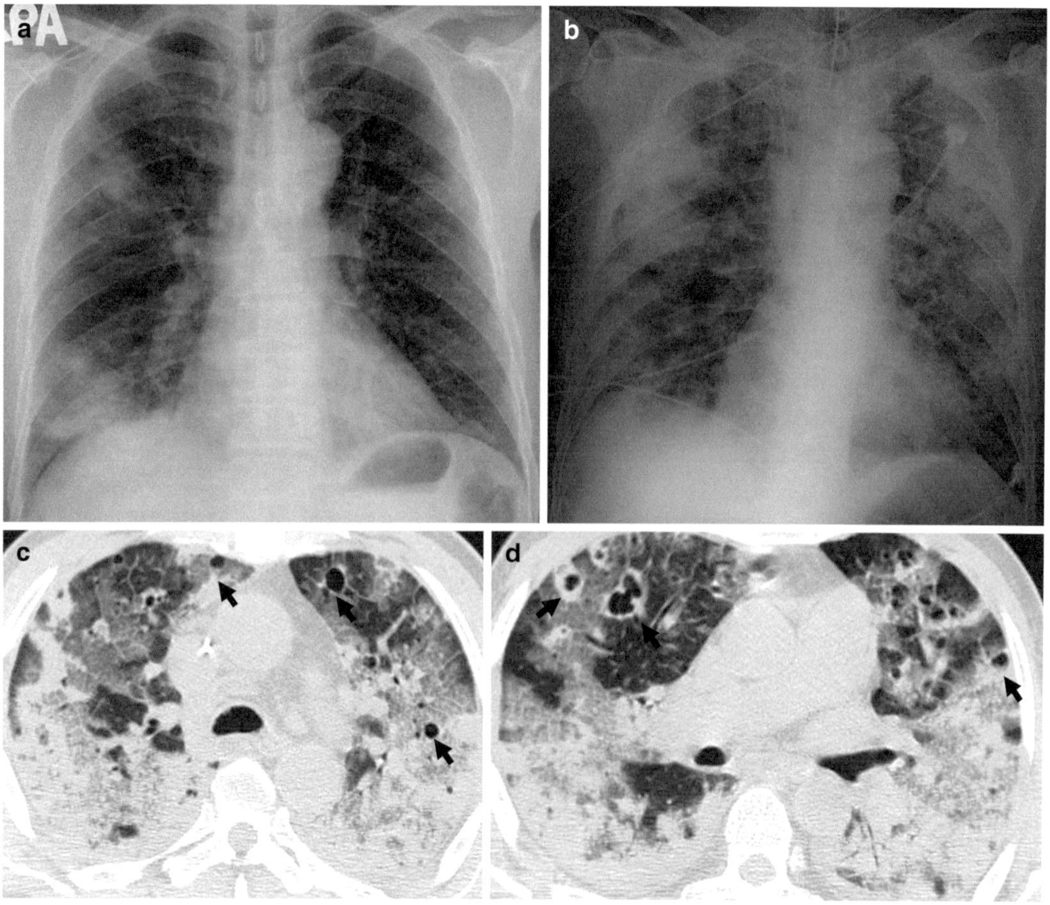

Fig. 8.10 Staphylococcus pneumonia in a 58-year-old man. (**a**) Chest radiograph obtained at admission shows nodular opacity in the right upper lung zone and mass-like consolidation in the right lower lung zone. (**b**) Chest radiograph obtained 3 days after **a** demonstrates extensive bilateral parenchymal opacity with a patchy distribution. An endotracheal intubation tube and central line are inserted. (**c**, **d**) Lung window images obtained at the levels of the tracheal carina (**c**) and bronchus intermedius (**d**) depict patchy and extensive consolidation in both lungs. Also note multiple cavitary lesions (arrows) in both lungs anteriorly

patients, predominantly patients necessitating mechanical ventilation [34].

8.3.3 Aspiration Pneumonia

Aspiration pneumonia is common in patients with decreased levels of consciousness (e.g., alcoholics), chronic debilitating diseases, and those with oropharyngeal or airway instrumentation (e.g., a feeding tube or mechanical ventilation). Aspirated materials may include sterile gastric secretions, gastric contents, or bacteria-laden oropharyngeal secretions. Most cases of bacterial pneumonia result from aspiration of infected materials from the oropharynx into the lower respiratory tract.

Approximately 90% of aspiration pneumonias are caused by anaerobic organisms [35]. In hospitalized patients, the stomach may become colonized with Gram-negative bacteria [36]. In these settings, intubation and mechanical ventilation may increase the incidence and extent of aspiration, with a resultant increase in the risk of pneumonia development. The location of pneumonia depends on a patient's position when aspiration occurs.

Radiographic manifestations usually consist of bilateral patchy areas of consolidation involving mainly the dependent regions (in supine patients, mainly the posterior and lateral basal segments of the lower lobes, superior segments of the lower lobes, and posterior segments of the upper lobes) (Fig. 8.11).

Patients with advanced periodontal disease are at increased risk for the development of aspiration pneumonia [35]. A distinct form of infection is caused by *Actinomyces israelii*, a low-virulence anaerobic bacteria, which is part of the normal flora in the mouths of subjects with poor oral hygiene. In this setting, aspiration of infected material results in localized or segmental pneumonia, usually in the dependent portions of the lung [1].

8.4 Pneumonia in Immunocompromised Patients

The number of immunocompromised patients has increased considerably in the last four decades, mainly for the following four reasons: (1) The acquired immunodeficiency syndrome (AIDS) epidemic, (2) Advances in cancer chemotherapy, (3) Expanded solid organ and hematopoietic stem cell transplantation (HSCT), and (4) Increased use of immunosuppressive therapy. Pneumonia is the most serious clinical problem in these patients. Mildly

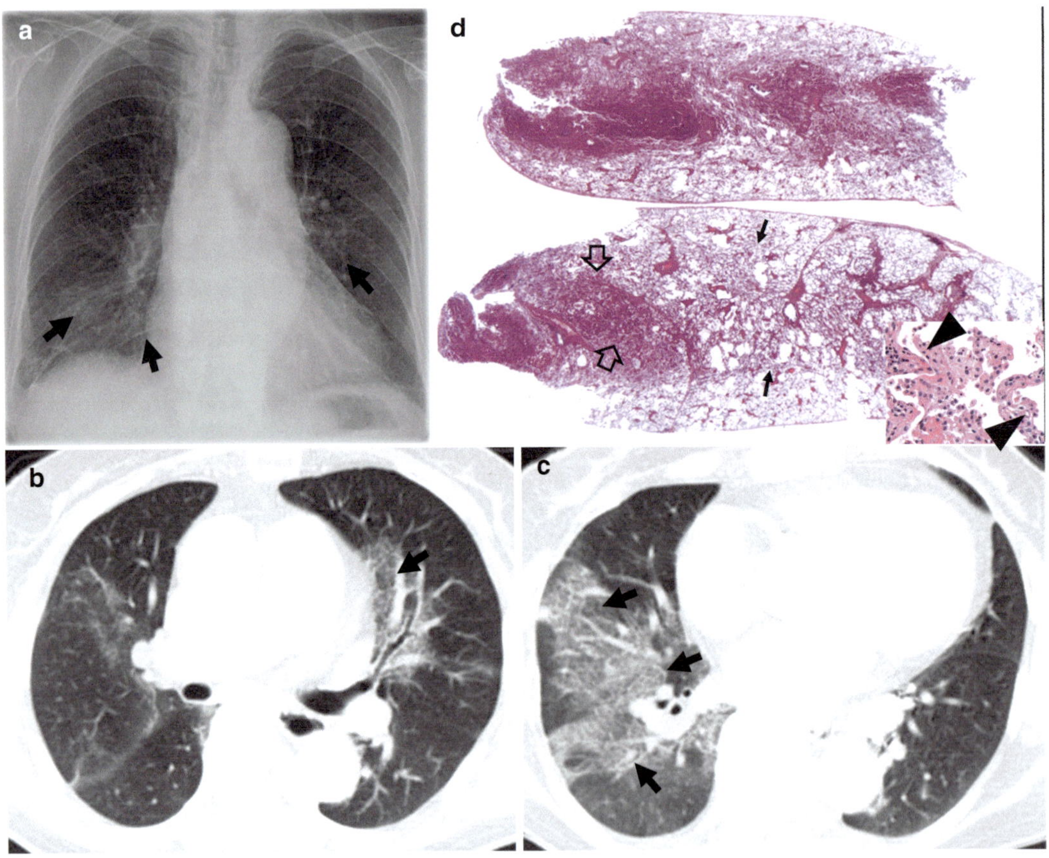

Fig. 8.11 Squalene aspiration pneumonia in a 73-year-old woman complaining of dyspnea and mild fever. (**a**) Chest radiograph shows patchy parenchymal opacity (arrows) in the right lower lung zone and left infrahilar area. The heart is enlarged. (**b**, **c**) Lung window of CT scans obtained at the levels of the bronchus intermedius (**b**) and right inferior pulmonary vein (**c**) demonstrate patchy areas (arrows) of crazy-paving appearance (linear densities within ground-glass opacity) in the right middle lobe, lingular division of left upper lobe, and right lower lobe. (**d**) A low-magnification view of a surgical lung biopsy specimen obtained from the right lower lobe discloses diffuse but mild interstitial thickening with loose fibrosis and inflammatory cell infiltration (arrows). Also note the alveolar spaces filled with inflammatory cells (open arrows). Inset: Many lipid-laden macrophages (arrowheads)

impaired host immunity in chronic disease states, diabetes mellitus, malnutrition, alcoholism, advanced age, prolonged corticosteroid use, and chronic obstructive lung disease are some common factor(s) predisposing individuals to pulmonary infection.

8.4.1 Category of Immune Deficiency and Organisms Involved

Immune deficiency may be subclassified into four categories, including neutrophil (phagocytosis) deficiency, reduced cell-mediated immunity, humoral (immunoglobulin or antibody) immune dysfunction, and complement deficiency. The common pathogens related to each category of immune deficiency differ from one another. For example, in neutrophil deficiency, aspergillosis and mucormycosis are well-known infection types. Fungi including *Pneumocystis*, viruses, and mycobacteria are frequently involved in reduced cell-mediated immunity. In humoral immune dysfunction and complement deficiency, encapsulated bacteria (*S. pneumoniae* and *H. influenzae*) are the most common organisms involved (Table 8.2) [37].

8.4.2 Causative Organisms Versus Imaging Patterns in Opportunistic Infection

Bacterial infection usually causes lobar- or bronchopneumonia. Viral infection in immunocompromised patients causes bilateral symmetric bronchopneumonia or interstitial pneumonia. Fungal infection appears as interstitial pneumonia (*Pneumocystis jirovecii*), nodules (invasive pulmonary aspergillosis and mucormycosis) and cavities or cysts (invasive pulmonary aspergillosis and mucormycosis). Mycobacterial infection leads to lobar consolidation, nodules or cavities, or cysts (Table 8.3).

8.4.3 Transplantation-Associated Pneumonia and Chronological Changes

In immune deficiency associated with hematopoietic stem cell transplantation, the amount of time that has elapsed since transplantation is closely correlated with the organisms involved in opportunistic infection. Within a month after transplantation, Gram-negative bacteria and *Aspergillus* (Fig. 8.12) are the two most impor-

Table 8.2 Type of immunodeficiency versus frequently involved organisms

Immunodeficiency	Pathogens
Neutrophils (phagocytes) (e.g., hematologic malignancy, HSCT, chemo-radiation therapy)	Bacteria, fungus – Gram-positive (e.g., *S aureus*), Gram-negative (e.g., *Klebsiella*, *P. aeruginosa*, *E. coli*) – *Aspergillus*, *Candida*, Mucormycosis
Cell-mediated immunity (e.g., AIDS, malignancy, organ transplantation, immunosuppressive therapy, prolonged steroid use)	Fungus, virus, intracellular bacteria, mycobacteria – *P. jirovecii*, *Aspergillus*, *Cryptococcus* etc. – CMV, *H. simplex*
Humoral-mediated immunity (Ig, Ab) (e.g., Immuosuppressive therapy, hematologic malignancy, chemo-radiation therapy, asplenia/splenectomy), Good's syndrome	Encapsulated bacteria – *St. pneumonia*, *H. influenza,* etc.
Complement (e.g., autoimmune disease)	Bacteria

HSCT hematopoietic stem cell transplantation; *AIDS* acquired immune deficiency syndrome; *Ig* immunoglobuline; *Ab* antibody; *CMV* cytomegalovirus

Table 8.3 Imaging patterns versus pathogenic organisms in opportunistic infection

	Lobar pneumonia	Bronchopneumonia	Interstitial pneumonia/GGO	Nodules	Cavities/cysts
Bacteria	+++[a]	+++[b]	+[c]	+[d]	+[e]
Virus	+	++	+++	+[f]	–
Fungus	+	+	++[g] (PJP)	+++	+++
Mycobacteria	+++	+	+	+++	++

Note: Community-acquired pneumonia-related organisms: [a]*Streptococcus*, *Chlamydia*, *Klebsiella*, and *Legionella*; [b]*Mycoplasma*, *H. influenzae*, *S. aureus*, and *Moraxella catarrhalis*; [c]*Mycoplasma*; [d]*Actinomycosis*; [e]*S. auerus*, *Klebsiella*, *Pseudomonas*, and *Actinomycosis*; [f]*Varicella zoster* virus; and [g]*Pneumocystis jiroveccii* pneumonia (PJP)

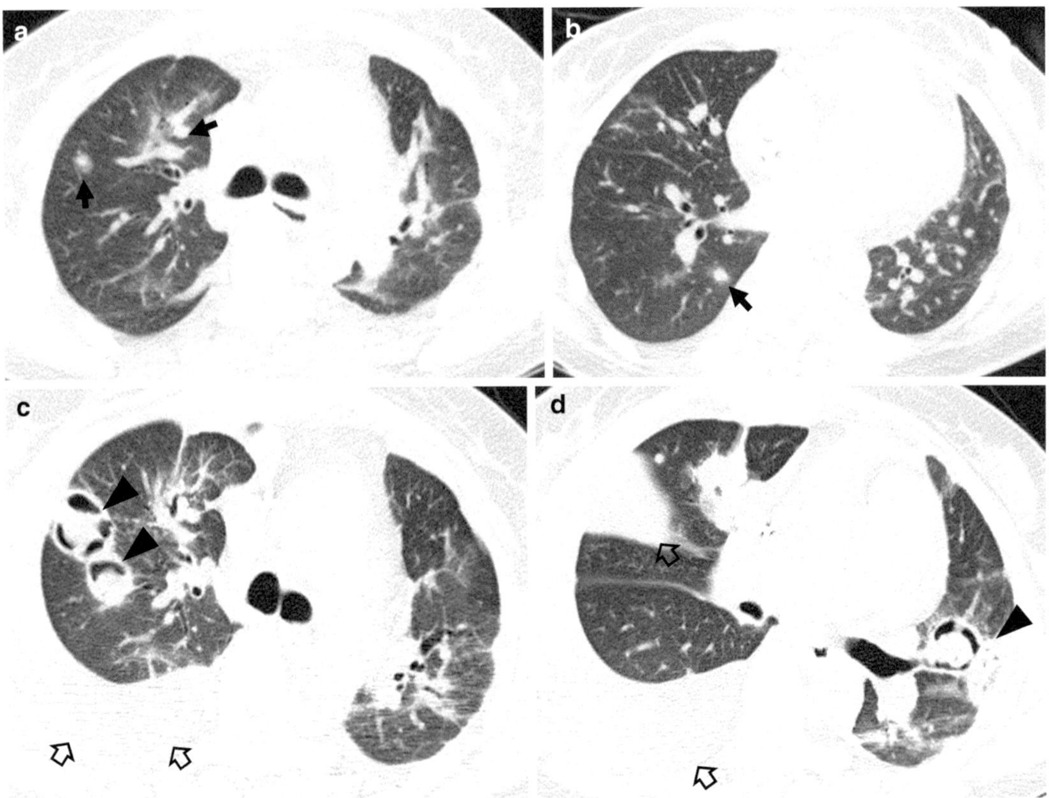

Fig. 8.12 Vascular invasive pulmonary aspergillosis in a 29-year-old woman with acute myeloid leukemia. (**a**, **b**) Lung window images obtained at the levels of the main bronchi (**a**) and right inferior pulmonary vein (**b**) show nodules with the halo sign (arrows) in the right lung (absolute neutrophil count, 110/μL). (**c**, **d**) CT images obtained at levels similar to (**a**, **b**) demonstrate CT-air crescent signs (arrowheads) where nodules with a halo sign were seen (absolute neutrophil count, 5570/μL). Also note the large right pleural effusion (open arrows)

tant organisms involved in infection. Between 1 and 3 months after transplantation, viruses (cytomegalovirus in particular) (Fig. 8.13) and *Pneumocystis* (Fig. 8.14) are often involved. After 100 days, opportunistic infection is relatively rare (Table 8.4). In solid organ transplantation, within a month after transplantation, bacterial pneumonia and reactivation of herpes simplex virus (HSV) infection are common. Between 1 and 6 months, viral (cytomegalovirus), fungal (*Aspergillus* and *Pneumocystis*), bacterial (*Nocardia* and *Listeria*), and mycobacterial (*M. tuberculosis*) infections are predominant. After 6 months, organisms similar to those

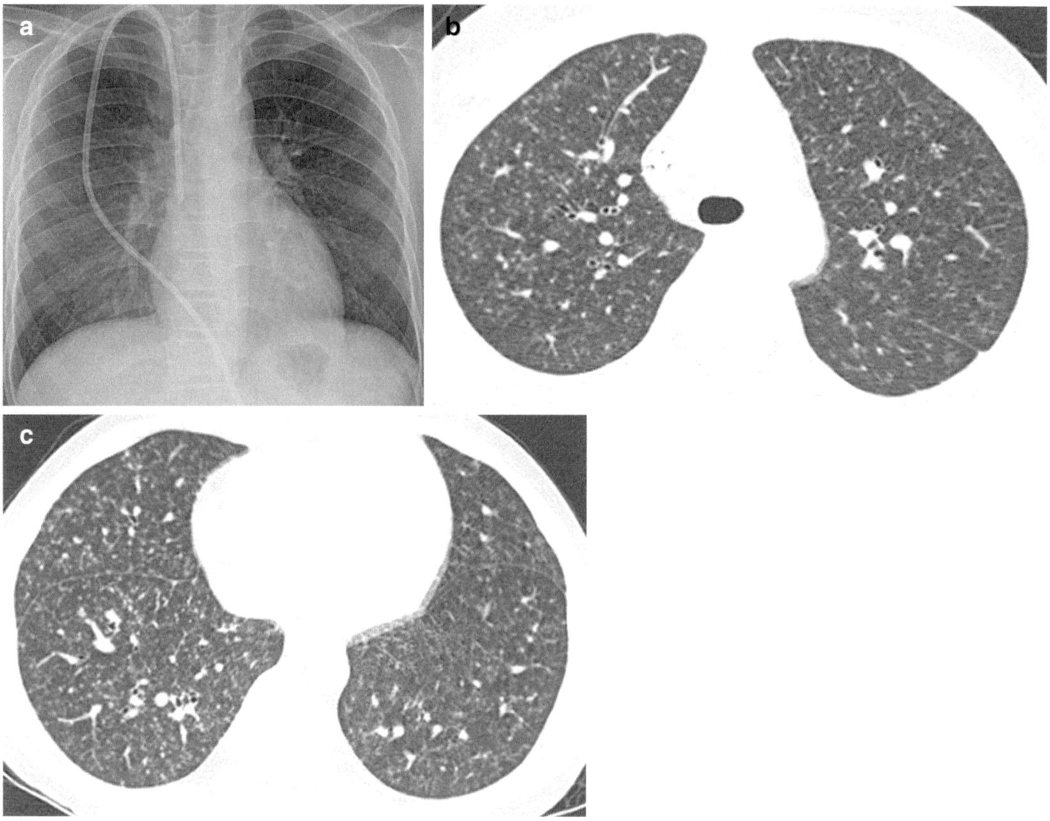

Fig. 8.13 Cytomegalovirus pneumonia manifesting as miliary lung disease in a 14-year-old man with AIDS who underwent hematopoietic stem cell transplantation. (**a**) Chest radiograph obtained 2 months after transplantation shows miliary lung nodules in both lungs. A central line has been inserted. (**b**, **c**) Lung window images of a thin-section specimen (1.5 mm thickness) obtained at the levels of the azygos arch (**b**) and suprahepatic inferior vena cava (**c**) demonstrate millet-sized small nodules in both lungs with random distribution (miliary lung disease)

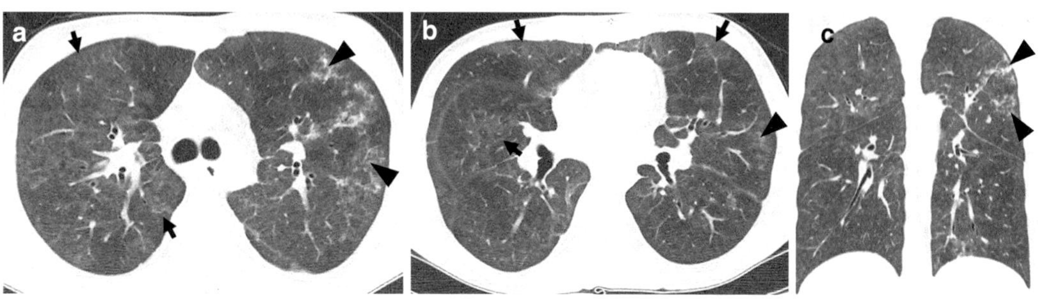

Fig. 8.14 *Pneumocystis jirovecii* pneumonia in a 25-year-old man who received lung transplantation for cystic fibrosis. (**a**, **b**) Lung window images obtained at the levels of the main bronchi (**a**) and superior segmental bronchi of both lower lobes (**b**) show patchy areas of ground-glass opacity (arrows) and branching nodular lesions with fluffy margin (arrowheads). (**c**) Coronal reformatted image also demonstrates patchy areas of ground-glass opacity and branching nodular lesion with fluffy margin (arrowheads)

Table 8.4 Chronology of organisms involved in opportunistic infection following hematopoietic stem cell transplantation

	<1 month (neutropenic phase)	1–3 months (100 days) (early phase)	> 100 Days (late phase)
HSCT	Bacterial—Gram-negative organisms Fungal—Aspergillus	Viral—CMV Pneumocystis pneumonia	Opportunistic infection, unusual

CMV cytomegalovirus
Modified from Jepson SL et al. *Clin Radiol* 2012;67:1001–1010

Table 8.5 Chronology of organisms involved in opportunistic infection following solid organ transplantation

	<1 month	1–6 months	>6 months
Solid organ transplantation	Bacterial pneumonia—commonly related to post-surgical complication and endotracheal intubation Reactivation HSV	Opportunistic infection Viral—CMV Fungal—Aspergillus, PJP Bacterial—Nocardia, Listeria Mycobacterial—M. TB	Similar organisms to CAP (unless issues with rejection and high-dose immunosuppression therapy)

CMV cytomegalovirus; *PJP Pneumocystis jirovecii* pneumonia. *M. TB Mycobacterium tuberculosis*; *CAP* community-acquired pneumonia
Modified from Jepson SL et al. *Clin Radiol* 2012;67:1001–1010

seen in CAP are involved in opportunistic infection (Table 8.5) [38].

8.4.4 AIDS and Pulmonary Infection

Since acquired immune deficiency syndrome (AIDS) was first reported in the 1980s, the condition has been related to increased susceptibility to opportunistic infection with resultant increases in morbidity and mortality. However, with the introduction of highly active antiretroviral therapy (HAART) in 1996, the rate of opportunistic infections in AIDS patients has dramatically decreased.

One of the most common opportunistic infections in HIV-infected patients is *Pneumocystis jirovecii* pneumonia (PJP). PJP usually occurs when a patient's CD4+ T cell count falls below 200 cells/μL [39]. As with other conditions in HIV-infected individuals, the incidence of PJP declined following the widespread use of HAART and prophylaxis. However, PJP is still the most common opportunistic pulmonary infection in HIV-infected patients; it is responsible for approximately 25% of cases of pneumonia during HIV infection [40]. PJP presents with an insidious onset of fever, dry cough, and worsening dyspnea, which are typically present for about 1 month prior to diagnosis, in contrast with the more acute presentation seen in other opportunistic infections. On chest radiographs (CXR), the infection appears as diffuse or perihilar fine reticular or poorly defined ground-glass opacity (GGO); over time, the opacity changes into diffuse homogeneous opacity with coarse internal reticulation. On TSCT, the abnormalities appear as scattered or diffuse GGO or consolidation with interlobular septal thickening. Small nodules or branching nodular lesions are seen in approximately 10% of patients, usually with areas of opacity. Pneumatoceles are found in up to one-third of patients; they can be single or multiple, present in any location, and usually resolve without any sequela. Pneumothorax is also common in such patients (Fig. 8.15) [41].

Cytomegalovirus (CMV) is the most common viral pathogen in AIDS patients. However, its significance as a pulmonary pathogen in HIV-infected patients is often unclear [42]. Widespread HAART use has reduced the incidence of CMV infection in AIDS patients. When present, CMV pneumonia typically affects those with advanced immune suppression (CD4+ count <100 cells/μL). Co-infection with PJP is common and is a poor prognostic sign [43, 44].

The incidence of bacterial pneumonia in HIV-infected patients is 25-fold higher than in the general population [45]. The most common pathogens involved are *S. pneumoniae*, *H. influenzae*, *S aureus*, and *Pseudomonas* spp., in declining order of frequency. The incidence of bacterial pneumonia increases in proportion to a decreased number of CD4+ lymphocytes.

Tuberculosis has reemerged as a global health problem with the advent of AIDS. An estimated one-third of HIV-infected patients are coinfected with tuberculosis [46]. Moreover, HIV-infected individuals have a 50- to 200-fold greater risk of tuberculosis than the general population [47]. Radiological manifestations mainly depend on immune status (CD4+ count). When the CD4+ count is greater than 200 cells/μL, the imaging features are typically small nodules with branching, larger nodules, or cavitation in the upper lobes or the superior segments of the lower lobes. In patients with CD4+ counts of less than 200 cells/μL, findings typically include lymphadenopathy, airspace consolidation, or pleural effusion. The risk of disseminated infection is proportional to decreasing CD4+ count (Fig. 8.16) [48].

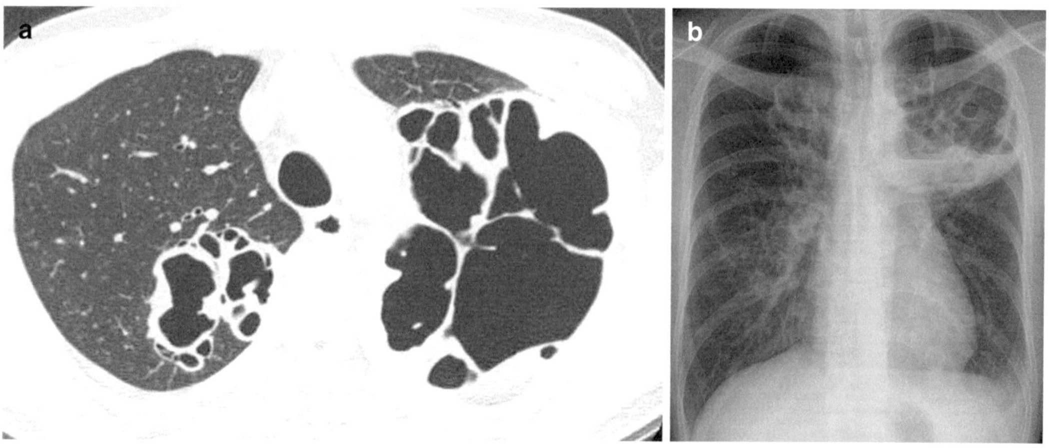

Fig. 8.15 *Pneumocystis jirovecii* pneumonia manifesting as cystic lesions in both lungs in a 29-year-old man with AIDS. (**a**) Lung window image obtained at the level of the aortic arch shows multi-septated air-filled cystic lesions in both lungs. (**b**) Follow-up radiograph demonstrates multiple air–fluid levels in cystic lesions in the left upper lung zone

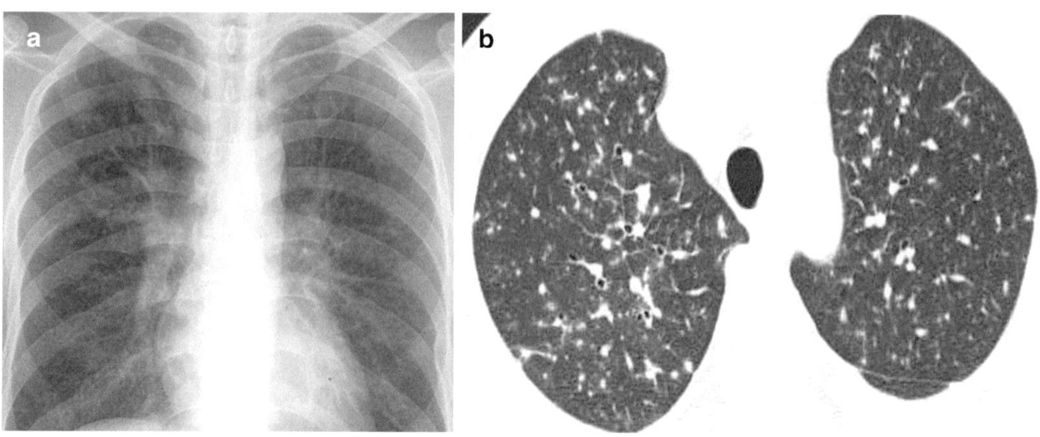

Fig. 8.16 Disseminated tuberculosis infection in a severely immunocompromised 42-year-old man with AIDS. (**a**) Chest radiograph shows small innumerable nodules in both lungs. (**b**) Lung window image of a CT scan obtained at the level of the aortic arch demonstrates random nodules in both lungs. (**c**) Mediastinal window image obtained at the level of the great vessels depicts enlarged lymph nodes showing central necrosis (arrows). (From Jeong YJ and Lee KS. *Am J Roentgenol* 2008;191:834–844, with permission)

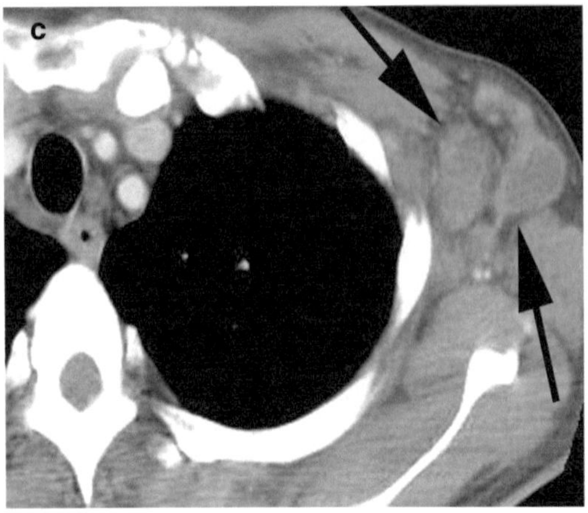

Fig. 8.16 (continued)

8.5 Differential Diagnosis

8.5.1 Acute Eosinophilic Pneumonia

Acute eosinophilic lung disease may imitate pulmonary infection, as both conditions are characterized clinically by acute febrile illness lasting 1–5 days accompanied by myalgia, pleuritic chest pain, and hypoxemic respiratory failure. On chest radiograph, acute eosinophilic lung disease manifests as diffuse bilateral opacity with some internal reticulation. On TSCT, ground-glass opacity (GGO) is observed in all patients with bilateral and random or patchy distribution. Smooth septal thickening is seen in two-thirds of patients. Bilateral pleural effusions are seen in more than half of patients. Frequently, smooth septal thickening or pleural effusions on TSCT help discriminate acute eosinophilic lung disease from acute pneumonia with an interstitial lung disease pattern and adult respiratory distress syndrome (Fig. 8.17) [49].

8.5.2 Cryptogenic Organizing Pneumonia, AFOP, and AIP (ARDS)

In patients with organizing pneumonia, low-grade fever, persistent but nonproductive cough, and shortness of breath are common. Imaging studies demonstrate parenchymal opacity or nodules along the bronchovascular bundles or subpleural lungs. Thus, the disease may be confused in terms of CT findings with those of infectious pneumonia. The distribution of parenchymal opacity or nodules in organizing pneumonia overlap with that seen in bilateral bronchopneumonia. However, in bilateral bronchopneumonia, branching small nodular lesions with fluffy margins are usually present, while in organizing pneumonia, branching nodular lesions are not seen [50].

Acute fibrinous and organizing pneumonia (AFOP) and acute interstitial pneumonia (AIP, the pathologic term for clinical adult respiratory distress syndrome) also demonstrate parenchymal opacity as the main lung lesion pattern. The branching nodular lesions with fluffy margins seen in infectious bilateral bronchopneumonia are not seen in these conditions. Moreover, the distribution of opacity is random or patchy in AFOP and AIP, whereas opacity appears along the bronchovascular bundles or subpleural lungs in infectious bronchopneumonia.

8.5.3 Pulmonary Tuberculosis Manifesting as ARDS or Cystic Lung Disease

Pulmonary tuberculosis may present with acute respiratory failure and is associated with a high mortality rate [51]. In this condition, early diagnosis and timely treatment with antituberculosis therapy may diminish morbidity and mortality [52]. Because thoracic imaging studies in this condition show diffusely increased lung opacity, the imaging findings may simulate diffuse interstitial lung disease. Chest radiographs most commonly demonstrate bilateral small nodular lesions mixed with consolidation or GGO, whereas TSCT has features of miliary or bronchogenic disseminate tuberculosis with diffuse areas of GGO (Fig. 8.18) [53].

In pulmonary tuberculosis, diffuse bilateral pulmonary opacity leading to acute respiratory failure and simulated acute interstitial pneumonia may evolve to show internal air-filled cystic lesions

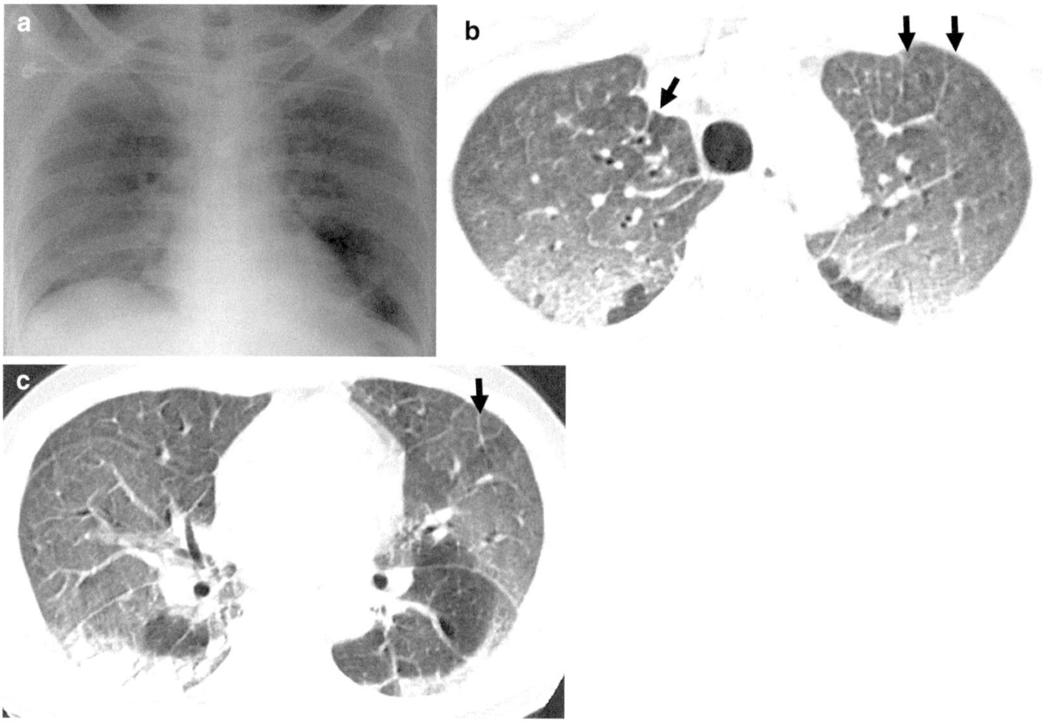

Fig. 8.17 Acute eosinophilic pneumonia in a 45-year-old male smoker who complained of dyspnea. (**a**) Chest radiograph shows diffuse ground-glass opacity in both lungs. (**b**, **c**) Lung window images obtained at the levels of the aortic arch (**b**) and right middle lobar bronchus (**c**) demonstrate wide and extensive areas of ground-glass opacity and consolidation in both lungs. Also note smooth interlobular thickening (arrows) in the anterior lungs

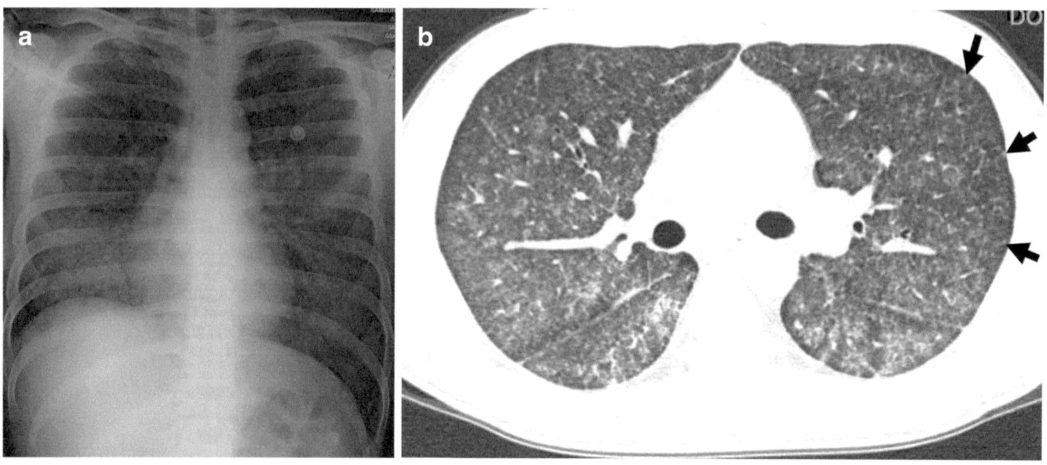

Fig. 8.18 Miliary tuberculosis in a 27-year-old man appearing as adult respiratory distress syndrome and involving air-filled cystic lesions within lesions. (**a**) Chest radiograph obtained in the emergency department shows diffuse ground-glass opacity containing millet-sized nodules within lesions. (**b**, **c**) Lung window images obtained at the levels of the distal main bronchi (**b**) and suprahepatic inferior vena cava (**c**) demonstrate diffuse ground-glass opacity in both lungs and inner miliary nodules (arrows). (**d**, **e**) CT scans obtained 10 days after (**b**, **c**) depict more clearly miliary nodules in both lungs. Also note air-filled cystic lesions (arrows) in the anterior segment of the left upper lobe and related pneumomediastinum (arrowheads) owing to ruptured cystic lesions

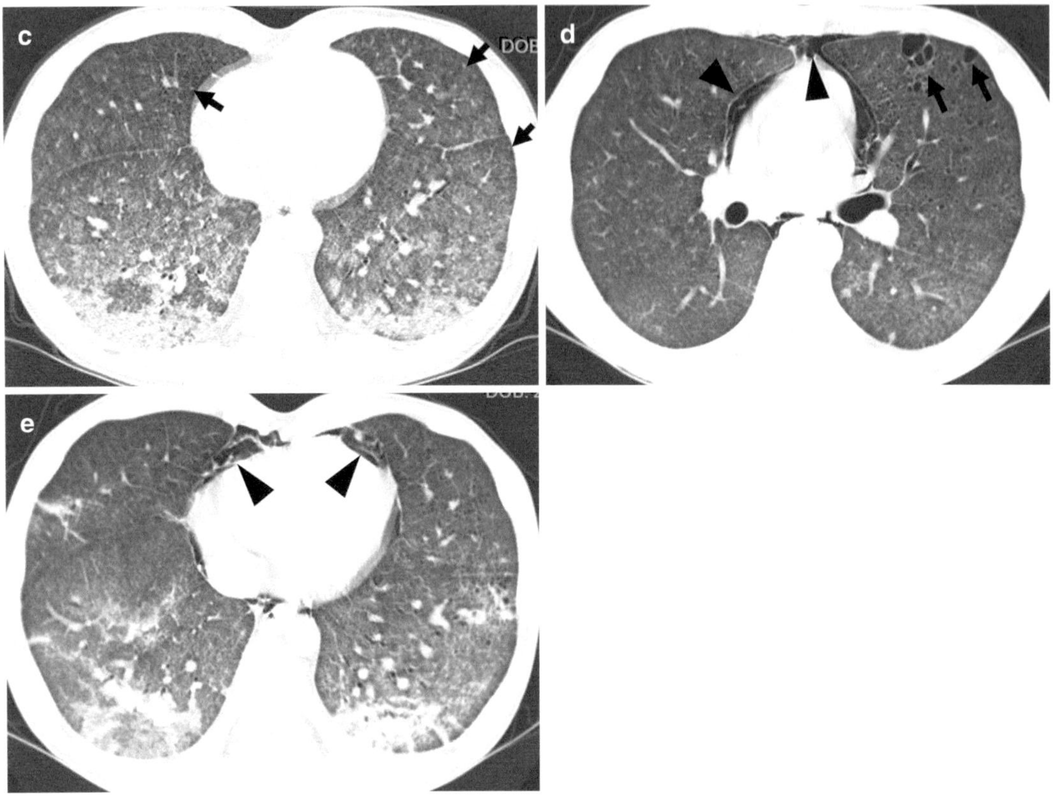

Fig. 8.18 (continued)

within the opacity. Both the opacity and air-filled cystic lung lesions disappear almost completely with anti-tuberculous chemotherapy [54].

8.6 The Role of Chest Radiographs and CT in Pneumonia

The main role of imaging lies in the detection or exclusion of the presence of pneumonia. Other roles include narrowing of differential diagnoses by identification of the causative organisms involved. An enlightened diagnostic approach can be chosen after observing initial imaging findings. The response to antibiotic therapy may be evaluated by observing follow-up imaging studies [31].

8.7 Summary and Key Points

In CAP, the organisms involved are closely related with patient age and the presence or absence of underlying comorbidity. In patients <60 years old without comorbidity, CAP is usually caused by *Streptococcus pneumoniae* (*S. pneumoniae*), *Mycoplasma pneumonia pneumoniae* (*M. pneumonia pneumoniae*), respiratory viruses, *Hemophilus influenzae*, *Chlamydia pneumoniae,* and *Legionella*. In those >60 years of age or with comorbidities, CAP is most often caused by *S. pneumoniae*, respiratory viruses, *H. influenzae*, anaerobic Gram-negative bacteria, and *Staphylococcus aureus* (*S. aureus*). Patients with CAP who require hospitalization have more extensive pneumonia with bilateral lung abnormalities and with signs and symptoms of infection.

In opportunistic infection, different organisms cause different patterns of pneumonia on imaging studies. Bacterial infection leads to a pattern of lobar or segmental pneumonia or bronchopneumonia. Viral infection is indicated by a pattern associated with bilateral bronchopneumonia or interstitial pneumonia. In fungal pneumonia, the abnormalities appear as the pattern of interstitial (*Pneumocystis*) pneumonia, as nodules, or as cavities. Mycobacterial infection appears as lobar or segmental consolidation, nodules, or cavities (Fig. 8.19) [37].

Nodules with a halo sign or consolidation with surrounding ground-glass opacity are frequently seen in invasive pulmonary aspergillosis and invasive mucormycosis, particularly when absolute neutrophil (ANC) count falls below 500 cells/μL (Fig. 8.12). The air-crescent sign with lung ball formation within the nodules or the areas of consolidation heralds improvement of such invasive fungal infection with recovery of ANC but is also a sign warning that resection surgery for the cavitary lesions is needed for fear of bleeding and resultant massive hemoptysis within the cavity [37, 55]. Airway invasive pulmonary aspergillosis is another invasive form of bronchopneumonia in which airway walls are destroyed by the fungal infection. CT findings include extensive bronchopneumonia showing diffuse bronchial wall thickening, tree-in-bud signs, peribronchial opacity, and presence of a mucosal sinus tract or fistula in the central airways [56].

Despite the nonspecific and overlapping signs and symptoms of SARS-CoV, MERS-CoV, and SARS-CoV-2 infections, the imaging findings have several important differences. Pleural effusion is rare in SARS-CoV-2 infection but occurs in 15% and 30% of SARS-CoV and MERS-CoV infections, respectively, usually during the first week of infection. Bilateral and random distributions of parenchymal opacity lesions are more common in SARS-CoV-2 than in SARS-CoV

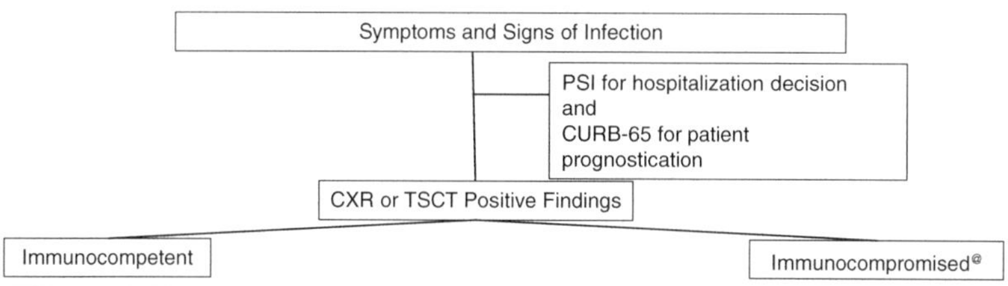

Immunocompetent

Organisms Involved / Patterns	Lobar	Bronchopn	Interstitial pn	Nodules	Cavities /cysts
Bacteria	$++^{\#}$	$+++^{+}$	—	—	—
Virus	—	$+++^{*}$	$+^{*\wedge}$	+	—
Fungus	+	$+^{\&}$	—	$+^{\&}$	±
Mycobacteria	+	+++	—	++	+

Immunocompromised@

Organisms Involved / Patterns	Lobar	Bronchopn	Interstitial pn	Nodules	Cavities /cysts
Bacteria	+++	+++	+	+	+
Virus	+	$++^{*}$	$+++^{*\wedge\wedge}$	+	—
Fungus	$+^{\&\&}$	+	$++^{\&\&\&}$	$+++^{\&\&}$	$+++^{\&\&}$
Mycobacteria	+++	+	+	+++	++

Notes. - # *St. pneumoniae, K. pneumoniae, and Leginonella pneumophila; + S. aureus, H. Influenza, P. aeruginosa,* Anaerobic bacteria, virus, *Mycoplasmsa pneumoniae pneumonia*; *Bilateral, ^CMV (Cytomegalovirus) & Hantavirus; ^^CMV; &Usually Crpytococcosis, Histoplasmosis & Blastomycosis, &&Invasive pulmonary aspergillosis and mucormycosis, &&&Pneumocystis, @Also refer to Table 3
Bronchopn = Bronchopneumonia, Pn= Pneumonia, CXR = Chest radiograph, TSCT = Thin-Section CT, PSI = Pneumonia Severity Index, CURB-65 includes C = Confusion, U = Urea Nitrogen, R = Respiration, and B = Blood pressure.

Fig. 8.19 Structured diagnostic approach to pulmonary infection in the emergency department in consideration of an individual's immune status. Notes: #*S. pneumoniae, K. pneumoniae*, and *Legionella pneumophila*; +*S. aureus, H. Influenza, P. aeruginosa*, anaerobic bacteria, viruses, and *Mycoplasmsa pneumoniae pneumonia*; *Bilateral, ^CMV (cytomegalovirus) and hantavirus; ^^CMV; &Usually crpytococcosis, histoplasmosis and blastomycosis; && Invasive pulmonary aspergillosis and mucormycosis; &&&Pneumocystis; @Refer to Table 8.3. Bronchopn = Bronchopneumonia, Pn = Pneumonia, CXR = Chest radiograph, TSCT = Thin-Section CT, PSI = Pneumonia Severity Index, CURB-65 includes C = Confusion, U = Urea Nitrogen, R = Respiration, and B = Blood pressure and MERS-CoV. The most common initial CXR and CT findings are GGO and consolidation with peripheral predominance; these lesions eventually spread to the bilateral lungs as the disease progresses and pulmonary fibrosis may develop on long-term follow-up. Crazy-paving signs are frequently seen within GGO lesions. One imaging feature that helps determine the clinical outcome or prognosis of coronavirus infection is the extent of parenchymal abnormalities. More extensive parenchymal abnormalities, especially in older patients or those with comorbidities, suggest a poorer prognosis, necessitating intensive care unit management or predicting mortality.

References

1. Niederman MS, McCombs JS, Unger AN, Kumar A, Popovian R. The cost of treating community-acquired pneumonia. Clin Ther. 1998;20:820–37.
2. Garibaldi RA. Epidemiology of community-acquired respiratory tract infections in adults. Incidence, etiology, and impact. Am J Med. 1985;78:32–7.
3. Plouffe JF, Martin DR. Pneumonia in the emergency department. Emerg Med Clin North Am. 2008;26:389–411.
4. Shah RM, Kaji AV, Ostrum BJ, Friedman AC. Interpretation of chest radiographs in AIDS patients: usefulness of CD4 lymphocyte counts. Radiographics. 1997;17:47–58. discussion 59-61
5. Fine MJ, Auble TE, Yealy DM, et al. A prediction rule to identify low-risk patients with community-acquired pneumonia. N Engl J Med. 1997;336:243–50.
6. Chalmers JD, Singanayagam A, Akram AR, et al. Severity assessment tools for predicting mortality in hospitalised patients with community-acquired pneumonia. Systematic review and meta-analysis. Thorax. 2010;65:878–83.
7. British Thoracic Society Standards of Care Committee. BTS guidelines for the management of community acquired pneumonia in adults. Thorax. 2001;56(Suppl 4):1–64.
8. Lim WS, Macfarlane JT, Boswell TC, et al. Study of community acquired pneumonia aetiology (SCAPA) in adults admitted to hospital: implications for management guidelines. Thorax. 2001;56:296–301.
9. Tanaka N, Matsumoto T, Kuramitsu T, et al. High resolution CT findings in community-acquired pneumonia. J Comput Assist Tomogr. 1996;20:600–8.
10. Lee JY, Lee KS, Jung KJ, et al. Pulmonary tuberculosis: CT and pathologic correlation. J Comput Assist Tomogr. 2000;24:691–8.
11. Ikezoe J, Takeuchi N, Johkoh T, et al. CT appearance of pulmonary tuberculosis in diabetic and immunocompromised patients: comparison with patients who had no underlying disease. AJR Am J Roentgenol. 1992;159:1175–9.
12. Reittner P, Muller NL, Heyneman L, et al. Mycoplasma pneumoniae pneumonia: radiographic and high-resolution CT features in 28 patients. AJR Am J Roentgenol. 2000;174:37–41.
13. Kang H, Lee KS, Jeong YJ, Lee HY, Kim KI, Nam KJ. Computed tomography findings of influenza A (H1N1) pneumonia in adults: pattern analysis and prognostic comparisons. J Comput Assist Tomogr. 2012;36:285–90.
14. Agarwal PP, Cinti S, Kazerooni EA. Chest radiographic and CT findings in novel swine-origin influenza A (H1N1) virus (S-OIV) infection. AJR Am J Roentgenol. 2009;193:1488–93.
15. Kim EA, Lee KS, Primack SL, et al. Viral pneumonias in adults: radiologic and pathologic findings. Radiographics. 2002;22:S137–49.
16. Moon JH, Kim EA, Lee KS, Kim TS, Jung KJ, Song JH. Cytomegalovirus pneumonia: high-resolution CT findings in ten non-AIDS immunocompromised patients. Korean J Radiol. 2000;1:73–8.
17. Franquet T, Lee KS, Muller NL. Thin-section CT findings in 32 immunocompromised patients with cytomegalovirus pneumonia who do not have AIDS. AJR Am J Roentgenol. 2003;181:1059–63.
18. Wu C, Chen X, Cai Y, et al. Risk factors associated with acute respiratory distress syndrome and death in patients with coronavirus disease 2019 pneumonia in Wuhan. JAMA Intern Med: China; 2020.
19. Assiri A, Al-Tawfiq JA, Al-Rabeeah AA, et al. Epidemiological, demographic, and clinical characteristics of 47 cases of Middle East respiratory syndrome coronavirus disease from Saudi Arabia: a descriptive study. Lancet Infect Dis. 2013;13:752–61.
20. Ko SF, Lee TY, Huang CC, et al. Severe acute respiratory syndrome: prognostic implications of chest radiographic findings in 52 patients. Radiology. 2004;233:173–81.
21. Hsieh SC, Chan WP, Chien JC, et al. Radiographic appearance and clinical outcome correlates in 26 patients with severe acute respiratory syndrome. AJR Am J Roentgenol. 2004;182:1119–22.
22. Das KM, Lee EY, Al Jawder SE, et al. Acute Middle East respiratory syndrome coronavirus: temporal lung changes observed on the chest radiographs of 55 patients. AJR Am J Roentgenol. 2015;205:W267–74.
23. Wong HYF, Lam HYS, Fong AH, et al. Frequency and distribution of chest radiographic findings in COVID-19 positive patients. Radiology. 2019; https://doi.org/10.1148/radiol.2020201160.
24. Franquet T, Jeong YJ, Lam HYS, et al. Imaging findings in coronavirus infections: SARS-CoV, MERS-CoV and SARS-CoV-2. Br J Radiol. 2020; https://doi.org/10.1259/bjr.20200515.
25. Ooi GC, Khong PL, Muller NL, et al. Severe acute respiratory syndrome: temporal lung changes at thin-section CT in 30 patients. Radiology. 2004;230:836–44.

26. Das KM, Lee EY, Enani MA, et al. CT correlation with outcomes in 15 patients with acute Middle East respiratory syndrome coronavirus. AJR Am J Roentgenol. 2015;204:736–42.
27. Wang Y, Dong C, Hu Y, et al. Temporal changes of CT findings in 90 patients with COVID-19 pneumonia: a longitudinal study. Radiology. 2020; https://doi.org/10.1148/radiol.2020200843.
28. Chung M, Bernheim A, Mei X, et al. CT imaging features of 2019 novel coronavirus (2019-nCoV). Radiology. 2020;295:202–7.
29. Chang YC, Yu CJ, Chang SC, et al. Pulmonary sequelae in convalescent patients after severe acute respiratory syndrome: evaluation with thin-section CT. Radiology. 2005;236:1067–75.
30. Jain S, Self WH, Wunderink RG, et al. Community-acquired pneumonia requiring hospitalization among U.S. adults. N Engl J Med. 2015;373:415–27.
31. Lee KS, Kim TJ, Peck KR, Han J. Infectious pneumonia in immunocompetent patients: updates in clinical and imaging features. Precis Future Med. 2018;2:79–94.
32. Craven DE. What is healthcare-associated pneumonia, and how should it be treated? Curr Opin Infect Dis. 2006;19:153–60.
33. Finch RG, Woodhead MA. Practical considerations and guidelines for the management of community-acquired pneumonia. Drugs. 1998;55:31–45.
34. Ibrahim EH, Ward S, Sherman G, Kollef MH. A comparative analysis of patients with early-onset vs late-onset nosocomial pneumonia in the ICU setting. Chest. 2000;117:1434–42.
35. Bartlett JG, Finegold SM. Anaerobic infections of the lung and pleural space. Am Rev Respir Dis. 1974;110:56–77.
36. Unger JD, Rose HD, Unger GF. Gram-negative pneumonia. Radiology. 1973;107:283–91.
37. Peck KR, Kim TJ, Lee MA, Lee KS, Han J. Pneumonia in immunocompromised patients: updates in clinical and imaging features. Precis Future Med. 2018;2:95–108.
38. Jepson SL, Pakkal M, Bajaj A, Raj V. Pulmonary complications in the non-HIV immunocompromised patient. Clin Radiol. 2012;67:1001–10.
39. Murray JF, Mills J. Pulmonary infectious complications of human immunodeficiency virus infection. Part II. Am Rev Respir Dis. 1990;141:1582–98.
40. Wolff AJ, O'Donnell AE. Pulmonary manifestations of HIV infection in the era of highly active antiretroviral therapy. Chest. 2001;120:1888–93.
41. Kuhlman JE, Kavuru M, Fishman EK, Siegelman SS. Pneumocystis carinii pneumonia: spectrum of parenchymal CT findings. Radiology. 1990;175:711–4.
42. Baughman RP. Cytomegalovirus: the monster in the closet? Am J Respir Crit Care Med. 1997;156:1–2.
43. Yu Q, Jia P, Su L, Zhao H, Que C. Outcomes and prognostic factors of non-HIV patients with *Pneumocystis jirovecii* pneumonia and pulmonary CMV co-infection: a retrospective cohort study. BMC Infect Dis. 2017;17:392.
44. Leoni MC, Mussa M, Chieffo G, et al. Aetiology and outcome of pneumoniae in HIV-positive patients in the antiretroviral era. Infect Dis (Lond). 2017;49:225–8.
45. Feikin DR, Feldman C, Schuchat A, Janoff EN. Global strategies to prevent bacterial pneumonia in adults with HIV disease. Lancet Infect Dis. 2004;4:445–55.
46. Dye C, Scheele S, Dolin P, Pathania V, Raviglione MC. Consensus statement. Global burden of tuberculosis: estimated incidence, prevalence, and mortality by country. WHO Global Surveillance and Monitoring Project. JAMA. 1999;282:677–86.
47. Markowitz N, Hansen NI, Hopewell PC, et al. Incidence of tuberculosis in the United States among HIV-infected persons. The pulmonary complications of HIV infection study group. Ann Intern Med. 1997;126:123–32.
48. Jeong YJ, Lee KS. Pulmonary tuberculosis: up-to-date imaging and management. AJR Am J Roentgenol. 2008;191:834–44.
49. Cheon JE, Lee KS, Jung GS, Chung MH, Cho YD. Acute eosinophilic pneumonia: radiographic and CT findings in six patients. AJR Am J Roentgenol. 1996;167:1195–9.
50. Lee KS, Kullnig P, Hartman TE, Muller NL. Cryptogenic organizing pneumonia: CT findings in 43 patients. AJR Am J Roentgenol. 1994;162:543–6.
51. Penner C, Roberts D, Kunimoto D, Manfreda J, Long R. Tuberculosis as a primary cause of respiratory failure requiring mechanical ventilation. Am J Respir Crit Care Med. 1995;151:867–72.
52. Bobrowitz ID. Active tuberculosis undiagnosed until autopsy. Am J Med. 1982;72:650–8.
53. Choi D, Lee KS, Suh GY, et al. Pulmonary tuberculosis presenting as acute respiratory failure: radiologic findings. J Comput Assist Tomogr. 1999;23:107–13.
54. Ko KS, Lee KS, Kim Y, Kim SJ, Kwon OJ, Kim JS. Reversible cystic disease associated with pulmonary tuberculosis: radiologic findings. Radiology. 1997;204:165–9.
55. Kim MJ, Lee KS, Kim J, Jung KJ, Lee HG, Kim TS. Crescent sign in invasive pulmonary aspergillosis: frequency and related CT and clinical factors. J Comput Assist Tomogr. 2001;25:305–10.
56. Logan PM, Primack SL, Miller RR, Muller NL. Invasive aspergillosis of the airways: radiographic, CT, and pathologic findings. Radiology. 1994;193:383–8.

9 Mediastinal and Spinal Infection

9.1 Introduction

Mediastinitis refers to inflammation of the tissues located in the mediastinum. It can be classified into acute and chronic forms. Acute mediastinitis is an uncommon but potentially life-threatening condition with a high mortality rate when diagnosis is delayed. Most cases are associated with esophageal rupture or with esophageal or cardiac surgery. The chronic form of mediastinitis is referred to as fibrosing mediastinitis. It can be classified into the granulomatous subtype, also known as the focal subtype, and the nongranulomatous subtype, also known as the diffuse or idiopathic subtype. The former is most often associated with chronic granulomatous infections, such as histoplasmosis or tuberculosis. Infectious spondylitis refers to infections of the spine which involve the vertebrae, intervertebral disc, paraspinal soft tissue, or epidural space. It is important to differentiate tuberculous spondylitis from pyogenic spondylitis because appropriate treatment differs and may reduce the rate of disability and functional impairment. Descending necrotizing mediastinitis is an acute infection of the mediastinum with a high mortality rate. Continuity of the fascial planes between the neck and mediastinum allows infection to spread from the oral cavities and neck into the mediastinum. These conditions demonstrate characteristic imaging findings that help in making a timely diagnosis and providing optimal patient management.

9.2 Acute Mediastinitis

9.2.1 Etiology and Pathophysiology

Acute mediastinitis refers to acute inflammation or infection of the tissues located in the mediastinum. It is a life-threatening condition with a high mortality rate, especially when diagnosis is delayed; therefore, the diagnosis of acute mediastinitis necessitates prompt use of broad-spectrum antibiotics, aggressive drainage procedures, and surgical intervention. According to its etiology, acute mediastinitis may be classified as (1) a direct injury to adjacent structures, including the esophagus (Figs. 9.1 and 9.2), tracheobronchial trees, sternum (Fig. 9.3), or cardiovascular structures; (2) a direct extension of infection of the head and neck (Fig. 9.4); or (3) a hematogenous spread of infection (Table 9.1) [1, 2].

Iatrogenic esophageal perforation following esophageal endoscopy or balloon dilatation is the most common cause of acute mediastinitis [3, 4]. The presence of esophageal injury is increasing with the widespread use of endoscopy in diagnostic and therapeutic procedures [5, 6]. Esophageal perforation may occur in esophageal cancer in association with tumor necrosis or radiation therapy [7, 8]. Other causes of esophageal rupture, including Boerhaave syndrome, are described in detail in Chap. 5: Traumatic and nontraumatic esophageal emergency.

T. J. Kim et al., *Emergency Chest Radiology*, https://doi.org/10.1007/978-981-33-4396-2_9

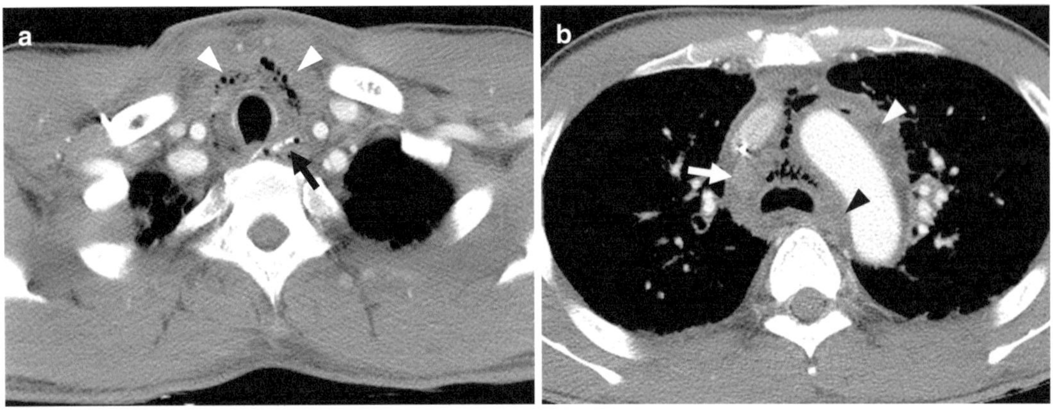

Fig. 9.1 Acute mediastinitis due to esophageal perforation by foreign body impaction (fish bone) in a 42-year-old man. (**a**) Mediastinal window image of a CT scan obtained at the level of the thoracic inlet shows a high-density foreign body (arrow) in the cervical esophagus and peritracheal air bubbles (arrowheads), suggesting esophageal perforation. The foreign body was removed by endoscopy. (**b**) Mediastinal window image of a CT scan obtained at the level of the aortic arch demonstrates increased soft tissue attenuation (arrowheads), pneumomediastinum, and lymphadenopathy (arrow), indicating acute mediastinitis secondary to esophageal perforation

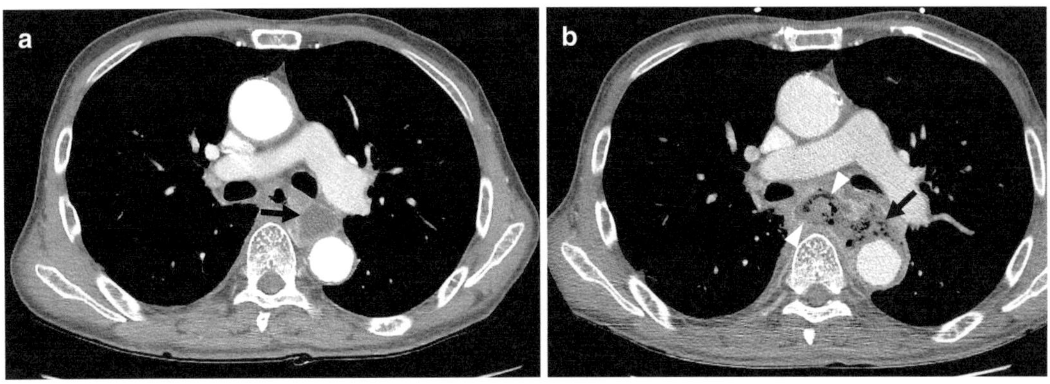

Fig. 9.2 Mediastinal abscess and subsequent perforation of the neoesophagus in a 60-year-old man with a history of Ivor Lewis operation due to esophageal cancer. (**a**) Mediastinal window image of a CT scan obtained at the level of the main pulmonary artery shows a mediastinal abscess (arrow) adjacent to the descending thoracic aorta. (**b**) CT image obtained 2 weeks after **a** shows a perforation of the neoesophagus (pulled-up stomach, arrowheads) with large abscess formation (arrow). The patient expired due to sepsis

Postoperative mediastinitis occurs in approximately 0.5% to 5% of patients who undergo median sternotomy for cardiovascular surgery [9–11]. The risk of mediastinitis is markedly increased in immunocompromised patients, patients with diabetes, obesity, and reoperation, and following the use of bilateral internal mammary arteries for coronary grafting [12]. Direct extension of a head and neck infection may result in the condition referred to as descending necrotizing mediastinitis, which is the most lethal form of mediastinitis; refer to Sect. 9.4. Descending necrotizing mediastinitis for more detail on this subject. Rarely, mediastinitis may also result from hematogenous spread of an extrathoracic infection, such as septic arthritis [13]. Acute mediastinitis from esophageal or oropharyngeal sources is usually a mixed infection, with aerobes and anaerobes acting together. The most common organisms involved include *Streptococcus*, *Pseudomonas,* and *Candida* [13, 14].

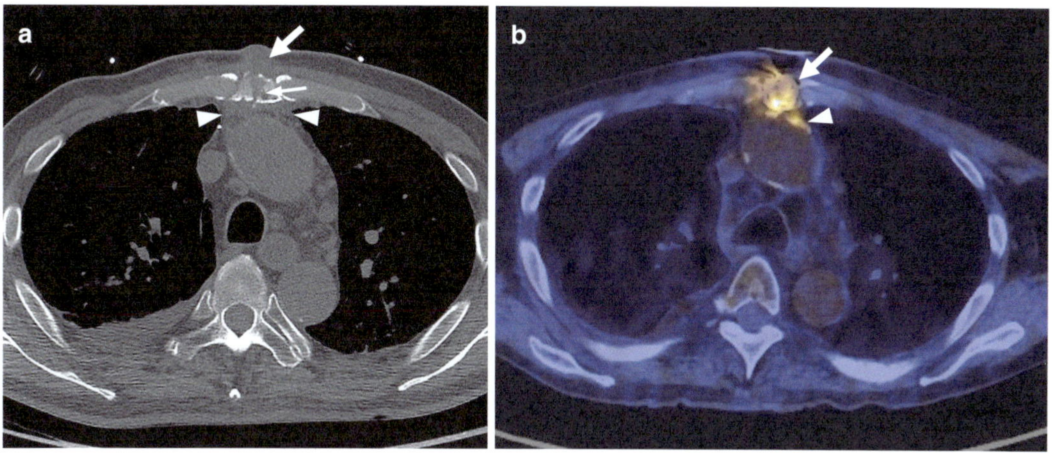

Fig. 9.3 Acute mediastinitis secondary to sternal osteomyelitis in a 62-year-old man. The patient underwent a median sternotomy for heart transplantation 3 weeks prior. (**a**) Bone window CT image demonstrates a midsternal lucency (thin arrow), suggesting sternal osteomyelitis. Also note the bulging soft tissue (thick arrow) at the surgical wound site, suggesting a draining sinus tract, and retrosternal soft tissue prominence (arrowheads), indicating poststernotomy mediastinitis. (**b**) ^{18}F-Fluorodeoxyglucose (FDG) positron emission tomography/CT demonstrates strong FDG avidity, representing active inflammation of the sternum (arrow) and anterior mediastinum (arrowhead)

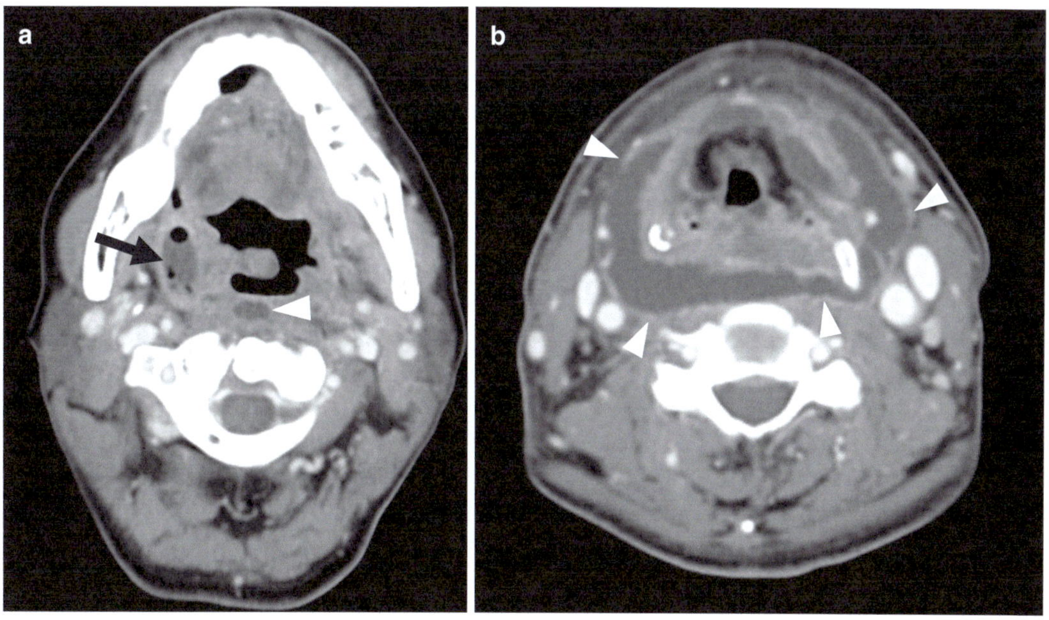

Fig. 9.4 Descending necrotizing mediastinitis in a 56-year-old man with abscesses in the oral cavity. (**a**) Axial contrast-enhanced CT image obtained at the level of the mandible shows multiple abscess pockets in the parapharyngeal space (arrow) and retropharyngeal space (arrowhead). (**b**) Axial contrast-enhanced CT image obtained at the level of the thyroid cartilage shows large fluid collection in the parapharyngeal and retropharyngeal space with peripheral rim-like enhancement (arrowheads). (**c**) Close-up view of a posteroanterior chest radiograph shows smooth widening of the upper mediastinum (arrows). (**d**) Mediastinal window image of a CT scan obtained at the level of the carina shows localized low-attenuation areas, consistent with abscess formation anterior to the main bronchi (arrows)

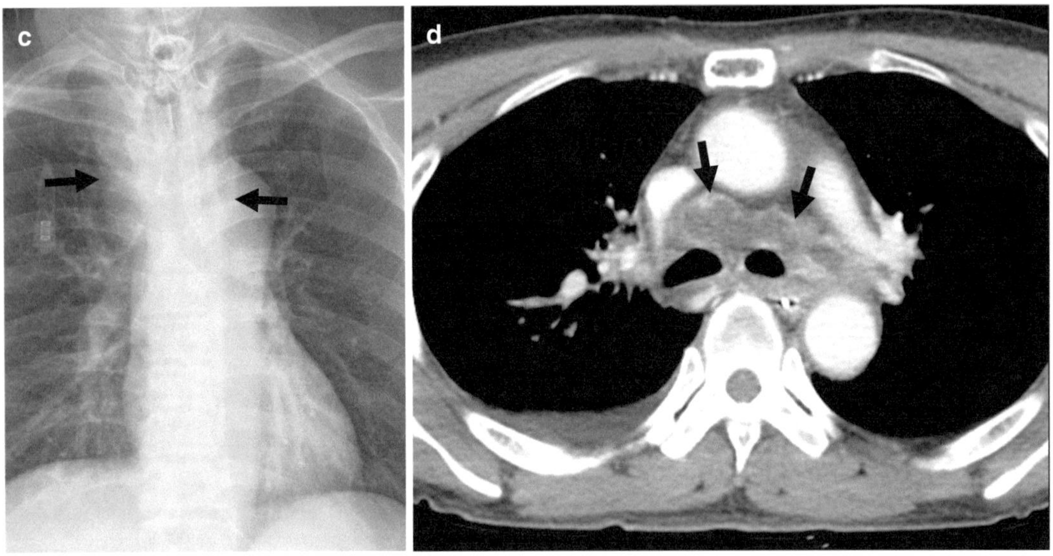

Fig. 9.4 (continued)

Table 9.1 Etiology of acute mediastinitis

Etiology
Esophageal rupture or perforation
Iatrogenic: diagnostic or therapeutic endoscopic procedures, balloon dilatation, surgery
Spontaneous rupture: Boerhaave syndrome, bronchial asthma, labor
Blunt or penetrating trauma
Foreign body impaction
Esophageal cancer: perforation, radiation therapy
Tracheobronchial perforation
Blunt or penetrating trauma
Iatrogenic: intubation, bronchoscopy, tracheostomy
Foreign body impaction
Vascular perforation
Iatrogenic: indwelling central venous catheter
Direct extension
Adjacent tissue: oropharyngeal, odontogenic, paraspinal, chest wall, retroperitoneal, and subphrenic infection

9.2.2 Clinical Presentations

The typical symptoms of acute mediastinitis are sudden-onset chills, high fever, tachycardia, and tachypnea. Retrosternal pain worsened by breathing or coughing may radiate to the neck. The Hamman sign, a loud crunching or clicking sound synchronous with the heartbeat on auscultation over the apex of the heart, maybe secondary to pneumomediastinum associated with acute mediastinitis [15]. Accurate diagnosis depends on the appropriate clinical suspicion based on an awareness of predisposing events or risk factors for mediastinitis. In most patients, a history of events with potential predispositions or disease processes may be available, but cases without such information may occur. In the latter situation, diagnosis may be delayed because the symptoms of mediastinitis may mimic those of myocardial infarction, aortic dissection, or pulmonary thromboembolism.

Patients with mediastinitis due to sternotomy present with fever and tachycardia and may report worsening sternal pain since surgery, drainage from the wound site, an audible click sound due to sternal nonunion, and progressive redness of the wound site. The development of sternal dehiscence that occurs 2 weeks after sternotomy is suggestive of mediastinitis (Fig. 9.3) [16, 17].

9.2.3 Imaging Diagnosis

In acute mediastinitis, the most common chest radiographic finding is widening of the mediastinum with a smooth, sharply defined margin, usually more evident in the superior mediastinum (Figs. 9.4 and 9.5). Air bubbles may be visible within the mediastinum (i.e., pneumomediasti-

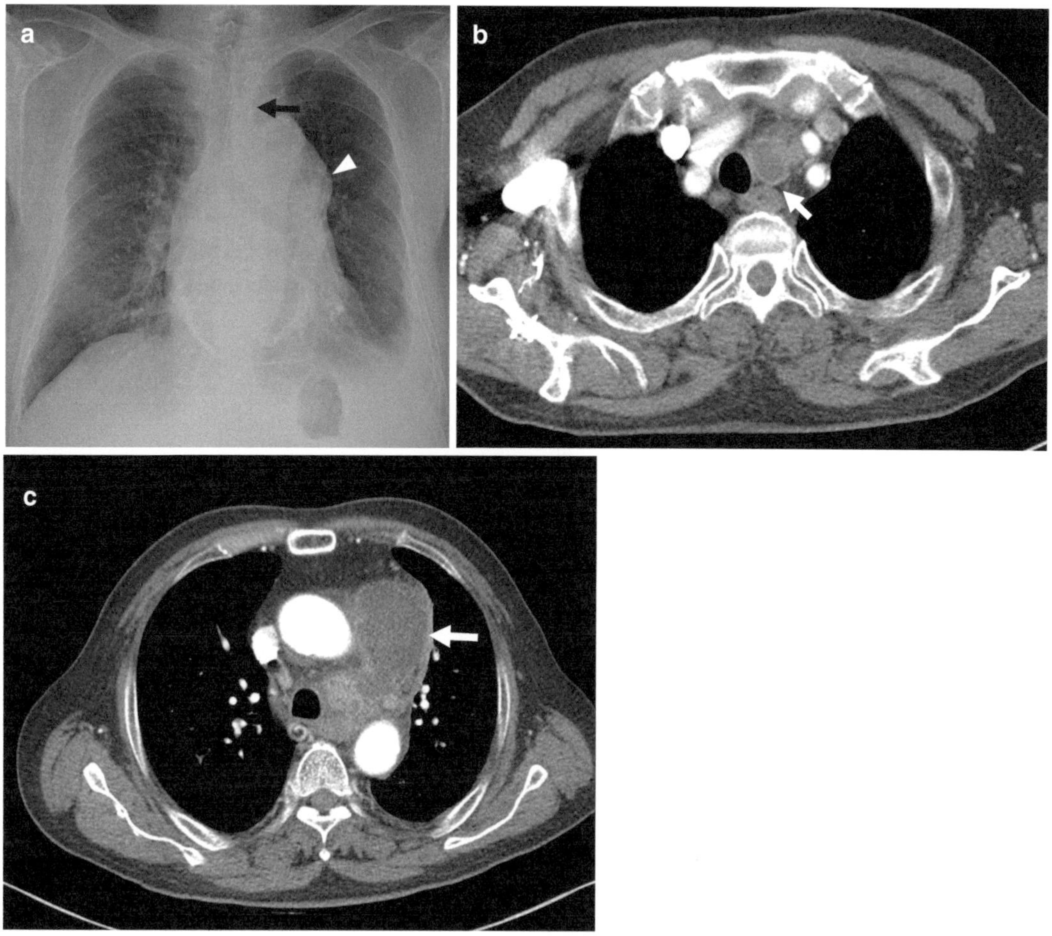

Fig. 9.5 Mediastinal abscess in a 45-year-old man who underwent endobronchial ultrasound-guided needle aspiration for an enlarged mediastinal lymph nodes 2 weeks prior. (**a**) Chest radiograph shows thickening of the left paratracheal stripe (arrow) and contour bulging at the aortopulmonary window (arrowhead). Note left pleural effusion. (**b**) Mediastinal window image of a CT scan obtained at the level of the left innominate vein shows an abscess in the left paratracheal area (arrow). (**c**) Mediastinal window image of a CT scan obtained at the level of the ascending aorta shows a large abscess in the aortopulmonary window (arrow)

num) as well as in the soft tissues of the neck [18, 19]. The details of imaging findings of pneumomediastinum are described in Chap. 2: Traumatic airway injury. Esophageal rupture, which is the most common cause of mediastinitis, is frequently accompanied by left pleural effusion and pneumothorax. However, right pleural effusion may occur in cases of midthoracic esophageal rupture [20]. Esophageal perforation can easily be demonstrated by esophagography. Extravasation of oral contrast media into the mediastinum or pleural space is an unequivocal sign of esophageal perforation. Radiographic findings of sternal dehiscence include displacement and rotation or disruption of the sternal wires on serial chest radiographs, and a midsternal lucent stripe thicker than 3 mm [21].

CT is the modality of choice for evaluating patients with suspected acute mediastinitis. CT findings in mediastinitis secondary to esophageal perforation include esophageal thickening, obliteration of fat planes, periesophageal areas of soft tissue or fluid attenuation, single or multiple abscesses, extraluminal gas, and extraluminal contrast [7, 22, 23]. CT also can be helpful in the evaluation of mediastinitis due to median sternotomy. The presence of a midsternal lucent strip on axial CT images that is thicker than 3 mm is suggestive of dehiscence (Fig. 9.3). CT findings of acute mediastinitis in patients with dehiscence include air or fluid collections and free air in the mediastinum. CT may also demonstrate pleural or pericardial effusions, enlarged lymph nodes, and sternal and lung parenchymal abnormalities. Because these findings are often present following esophageal or cardiovascular surgery, it may be difficult to distinguish normal postoperative findings from those of mediastinitis. The presence of mediastinal gas and fluid collections on CT after postoperative day 14 has a sensitivity and specificity of approximately 100% for the diagnosis of acute mediastinitis [11]. CT can also help guide diagnostic or therapeutic aspiration or drainage of fluid collections or abscesses [24, 25].

9.3 Fibrosing Mediastinitis

9.3.1 Etiology and Pathophysiology

Fibrosing mediastinitis, also known as chronic sclerosing mediastinitis or idiopathic mediastinal fibrosis, is a rare but potentially life-threatening condition characterized by progressive proliferation of dense infiltrative fibrous tissue into the mediastinum. This progressive fibrosis may cause compression or obstruction of adjacent mediastinal and hilar structures, including vessels, airways, and the esophagus, and result in a variety of clinical and radiological manifestations. There are two subtypes of fibrosing mediastinitis: the granulomatous subtype, also known as the focal subtype, and the nongranulomatous subtype, also known as the diffuse or idiopathic subtype [26, 27]. The granulomatous subtype is most commonly associated with antigen exposure of *Histoplasma capsulatum,* which is endemic to the Mississippi and Ohio River valleys in the United States. Other infections, including tuberculosis (Fig. 9.6) [28], aspergillosis, mucormycosis, blastomycosis [29], and cryptococcosis [30] are associated with fibrosing mediastinitis. This is the most common form of fibrosing mediastinitis, comprising approximately 80%–90% of all cases of fibrosing mediastinitis. The precise pathogenesis of progressive mediastinal fibrosis in patients who have these infections is not clear. It has been hypothesized that spillage of necrotic material from an affected lymph node results in mediastinal infection and secondary fibrosis [31]. The nongranulomatous subtype may be idiopathic or related to underlying autoimmune disorders, drug exposure, or prior radiation therapy [30, 32–34] (Fig. 9.7 and

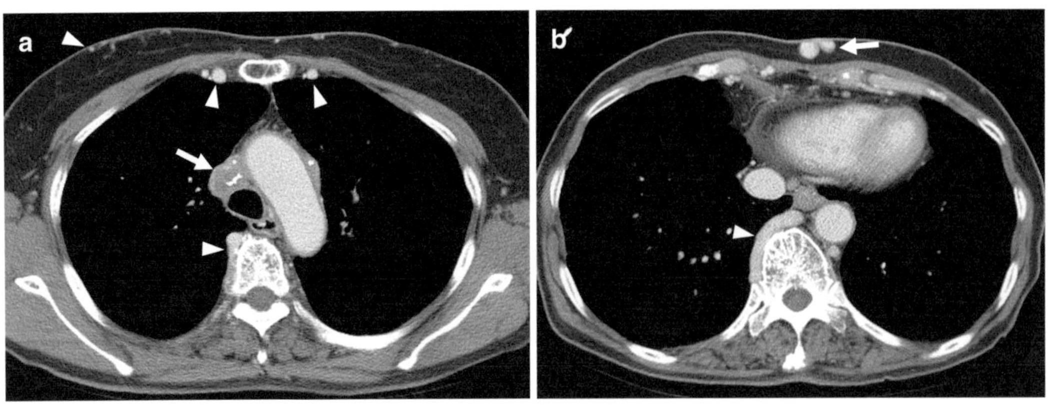

Fig. 9.6 Superior vena cava (SVC) obstruction in focal fibrosing mediastinitis secondary to tuberculosis in a 74-year-old woman with facial swelling. (**a**) Mediastinal window image of a CT scan obtained at the level of the aortic arch shows an enlarged and calcified right paratracheal lymph node (arrow) obstructing the SVC. Also note the dilated collateral veins (arrowheads). (**b**) Mediastinal window image of a CT scan obtained at the level of the cardiac apex shows collateral circulation in the anterior subcutaneous tissue (arrow) and a dilated intercostal vein (arrowhead) due to SVC obstruction

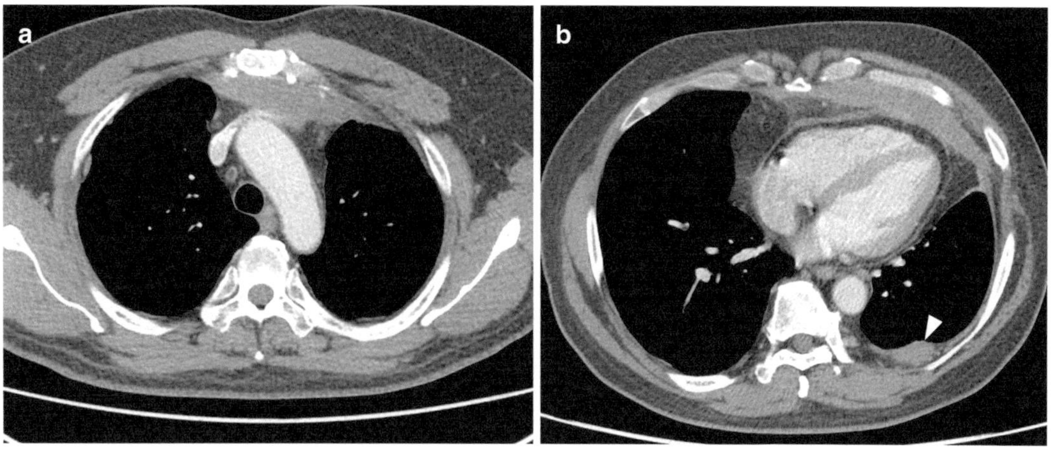

Fig. 9.7 Idiopathic fibrosing mediastinitis in a 55-year-old man with chest pain. (**a**) Mediastinal window image of a CT scan obtained at the level of the aortic arch shows a soft tissue-attenuation mass in the anterior mediastinum. (**b**) Mediastinal window image of a CT scan obtained at the level of the interventricular septum shows a soft tissue-attenuation mass in the anterior mediastinum. Also note a soft tissue mass in the left posterior chest wall (arrowhead). A CT-guided biopsy specimen revealed fibrosing mediastinitis

Table 9.2 Etiology of fibrosing mediastinitis

Infection
Histoplasmosis
Tuberculosis
Actinomycosis
Blastomycosis
Aspergillosis
Cryptococcosis
Mucormycosis
Autoimmune
Bechet disease
Drugs: methysergide
IgG4-related sclerosing disease
Rheumatoid arthritis
Sarcoidosis
Systemic lupus erythematosus
Radiation therapy
Malignancy and associated treatment

Table 9.2). This subtype represents approximately 10%–20% of all cases of fibrosing mediastinitis. The histopathologic diagnosis of fibrosing mediastinitis is based on the finding of a predominance of extensive pauci-cellular fibrous tissue (keloid scar tissue) infiltrating and obliterating adipose tissue, with or without patchy infiltration of mononuclear cells, in the absence of malignancy [35].

A subset of patients with the nongranulomatous subtype of fibrosing mediastinitis has other conditions, such as retroperitoneal fibrosis, Riedel's thyroiditis, and autoimmune pancreatitis, all of which have been associated with immunoglobulin G4-related disease (IgG4-RD). Additionally, it has been suggested that a subset of patients with the granulomatous subtype of fibrosing mediastinitis exhibit immunologic and histopathologic features that meet the criteria for IgG4-RD (Fig. 9.8) [36, 37].

9.3.2 Clinical Presentations

Patients with fibrosing mediastinitis are typically young at presentation but a wide range of ages has been reported, without a sex predilection [38]. The symptoms and signs of fibrosing mediastinitis vary widely depending on the involved organs and the degree and extent of fibrosis.

Respiratory symptoms resulting from airway involvement include dyspnea, cough, and hemoptysis. Bronchial stenosis related to fibrosing mediastinitis may result in recurrent or chronic obstructive pneumonia [31, 32, 35, 39]. Fibrous encasement or compression of the central pulmo-

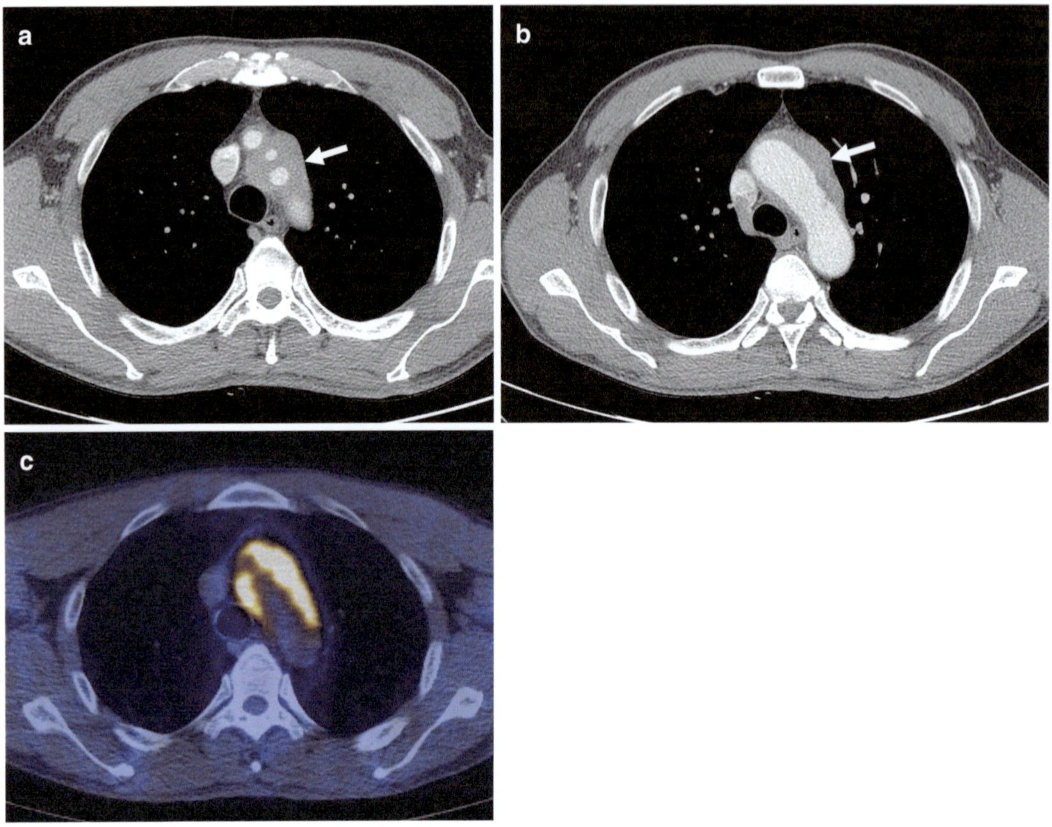

Fig. 9.8 Biopsy-proven IgG4-related fibrosing mediastinitis in a 62-year-old man. (**a**) Mediastinal window image of a CT scan shows an infiltrative soft tissue mass (arrow) encasing the arch vessels. (**b**) Mediastinal window image of a CT scan shows an infiltrative paraaortic soft tissue mass (arrow). (**c**) ^{18}F-Fluorodeoxyglucose (FDG) positron emission tomography/CT demonstrates strong FDG avidity in paraaortic soft tissues

nary arteries or veins may result in pulmonary congestion, pulmonary infarct, and pulmonary hypertension with symptoms similar to those of patients with chronic thromboembolic pulmonary hypertension [40–42]. Fibrosing mediastinitis is the second most common etiology of benign obstruction of the superior vena cava following the use of intravascular devices (Fig. 9.7) [40, 41, 43]. The most frequent signs and symptoms are swelling of the face or neck, swelling of the upper extremities, dyspnea, cough, and dilatation of chest vein collaterals. Dyspnea at rest, cough, and chest pain were less frequent than in patients with malignancy [43]. Involvement of nerves of the thorax may result in hoarseness (recurrent laryngeal nerve), diaphragmatic palsy (phrenic nerve), and Horner syndrome (sympathetic ganglion or nerves) [44]. Other intrathoracic manifestations of fibrosing mediastinitis include pleural thickening and pleural effusion, chylothorax, and constrictive pericarditis [26, 38, 44, 45].

9.3.3 Imaging Diagnosis

The radiologic features of fibrosing mediastinitis are often nonspecific, subtle, and easily underestimated [46]. The most common radiographic abnormality seen in nongranulomatous fibrosing mediastinitis is the widening of the mediastinum with obliteration or distortion of normal mediastinal interfaces, stripes, and lines. Focal lesions in granulomatous fibrosing mediastinitis most commonly involve the right paratracheal region (Fig. 9.6), followed by, in decreasing frequency, the subcarinal, left paratracheal, and posterior mediastinal regions [47–49]. Calcification within the mediastinum or hila is often present in granulomatous fibrosing mediastinitis (Fig. 9.6) [38]. CT is the mainstay of diagnostic evaluation for patients with suspected fibrosing mediastinitis. CT images can be used to accurately identify the specific mediastinal or hilar structures affected and estimate the extent of soft tissue involvement and the severity of the disease. Calcifications are more readily identified on CT than chest radiography, and the presence of calcification in a localized mediastinal soft tissue mass is a clear diagnostic marker of fibrosing mediastinitis [47]. The localized or infiltrative soft tissue in fibrosing mediastinitis may show variable heterogeneous enhancement after administration of intravenous contrast material. In nongranulomatous fibrosing mediastinitis, calcifications are typically absent (Figs. 9.7 and 9.8) [50].

Radiographic and CT findings in fibrosing mediastinitis greatly depend on the involved mediastinal or hilar structures. Airway involvement is frequently associated with obstructive pneumonia or atelectasis. The right main bronchus is the most commonly involved site, followed by the left main bronchus and the bronchus intermedius. Superior vena cava obstruction may show widening of the superior mediastinum due to dilated collateral veins on chest radiography. These collateral vessels are readily identified on contrast-enhanced CT as enhancing serpentine structures or varicosities in the mediastinum or chest wall (Fig. 9.6). Pulmonary arterial obstruction in fibrosing mediastinitis is usually unilateral and may result in localized areas of hypoperfusion on CT. Systemic collateral vessels such as bronchial artery or transpleural vessels may be seen in cases of long-standing pulmonary artery stenosis or occlusion [51]. Pulmonary venous obstruction may show findings of pulmonary venous congestion, such as peribronchial cuffing, septal thickening, and localized edema on chest radiography [52]. CT may demonstrate ground-glass opacity, interlobular septal thickening, bronchial wall thickening, and pleural effusion [51]. Chronic obstruction of the pulmonary artery or vein can also cause pulmonary infarction, and patients may have symptoms and signs similar to those of chronic thromboembolic pulmonary hypertension. Long-standing pulmonary vascular obstruction may lead to secondary pulmonary arterial hypertension and right-sided heart failure, which are the substantial causes of morbidity and mortality in patients with fibrosing mediastinitis [38, 40, 51].

Magnetic resonance (MR) imaging is equivalent to CT for assessment of the extent of disease and airway involvement but does not offer optimal identification of calcifications, which is important to arrive at a diagnosis of fibrosing mediastinitis. On MR, fibrosing mediastinitis usually shows intermediate signal intensity on T1-weighted images and variable signal intensity (sometimes low signal intensity due to its fibrous content) on T2-weighted images, and variable heterogeneous contrast material enhancement [38, 50].

^{18}F-Fluorodeoxyglucose positron emission tomography/CT (^{18}F-FDG–PET/CT) is not helpful for differentiation of fibrosing mediastinitis from malignancy because fibrosing mediastinitis also shows a variable degree of FDG avidity which represents inflammatory activity (Fig. 9.8c). It has been suggested that FDG uptake may be used to monitor treatment response in cases of proven fibrosing mediastinitis [53].

9.4 Descending Necrotizing Mediastinitis

9.4.1 Etiology and Pathophysiology

Descending necrotizing mediastinitis is an acute polymicrobial infection caused by the downward spread of oropharyngeal, cervical, and odontogenic infections along the fascial planes into the mediastinum. It is a potentially life-threatening condition, with a reported mortality rate ranging from 11% to 35% [54]. Anatomical continuity of the fascial planes between the neck and mediastinum leads to mediastinal extension of a deep neck infection. There are three potential major pathways along which an infection can spread from the neck to the mediastinum: (1) the pretracheal route to the anterior mediastinum, (2) the lateral pharyngeal route to the middle mediastinum, and (3) the retropharyngeal-retrovisceral route to the posterior mediastinum, which is the most common route (Figs. 9.4 and 9.9) [55]. The danger space is located posterior to the retropharyngeal space, separated by the alar fascia. This space extends from the base of the skull to the diaphragm, thus providing a pathway into the posterior mediastinum and pleural space. The most common cause of infection in the danger space is the rupture of a retropharyngeal abscess through the alar fascia [56].

9.4.2 Imaging Diagnosis

Neck or chest radiography may demonstrate subcutaneous emphysema, prevertebral soft tissue swelling pushing the trachea anteriorly, air in the mediastinum, and widening of the mediastinum [55]. Contrast-enhanced CT of the neck and chest should be performed in patients with oropharyngeal or dental infection with clinical suspicion of mediastinitis. CT allows for accurate diagnosis of descending necrotizing mediastinitis and may depict both the source of infection and the route of spread [57]. Neck CT findings include thickening of the subcutaneous tissues, thickening and enhancement of the muscles and fasciae, fluid collection, lymphadenopathy, and vascular thrombosis (Fig. 9.4). Chest CT findings include thickening and enhancement of the mediastinal fat, fluid collections with or without gas, pericardial effusion, and pleural effusion (Fig. 9.9) [55]. CT plays a key role in guiding patient management. It has been suggested that superior mediastinal drainage through a cervical approach is adequate for mediastinitis that is limited to the upper mediastinum above the carina, and complete mediastinal drainage via thoracotomy should be performed for mediastinitis extending below the carina [58].

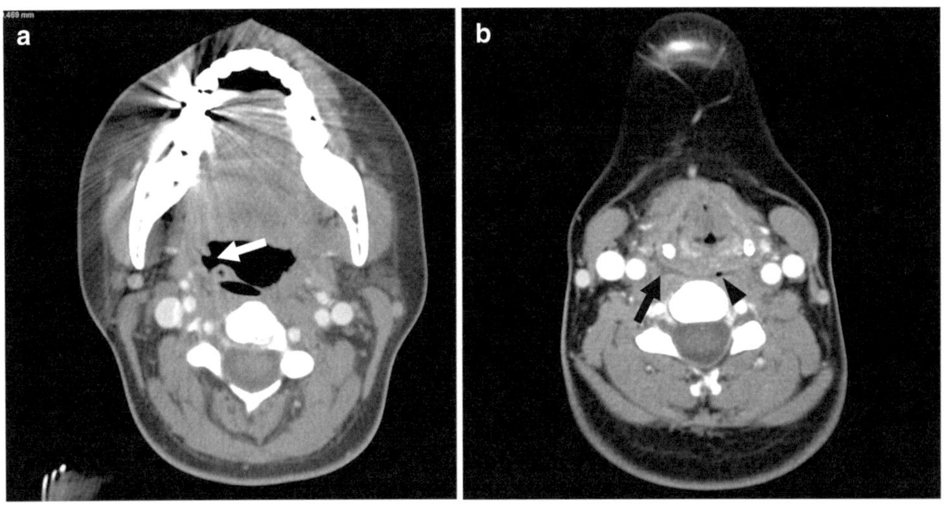

Fig. 9.9 Descending necrotizing mediastinitis secondary to hypopharyngeal perforation in an 18-year-old woman. (**a**) Contrast-enhanced neck CT scan demonstrates a perforation site at the right hypopharynx (arrow). (**b**) Mediastinal window image of a CT scan at the level of the cricoid cartilage demonstrates fluid collection (arrow) and an air bubble (arrowhead) in the retropharyngeal space. (**c**) Mediastinal window image of a CT scan at the level of the aortic arch shows multiple air bubbles and enlarged lymph nodes, indicating mediastinitis. Note the right pleural effusion. (**d**) Mediastinal window image of a CT scan at the level of the left ventricle shows air bubbles and fluid collection in the periaortic area. Also note the large amount of right pleural effusion and pleural enhancement, findings suggestive of empyema. (**e**) Esophagography using a water-soluble contrast agent (gastrografin) demonstrates contrast leakage through the hypopharyngeal defect (arrow). (**f**) Unenhanced CT obtained after esophagography demonstrates contrast spillage into the pleural space (arrows), indicating a mediastino-pleural fistula due to mediastinitis. Note a chest tube (arrowhead) in the right thorax

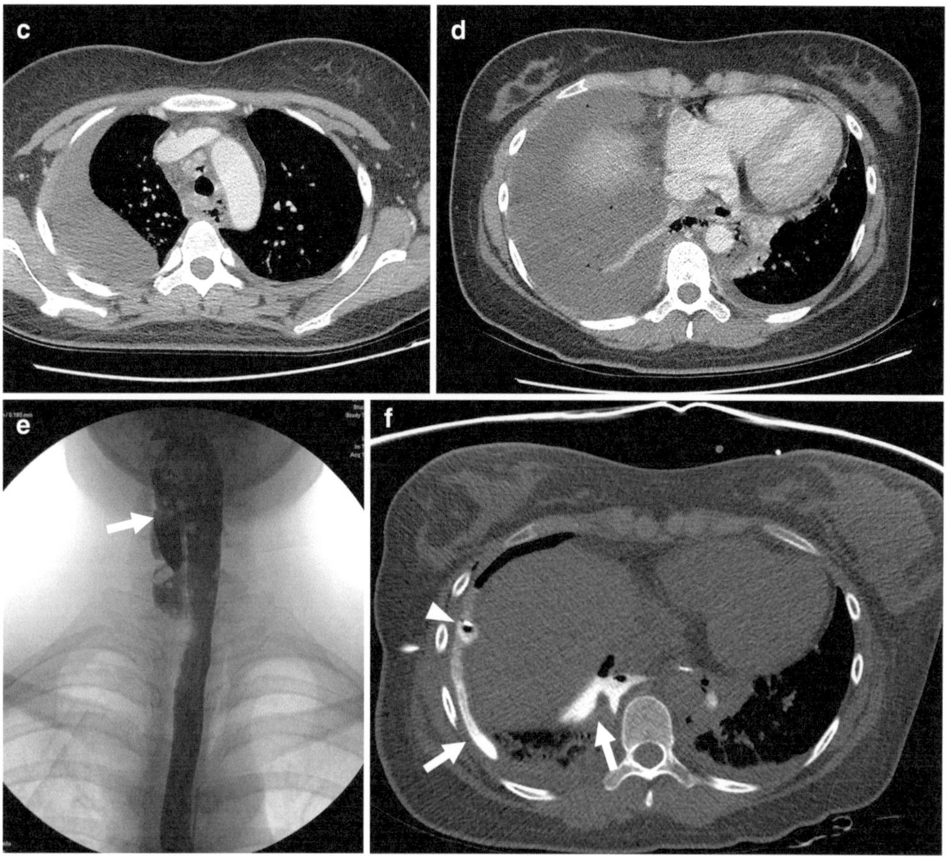

Fig. 9.9 (continued)

9.5 Infectious Spondylitis

9.5.1 Tuberculous Spondylitis

Tuberculous spondylitis most commonly involves the thoracic spine. Owing to the substantial overlap of clinical and radiological findings, it is often difficult to differentiate between tuberculous and pyogenic spondylitis. A history of chronicity, insidious progression, and the absence of leukocytosis are suggestive of tuberculous spondylitis rather than pyogenic spondylitis [59]. Tuberculous spondylitis most often starts in the anterior spine and progresses posteriorly. It has been suggested that a lack of proteolytic enzymes in *Mycobacterium* species as compared with pyogenic infection may result in preservation of intervertebral discs and subligamentous spread of the disease [60].

MR imaging is helpful in differentiating tuberculous spondylitis from pyogenic spondylitis. A well-defined paraspinal lesion with abnormal signal intensity, a thin, smooth abscess wall, subligamentous spread to three or more vertebral levels, and multiple vertebral or entire-body involvement are more suggestive of tuberculous spondylitis than pyogenic spondylitis (Fig. 9.10) [61, 62]. The presence of skip lesions and a large paraspinal cold abscess also suggest tuberculous spondylitis rather than pyogenic spondylitis [63]. The differential imaging features of tuberculous and pyogenic spondylitis are summarized in Table 9.3.

9.5.2 Pyogenic Spondylitis

The most common organisms that cause pyogenic spondylitis are *Staphylococcus aureus* and

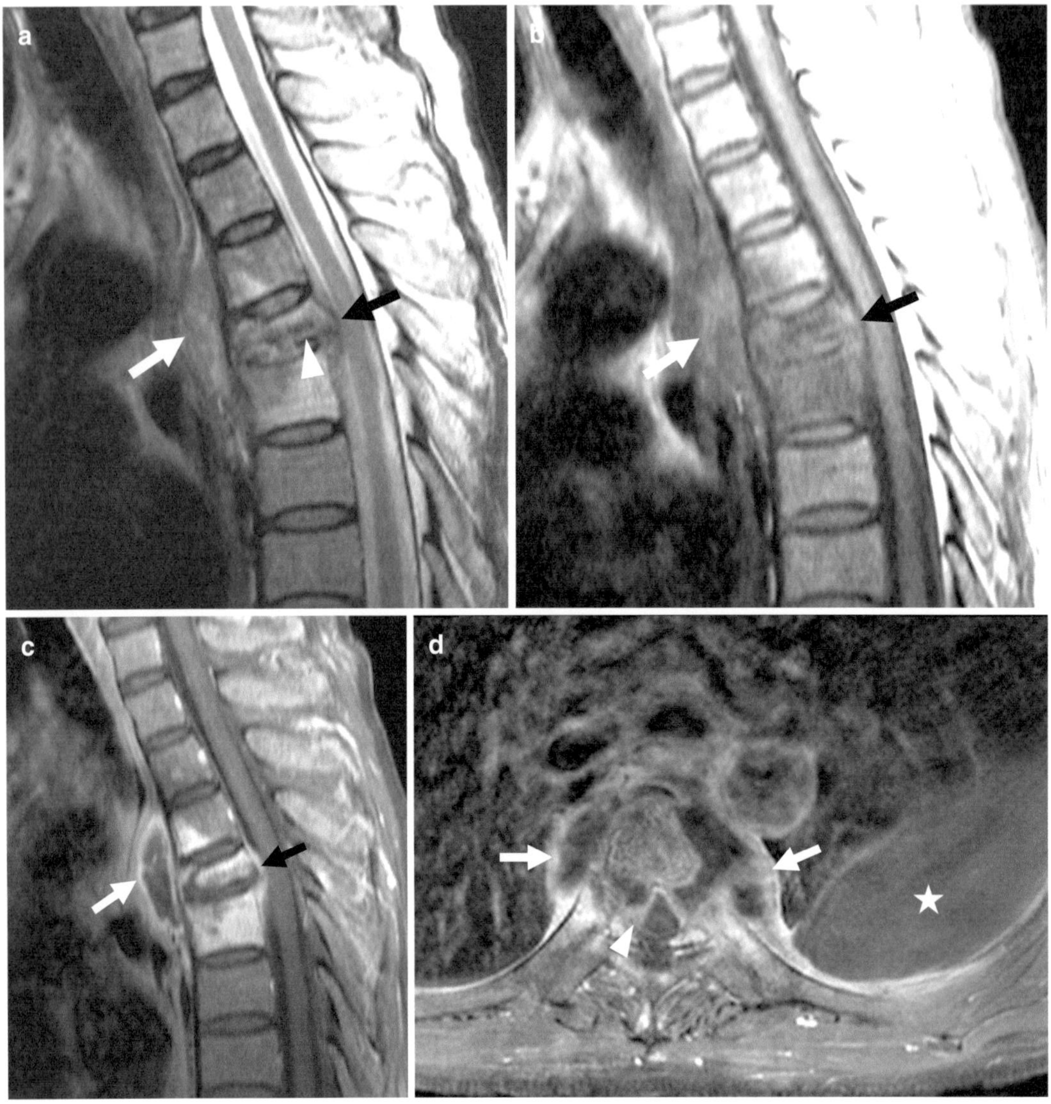

Fig. 9.10 Tuberculous spondylitis in a 45-year-old woman with back pain. (**a**) Sagittal T2-weighted MR image shows increased bone marrow signal intensity in the T3, T4, and T5 vertebral bodies, vertebral destruction (arrowhead), and formation of paraspinal (white arrow) and epidural abscesses (black arrow). (**b**) Sagittal T1-weighted MR image shows decreased bone marrow signal intensity in the T3, T4, and T5 vertebral bodies and paraspinal (white arrow) and epidural abscesses (black arrow). (**c**) Sagittal fat-suppressed contrast-enhanced T1-weighted MR image shows paraspinal (white arrow) and epidural (black arrow) abscesses with rim-like enhancement and enhancement of vertebral bodies. (**d**) Axial fat-suppressed contrast-enhanced T1-weighted MR image shows bilateral paraspinal abscesses (arrows) and epidural soft tissue (arrowhead). Note left pleural effusion due to tuberculous pleurisy (asterisk)

Streptococcus species, which account for more than 50% of cases [64, 65]. Pyogenic spondylitis commonly arises from arterial hematogenous spread of bacteria from distant septic foci. Pyogenic spondylitis typically involves two adjacent vertebrae and the intervertebral disc, as the same segmental artery supplies an intervertebral disc, the lower portion of the upper vertebra, and the upper portion of the lower vertebra [66]. The most common site of pyogenic spondylitis is the lumbar spine (45%–50%), followed by the thoracic (35%), cervical (3%–20%), and sacral

Table 9.3 MR imaging features of tuberculous and pyogenic spondylitis

	Tuberculous	Pyogenic
Thoracic spine involvement	+++	+
Multiple vertebral segments	+++	+
Subligamentous spread ≥3 vertebral bodies	+++	+
Skip lesion	+++	+
Disc preservation	Normal to mild destruction	Moderate to complete destruction
Paraspinal abnormal signal margin	Well-defined	Ill-defined
Vertebral body enhancement	Heterogeneous or focal	Homogenous
Paraspinal or intraosseous abscess	+++	+
Abscess calcification	+++	+
Anterior erosion	+++	+
Kyphosis	+++	+
Aggressiveness	+	+++

regions [67]. MR imaging demonstrates edematous changes of the vertebrae, which produces a low signal on T1-weighted images and a high signal on T2-weighted images (Fig. 9.11). Signal alterations can occur depending on the stage of the disease process, such as bone destruction, fibrosis, sclerosis, and fatty marrow changes after healing [68]. Intravenous administration of contrast material demonstrates enhancement of the infected disc, bone marrow, and nonosseous components of the spine and paravertebral area (Fig. 9.11). MR imaging is also useful in differentiating cellulitis from abscess formation, which requires immediate surgical intervention to prevent neurological complications [68]. Compared to tuberculous spondylitis, pyogenic spondylitis is characterized by its aggressive nature, which is caused by an array of enzymes that allow for the destruction of tissues with no regard for natural tissue barriers. This leads to rapid spread, extensive destruction, and more obvious clinical findings [68].

9.6 Summary

Mediastinitis can be classified into acute and chronic forms. Acute mediastinitis is a rare but potentially life-threatening condition. Esophageal rupture and esophageal or cardiac surgeries are the most common cause of acute mediastinitis. Common CT findings of acute mediastinitis include increased attenuation of mediastinal fat, air bubbles in the mediastinum, mediastinal fluid collection, and abscess formation. Fibrosing mediastinitis can be categorized into a granulomatous, or focal, subtype and a nongranulomatous (idiopathic), or diffuse, subtype. The granulomatous subtype is most often associated with histoplasmosis or tuberculosis. The nongranulomatous subtype is usually associated with autoimmune disorders and a subset of IgG4-related diseases. The characteristic imaging features of fibrosing mediastinitis include infiltrative soft tissue in the mediastinum (with or without calcifications) with compression or obstruction of various mediastinal structures. Descending necrotizing mediastinitis is a rare infectious condition that involves spread from the neck to the mediastinum via potential pathways. CT plays a key role in early diagnosis and proper management of this potentially life-threatening condition. Awareness of various mediastinal infections and their imaging features is crucial to ensure accurate and timely diagnosis and appropriate patient management.

Key Points

- Esophageal perforation secondary to diagnostic and therapeutic endoscopic procedures is the most common cause of acute mediastinitis.
- In acute mediastinitis, CT is the mainstay imaging technique for evaluation of the etiology and extent of disease and is also useful to help guide aspiration or drainage of mediastinal fluid collections or abscesses.
- Granulomatous fibrosing mediastinitis typically manifests as localized or infiltrative soft tissue with calcifications. The most commonly

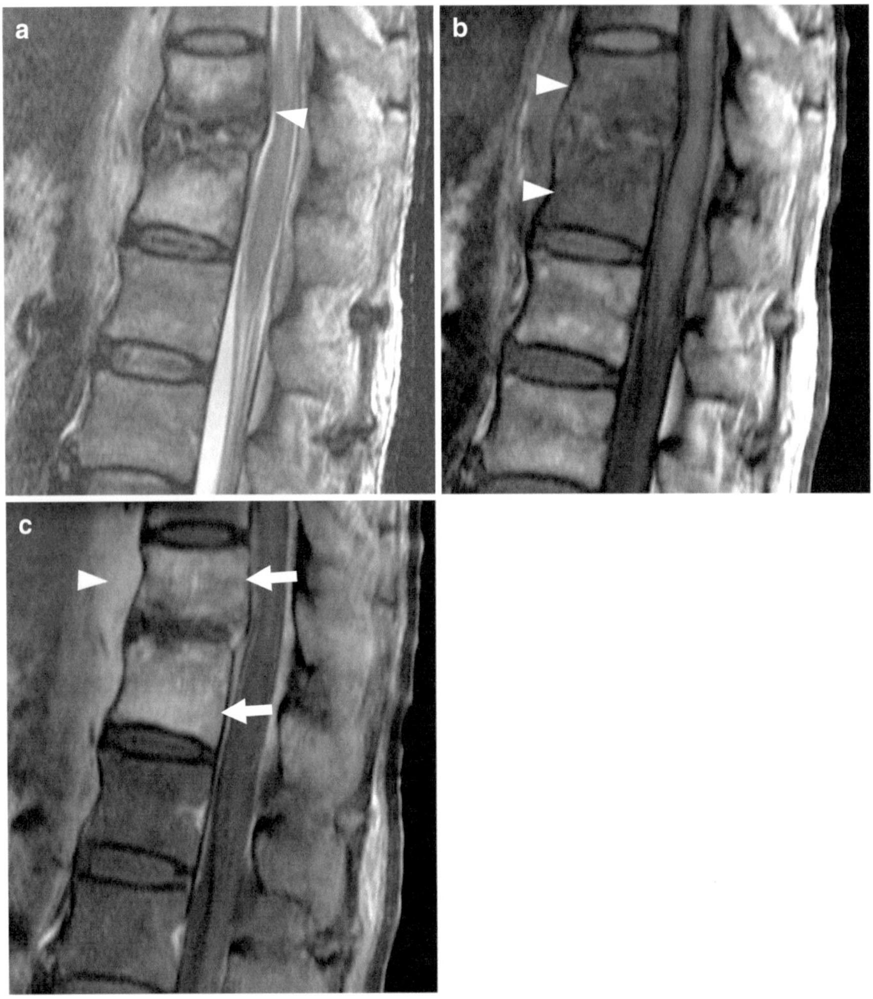

Fig. 9.11 Pyogenic spondylitis in a 69-year-old man with back pain. (**a**) Sagittal T2-weighted MR image shows increased signal intensity with endplate disruption in the T11 and T12 vertebral bodies. Also note anterior paravertebral and epidural abscesses with mild cord compression (arrowhead). (**b**) Sagittal T1-weighted MR image shows decreased signal intensity in the T11 and T12 vertebral bodies (arrowheads). (**c**) Sagittal fat-suppressed contrast-enhanced T1-weighted MR image shows diffuse enhancement of the T11 and T12 vertebral bodies (arrow) and anterior paravertebral abscess (arrowhead). Biopsy results confirmed the presence of an infection caused by *Klebsiella pneumoniae*

involved areas are the right paratracheal and subcarinal regions.

- Nongranulomatous fibrosing mediastinitis often manifests as infiltrative soft tissue involving multiple regions in the mediastinum and hila, usually without calcifications.
- Among the three potential routes for the spread of infection from the neck to the mediastinum, the retropharyngeal-retrovisceral route is the most common pathway involved in descending necrotizing mediastinitis.
- MR imaging findings suggestive of tuberculous spondylitis include a well-defined paraspinal lesion with abnormal signal intensity, a thin, smooth abscess wall, subligamentous spread to three or more vertebral levels, multiple vertebral or entire-body involvement, presence of skip lesions, and a large paraspinal cold abscess.

References

1. Katabathina VS, Restrepo CS, Martinez-Jimenez S, Riascos RF. Nonvascular, nontraumatic mediastinal emergencies in adults: a comprehensive review of imaging findings. Radiographics. 2011;31(4):1141–60. https://doi.org/10.1148/rg.314105177.
2. Akman C, Kantarci F, Cetinkaya S. Imaging in mediastinitis: a systematic review based on aetiology. Clin Radiol. 2004;59(7):573–85. https://doi.org/10.1016/j.crad.2003.12.001.
3. LaBerge JM, Kerlan RK Jr, Pogany AC, Ring EJ. Esophageal rupture: complication of balloon dilatation. Radiology. 1985;157(1):56. https://doi.org/10.1148/radiology.157.1.4034978.
4. Burnett CM, Rosemurgy AS, Pfeiffer EA. Life-threatening acute posterior mediastinitis due to esophageal perforation. Ann Thorac Surg. 1990;49(6):979–83. https://doi.org/10.1016/0003-4975(90)90882-7.
5. Costamagna G, Marchese M. Management of esophageal perforation after therapeutic endoscopy. Gastroenterol Hepatol (N Y). 2010;6(6):391–2.
6. Quine MA, Bell GD, McCloy RF, Matthews HR. Prospective audit of perforation rates following upper gastrointestinal endoscopy in two regions of England. Br J Surg. 1995;82(4):530–3. https://doi.org/10.1002/bjs.1800820430.
7. Gimenez A, Franquet T, Erasmus JJ, Martinez S, Estrada P. Thoracic complications of esophageal disorders. Radiographics. 2002; https://doi.org/10.1148/radiographics.22.suppl_1.g02oc18s247.
8. Vanagunas A, Jacob P, Olinger E. Radiation-induced esophageal injury: a spectrum from esophagitis to cancer. Am J Gastroenterol. 1990;85(7):808–12.
9. Grossi EA, Culliford AT, Krieger KH, et al. A survey of 77 major infectious complications of median sternotomy: a review of 7,949 consecutive operative procedures. Ann Thorac Surg. 1985;40(3):214–23. https://doi.org/10.1016/s0003-4975(10)60030-6.
10. Ottino G, De Paulis R, Pansini S, et al. Major sternal wound infection after open-heart surgery: a multivariate analysis of risk factors in 2,579 consecutive operative procedures. Ann Thorac Surg. 1987;44(2):173–9. https://doi.org/10.1016/s0003-4975(10)62035-8.
11. Jolles H, Henry DA, Roberson JP, Cole TJ, Spratt JA. Mediastinitis following median sternotomy: CT findings. Radiology. 1996;201(2):463–6. https://doi.org/10.1148/radiology.201.2.8888241.
12. Zacharias A, Habib RH. Factors predisposing to median sternotomy complications. Deep vs superficial infection. Chest. 1996;110(5):1173–8. https://doi.org/10.1378/chest.110.5.1173.
13. Swensen SJ, Aughenbaugh GL, Brown LR. Chest case of the day. Mediastinal abscess. AJR Am J Roentgenol. 1993;160(6):1318. https://doi.org/10.2214/ajr.160.6.8498244.
14. Brook I, Frazier EH. Microbiology of mediastinitis. Arch Intern Med. 1996;156(3):333–6.
15. Baumann MH, Sahn SA. Hamman's sign revisited. pneumothorax or pneumomediastinum? Chest. 1992;102(4):1281–2. https://doi.org/10.1378/chest.102.4.1281.
16. Boiselle PM, Mansilla AV, Fisher MS, McLoud TC. Wandering wires: frequency of sternal wire abnormalities in patients with sternal dehiscence. AJR Am J Roentgenol. 1999;173(3):777–80. https://doi.org/10.2214/ajr.173.3.10470922.
17. Boiselle PM, Mansilla AV, White CS, Fisher MS. Sternal dehiscence in patients with and without mediastinitis. J Thorac Imaging. 2001;16(2):106–10. https://doi.org/10.1097/00005382-200104000-00008.
18. Appleton DS, Sandrasagra FA, Flower CD. Perforated oesophagus: review of twenty-eight consecutive cases. Clin Radiol. 1979;30(5):493–7. https://doi.org/10.1016/s0009-9260(79)80178-6.
19. Christoforidis A, Nelson SW. Spontaneous rupture of esophagus with emphasis on the roentgenologic diagnosis. Am J Roentgenol Radium Ther Nucl Med. 1957;78(4):574–80.
20. Han SY, McElvein RB, Aldrete JS, Tishler JM. Perforation of the esophagus: correlation of site and cause with plain film findings. AJR Am J Roentgenol. 1985;145(3):537–40. https://doi.org/10.2214/ajr.145.3.537.
21. Boiselle PM, Mansilla AV. A closer look at the midsternal stripe sign. AJR Am J Roentgenol. 2002;178(4):945–8. https://doi.org/10.2214/ajr.178.4.1780945.
22. Exarhos DN, Malagari K, Tsatalou EG, et al. Acute mediastinitis: spectrum of computed tomography findings. Eur Radiol. 2005;15(8):1569–74. https://doi.org/10.1007/s00330-004-2538-3.
23. White CS, Templeton PA, Attar S. Esophageal perforation: CT findings. AJR Am J Roentgenol. 1993;160(4):767–70. https://doi.org/10.2214/ajr.160.4.8456662.
24. Gobien RP, Stanley JH, Gobien BS, Vujic I, Pass HI. Percutaneous catheter aspiration and drainage of suspected mediastinal abscesses. Radiology. 1984;151(1):69–71. https://doi.org/10.1148/radiology.151.1.6701339.
25. Breatnach E, Nath PH, Delany DJ. The role of computed tomography in acute and subacute mediastinitis. Clin Radiol. 1986;37(2):139–45. https://doi.org/10.1016/s0009-9260(86)80383-x.
26. McNeeley MF, Chung JH, Bhalla S, Godwin JD. Imaging of granulomatous fibrosing mediastinitis. AJR Am J Roentgenol. 2012;199(2):319–27. https://doi.org/10.2214/AJR.11.7319.
27. Parish JM, Rosenow EC. Mediastinal granuloma and mediastinal fibrosis. Semin Respir Crit Care Med. 2002;23(2):135–43. https://doi.org/10.1055/s-2002-25302.
28. Lee JY, Kim Y, Lee KS, Chung MP. Tuberculous fibrosing mediastinitis: radiologic findings. AJR Am J Roentgenol. 1996;167(6):1598–9. https://doi.org/10.2214/ajr.167.6.8956619.

29. Lagerstrom CF, Mitchell HG, Graham BS, Hammon JW Jr. Chronic fibrosing mediastinitis and superior vena caval obstruction from blastomycosis. Ann Thorac Surg. 1992;54(4):764–5. https://doi.org/10.1016/0003-4975(92)91025-5.
30. Mole TM, Glover J, Sheppard MN. Sclerosing mediastinitis: a report on 18 cases. Thorax. 1995;50(3):280–3. https://doi.org/10.1136/thx.50.3.280.
31. Dines DE, Payne WS, Bernatz PE, Pairolero PC. Mediastinal granuloma and fibrosing mediastinitis. Chest. 1979;75(3):320–4. https://doi.org/10.1378/chest.75.3.320.
32. Dechambre S, Dorzee J, Fastrez J, Hanzen C, Van Houtte P, d'Odemont JP. Bronchial stenosis and sclerosing mediastinitis: an uncommon complication of external thoracic radiotherapy. Eur Respir J. 1998;11(5):1188–90. https://doi.org/10.1183/09031936.98.11051188.
33. Kanne JP, Mohammed TL. Fibrosing mediastinitis associated with Behcet's disease: CT findings. Clin Radiol. 2007;62(11):1124–6. https://doi.org/10.1016/j.crad.2007.07.007.
34. Harman M, Sayarlioglu M, Arslan H, Ayakta H, Harman E. Fibrosing mediastinitis and thrombosis of superior vena cava associated with Behcet's disease. Eur J Radiol. 2003;48(2):209–12. https://doi.org/10.1016/S0720-048X(03)00006-8.
35. Peikert T, Colby TV, Midthun DE, et al. Fibrosing mediastinitis: clinical presentation, therapeutic outcomes, and adaptive immune response. Medicine (Baltimore). 2011;90(6):412–23. https://doi.org/10.1097/MD.0b013e318237c8e6.
36. Umehara H, Okazaki K, Masaki Y, et al. Comprehensive diagnostic criteria for IgG4-related disease (IgG4-RD), 2011. Mod Rheumatol. 2012;22(1):21–30. https://doi.org/10.1007/s10165-011-0571-z.
37. Peikert T, Shrestha B, Aubry MC, et al. Histopathologic overlap between fibrosing mediastinitis and IgG4-related disease. Int J Rheumatol. 2012;2012:207056. https://doi.org/10.1155/2012/207056.
38. Rossi SE, McAdams HP, Rosado-de-Christenson ML, Franks TJ, Galvin JR. Fibrosing mediastinitis. Radiographics. 2001;21(3):737–57. https://doi.org/10.1148/radiographics.21.3.g01ma17737.
39. Mathisen DJ, Grillo HC. Clinical manifestation of mediastinal fibrosis and histoplasmosis. Ann Thorac Surg. 1992;54(6):1053–7.; discussion 1057-1058. https://doi.org/10.1016/0003-4975(92)90069-g.
40. Williamson WA, Tronic BS, Levitan N, Webb-Johnson DC, Shahian DM, Ellis FH Jr. Pulmonary venous infarction. Chest. 1992;102(3):937–40. https://doi.org/10.1378/chest.102.3.937.
41. Toonkel RL, Borczuk AC, Pearson GD, Horn EM, Thomashow BM. Sarcoidosis-associated fibrosing mediastinitis with resultant pulmonary hypertension: a case report and review of the literature. Respiration. 2010;79(4):341–5. https://doi.org/10.1159/000243786.
42. Berry DF, Buccigrossi D, Peabody J, Peterson KL, Moser KM. Pulmonary vascular occlusion and fibrosing mediastinitis. Chest. 1986;89(2):296–301. https://doi.org/10.1378/chest.89.2.296.
43. Rice TW, Rodriguez RM, Light RW. The superior vena cava syndrome: clinical characteristics and evolving etiology. Medicine (Baltimore). 2006;85(1):37–42. https://doi.org/10.1097/01.md.0000198474.99876.f0.
44. Schowengerdt CG, Suyemoto R, Main FB. Granulomatous and fibrous mediastinitis. A review and analysis of 180 cases. J Thorac Cardiovasc Surg. 1969;57(3):365–79.
45. Hanley PC, Shub C, Lie JT. Constrictive pericarditis associated with combined idiopathic retroperitoneal and mediastinal fibrosis. Mayo Clin Proc. 1984;59(5):300–4. https://doi.org/10.1016/s0025-6196(12)61424-4.
46. McAdams HP. Chest case of the day. Fibrosing mediastinitis. AJR Am J Roentgenol. 1995;165(1):189–90. https://doi.org/10.2214/ajr.165.1.7785585.
47. Weinstein JB, Aronberg DJ, Sagel SS. CT of fibrosing mediastinitis: findings and their utility. AJR Am J Roentgenol. 1983;141(2):247–51. https://doi.org/10.2214/ajr.141.2.247.
48. Kountz PD, Molina PL, Sagel SS. Fibrosing mediastinitis in the posterior thorax. AJR Am J Roentgenol. 1989;153(3):489–90. https://doi.org/10.2214/ajr.153.3.489.
49. Dunn EJ, Ulicny KS Jr, Wright CB, Gottesman L. Surgical implications of sclerosing mediastinitis. A report of six cases and review of the literature. Chest. 1990;97(2):338–46. https://doi.org/10.1378/chest.97.2.338.
50. Rodriguez E, Soler R, Pombo F, Requejo I, Montero C. Fibrosing mediastinitis: CT and MR findings. Clin Radiol. 1998;53(12):907–10. https://doi.org/10.1016/s0009-9260(98)80218-3.
51. Chazova I, Robbins I, Loyd J, et al. Venous and arterial changes in pulmonary veno-occlusive disease, mitral stenosis and fibrosing mediastinitis. Eur Respir J. 2000;15(1):116–22. https://doi.org/10.1183/09031936.00.15111600.
52. Wieder S, Rabinowitz JG. Fibrous mediastinitis: a late manifestation of mediastinal histoplasmosis. Radiology. 1977;125(2):305–12. https://doi.org/10.1148/125.2.305.
53. Takalkar AM, Bruno GL, Makanjoula AJ, El-Haddad G, Lilien DL, Payne DK. A potential role for F-18 FDG PET/CT in evaluation and management of fibrosing mediastinitis. Clin Nucl Med. 2007;32(9):703–6. https://doi.org/10.1097/RLU.0b013e318125035b.
54. Ridder GJ, Maier W, Kinzer S, Teszler CB, Boedeker CC, Pfeiffer J. Descending necrotizing mediastinitis: contemporary trends in etiology, diagnosis, management, and outcome. Ann Surg. 2010;251(3):528–34. https://doi.org/10.1097/SLA.0b013e3181c1b0d1.
55. Pinto A, Scaglione M, Scuderi MG, Tortora G, Daniele S, Romano L. Infections of the neck leading to descending necrotizing mediastinitis: role

of multi-detector row computed tomography. Eur J Radiol. 2008;65(3):389–94. https://doi.org/10.1016/j.ejrad.2007.09.024.
56. Smith JK, Armao DM, Specter BB, Castillo M. Danger space infection: infection of the neck leading to descending necrotizing mediastinitis. Emerg Radiol. 1999;6(3):129–32.
57. Capps EF, Kinsella JJ, Gupta M, Bhatki AM, Opatowsky MJ. Emergency imaging assessment of acute, nontraumatic conditions of the head and neck. Radiographics. 2010;30(5):1335–52. https://doi.org/10.1148/rg.305105040.
58. Endo S, Murayama F, Hasegawa T, et al. Guideline of surgical management based on diffusion of descending necrotizing mediastinitis. Jpn J Thorac Cardiovasc Surg. 1999;47(1):14–9. https://doi.org/10.1007/BF03217934.
59. Moore SL, Rafii M. Imaging of musculoskeletal and spinal tuberculosis. Radiol Clin N Am. 2001;39(2):329–42. https://doi.org/10.1016/s0033-8389(05)70280-3.
60. Gouliamos AD, Kehagias DT, Lahanis S, et al. MR imaging of tuberculous vertebral osteomyelitis: pictorial review. Eur Radiol. 2001;11(4):575–9. https://doi.org/10.1007/s003300000631.
61. Jung NY, Jee WH, Ha KY, Park CK, Byun JY. Discrimination of tuberculous spondylitis from pyogenic spondylitis on MRI. AJR Am J Roentgenol. 2004;182(6):1405–10. https://doi.org/10.2214/ajr.182.6.1821405.
62. Hong SH, Choi JY, Lee JW, Kim NR, Choi JA, Kang HS. MR imaging assessment of the spine: infection or an imitation? Radiographics. 2009;29(2):599–612. https://doi.org/10.1148/rg.292085137.
63. Moorthy S, Prabhu NK. Spectrum of MR imaging findings in spinal tuberculosis. AJR Am J Roentgenol. 2002;179(4):979–83. https://doi.org/10.2214/ajr.179.4.1790979.
64. Yee DK, Samartzis D, Wong YW, Luk KD, Cheung KM. Infective spondylitis in southern Chinese: a descriptive and comparative study of ninety-one cases. Spine (Phila Pa 1976). 2010;35(6):635–41. https://doi.org/10.1097/BRS.0b013e3181cff4f6.
65. Govender S. Spinal infections. J Bone Joint Surg Br. 2005;87(11):1454–8. https://doi.org/10.1302/0301-620X.87B11.16294.
66. Sapico FL, Montgomerie JZ. Vertebral osteomyelitis. Infect Dis Clin N Am. 1990;4(3):539–50.
67. Jaramillo-de la Torre JJ, Bohinski RJ, Kuntz C. Vertebral osteomyelitis. Neurosurg Clin N Am. 2006;17(3):339–51., vii. https://doi.org/10.1016/j.nec.2006.05.003.
68. Tins BJ, Cassar-Pullicino VN, Lalam RK. Magnetic resonance imaging of spinal infection. Top Magn Reson Imaging. 2007;18(3):213–22. https://doi.org/10.1097/RMR.0b013e3180f60c3f.

10 Pulmonary Embolism

10.1 Introduction

Pulmonary embolism (PE) is the third most common cause of cardiovascular-related death [1]. Untreated or missed PE can lead to death [2], and PE is associated with a high potential risk for a future venous thromboembolism. Prompt diagnosis and treatment are required to reduce morbidity and mortality [3]. In this chapter, we will discuss the imaging findings of acute and chronic PE on CT pulmonary angiography, the severity of patients with PE, and the additional value of iodine maps. In addition, representative cases of non-thrombotic PE will be described.

10.2 Thrombotic Pulmonary Embolism

As the clinical manifestations of acute PE are broad and often nonspecific, suspicion of PE should be assessed carefully, especially when a patient has underlying risk factors. At the same time, it should be remembered that overdiagnosis of PE can be as harmful as underdiagnosis [4, 5]. False-positive results and subsequent anticoagulation treatment can result in severe complications [5].

10.2.1 CT Pulmonary Angiography

In most centers, CT pulmonary angiography is the first-line test in patients with a high clinical probability of PE. CT pulmonary angiography is considered indicative of PE when it shows a clot at least at the segmental level of the pulmonary arterial tree. It can also suggest alterative diagnoses in patients without PE. In the Prospective Investigation On Pulmonary Embolism Diagnosis II study, CT pulmonary angiography (mainly four-detector) showed a sensitivity of 83% and a specificity of 96% for PE diagnosis [6]. The clinical validity of negative results on CT angiography in excluding acute PE is well-established, with a negative predictive value of 99% [7]. False-negative results on CT pulmonary angiography have been reported in patients with a high clinical probability of PE [6]; however, such discrepancies are infrequent and the 3-month thromboembolic risk is low in these patients [8].

10.2.1.1 Imaging Findings

On CT pulmonary angiography, PE appears as an intraluminal low-attenuating filling defect within an opacified pulmonary artery. The thrombus may completely obstruct the lumen (Fig. 10.1) or partially obstruct flow in a central or eccentric

T. J. Kim et al., *Emergency Chest Radiology*, https://doi.org/10.1007/978-981-33-4396-2_10

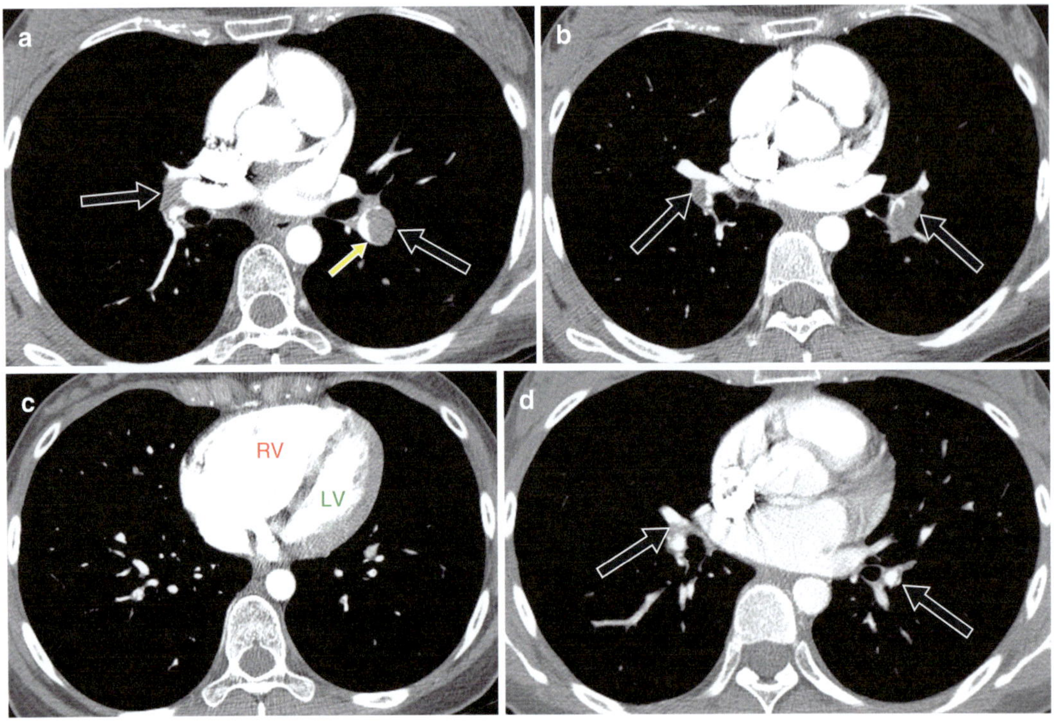

Fig. 10.1 Acute and chronic pulmonary thromboembolism. (**a**, **b**) Chest CT shows acute pulmonary thromboembolism in the bilateral pulmonary arteries (arrows). Note that the diameter of the pulmonary arteries is increased and filling defects form acute angles (yellow arrow) with respect to the vessel wall. (**c**) Enlargement of right ventricle and flattening of the interventricular septum are suggestive of right ventricle pressure overload. (**d**) Chest CT performed 3 months later shows chronic pulmonary thromboembolism in the bilateral pulmonary arteries (arrows). Note that the diameter of the pulmonary arteries has decreased and a web-like filling defect is present, suggestive of chronic pulmonary thromboembolism

location. Several CT imaging findings can be used to help differentiate acute and chronic thromboembolic disease [9]. In acute PE, the diameter of the pulmonary artery may be increased because of impaction of the thrombus by pulsatile flow. Non-obstructing eccentric filling defects form acute angles with respect to the vessel wall (Fig. 10.1). Acute PE occasionally leads to pulmonary infarction (Fig. 10.2), which is seen as a wedge-shaped pleural-based opacity in the territory of a thrombosed pulmonary artery [10]. Peripheral rather than central pulmonary emboli tend to cause infarction because the bronchial arteries play a less prominent role in perfusing the peripheral lung [11]. Central lucencies in peripheral consolidations are highly suggestive of pulmonary infarction [12]. In one previous study, central lucencies in peripheral consolidation were observed in 46% (23 of 50) of patients with pulmonary infarction [12]. Central lucencies on CT correspond to areas of central necrosis and peripheral consolidation corresponds to inflammatory reaction and alveolar filling with blood [12].

The majority of cases of acute PE resolve without sequelae. In a small percentage of patients, particularly those with large emboli, the emboli undergo organization, recanalization, and retraction. The end result is vascular stenosis, which may lead to severe pulmonary hypertension and cor pulmonale [13, 14]. In cases of chronic PE, the vessel diameter may permanently decrease due to contraction of a thrombus (Fig. 10.3). The organized thrombus can cause

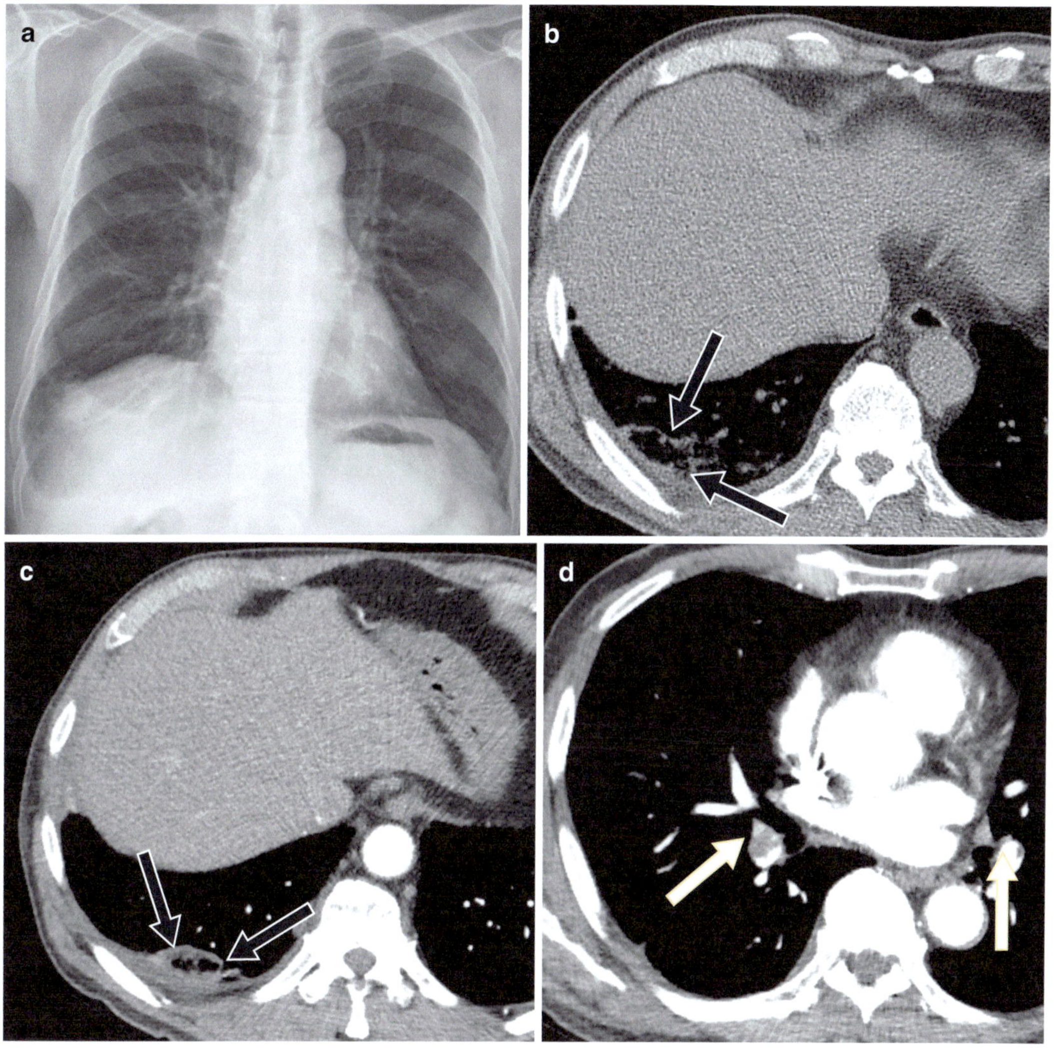

Fig. 10.2 Pulmonary infarction suspected on non-contrast CT in a 78-year-old man who complained of chest pain and cough. (**a**) There is a small amount of right pleural effusion and patchy increased opacity in the right lower lung base. (**b**) Non-contrast CT shows ill-defined ground-glass opacity (black arrows) in the right lower lobe. Note that central lucency is suspected inside the right lower lobe lesion, which suggests pulmonary infarction. Contrast-enhanced chest CT was recommended for further evaluation. (**c**, **d**) Contrast-enhanced chest CT confirms the presence of pulmonary thromboembolism (white arrows) and associated pulmonary infarction (black arrows) in the right lower lobe. Central lucency reflects central necrosis due to pulmonary infarction

intimal irregularities, bands and webs, and abrupt vessel narrowing; any of these can lead to pulmonary artery stenosis. The thrombus forms obtuse angles with the vessel wall (Fig. 10.4) and may contain calcifications (Figs. 10.4 and 10.5). In addition, there may be a mosaic perfusion pattern in the lung parenchyma (Fig. 10.3). Distinction of a mosaic perfusion pattern due to chronic PE from a similar pattern due to small airway disease can be accomplished by assessing the diameter of the main pulmonary artery. The main pulmonary artery is typically enlarged in chronic PE, a finding that reflects the presence of pulmonary hypertension, whereas the main pulmonary artery in patients with airway disease is usually normal [14, 15].

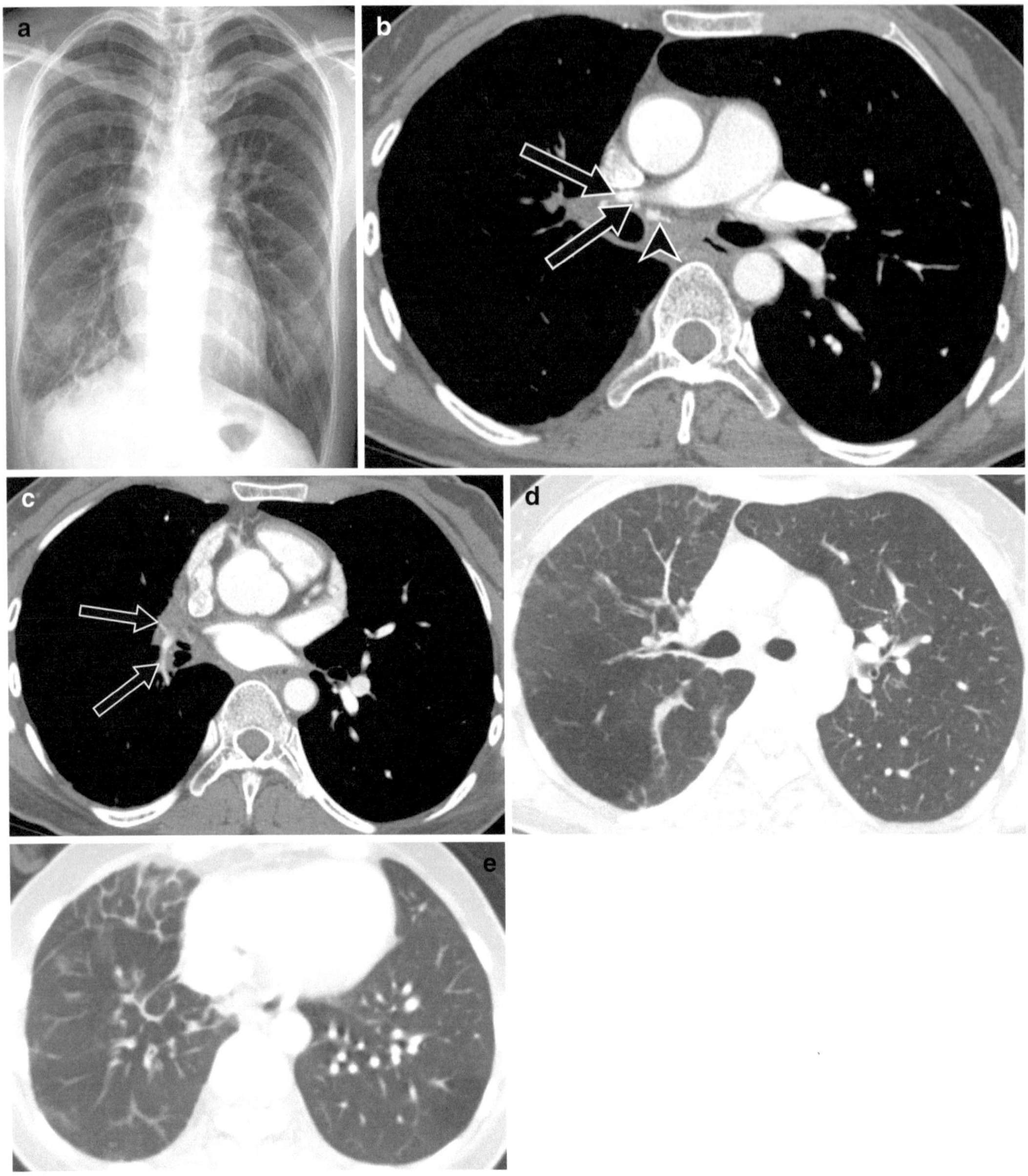

Fig. 10.3 Chronic pulmonary thromboembolism. (**a**) There is a volume decrease in the right hemithorax and reticular opacities in the right lower lung. (**b**) The diameter of the right main pulmonary artery is decreased (arrow) and right bronchial artery hypertrophy (arrowheads) has occurred. (**c**) The diameters of the right middle lobar and right lower lobar pulmonary arteries are decreased (arrows). There is compensatory hypertrophy in the left pulmonary artery. (**d**) There is mosaic attenuation in the right lung. Note the decrease in the number and diameter of pulmonary vessels in the right lung. (**e**) Septal and bundle thickening in the right lower lobe may be sequelae of previous ischemic changes

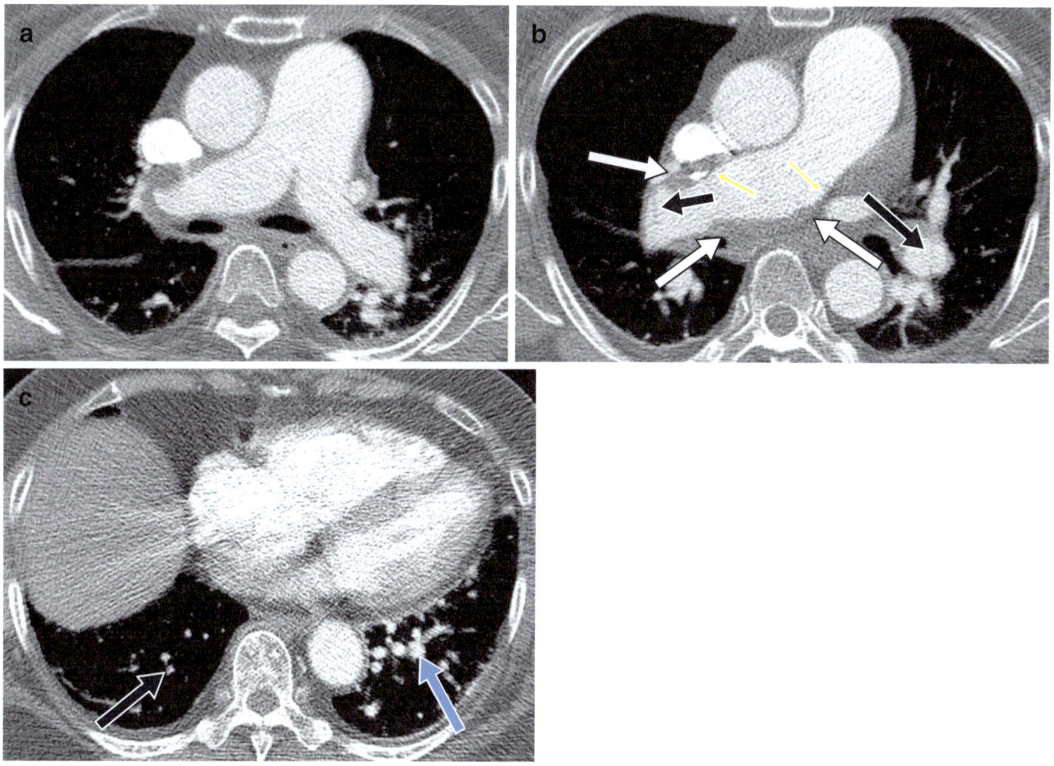

Fig. 10.4 Chronic pulmonary thromboembolism. (**a**) There is a pulmonary trunk dilatation, suggestive of pulmonary hypertension. (**b**) There are eccentric filling defects with calcifications (white arrows) and web-like filling defects (black arrows) in both pulmonary arteries. The thrombus forms obtuse angles (yellow arrows) with the vessel wall. These are imaging findings of chronic pulmonary thromboembolism. (**c**) Note that the diameters of the right pulmonary arteries (black arrow) are decreased when compared with those of the left pulmonary arteries (blue arrow)

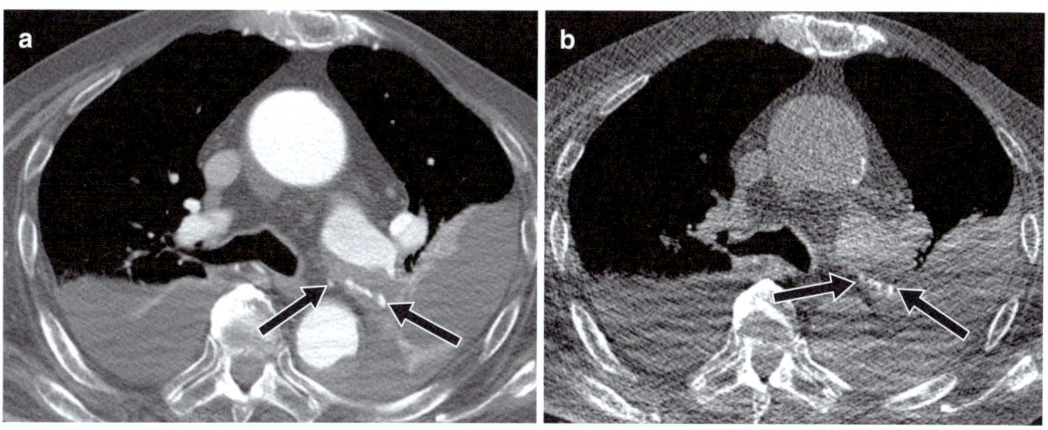

Fig. 10.5 Chronic pulmonary thromboembolism. (**a**, **b**) Chronic pulmonary thromboembolism may show calcifications (arrows) on chest CT

10.2.1.2 Severity and Right Ventricle Strain

The severity of PE can be stratified into high-risk/massive (PE causing hemodynamic compromise), intermediate-risk/sub-massive (no hemodynamic instability, PE causing right ventricular [RV] dysfunction demonstrated by echocardiography, CT, or elevated cardiac biomarkers), and low-risk/non-massive (PE without evidence of RV dysfunction or hemodynamic compromise) [16, 17]. High-risk PE warrants reperfusion treatment and hemodynamic support. Intermediate-risk PE requires hospitalization and monitoring, and rescue reperfusion may be considered if cardiopulmonary status deteriorates. Low-risk PE can be treated with standard anticoagulation medication on an outpatient basis.

RV failure due to acute pressure overload is considered the primary cause of death in severe PE and a critical determinant of outcome in acute PE. It is defined as a rapidly progressive syndrome with systemic congestion resulting from impaired RV filling and/or reduced RV flow output [18]. In patients without hemodynamic instability, a combination of RV dysfunction on an echocardiogram (or CT pulmonary angiography) (Fig. 10.6) with a positive cardiac troponin test is used to differentiate between intermediate- and

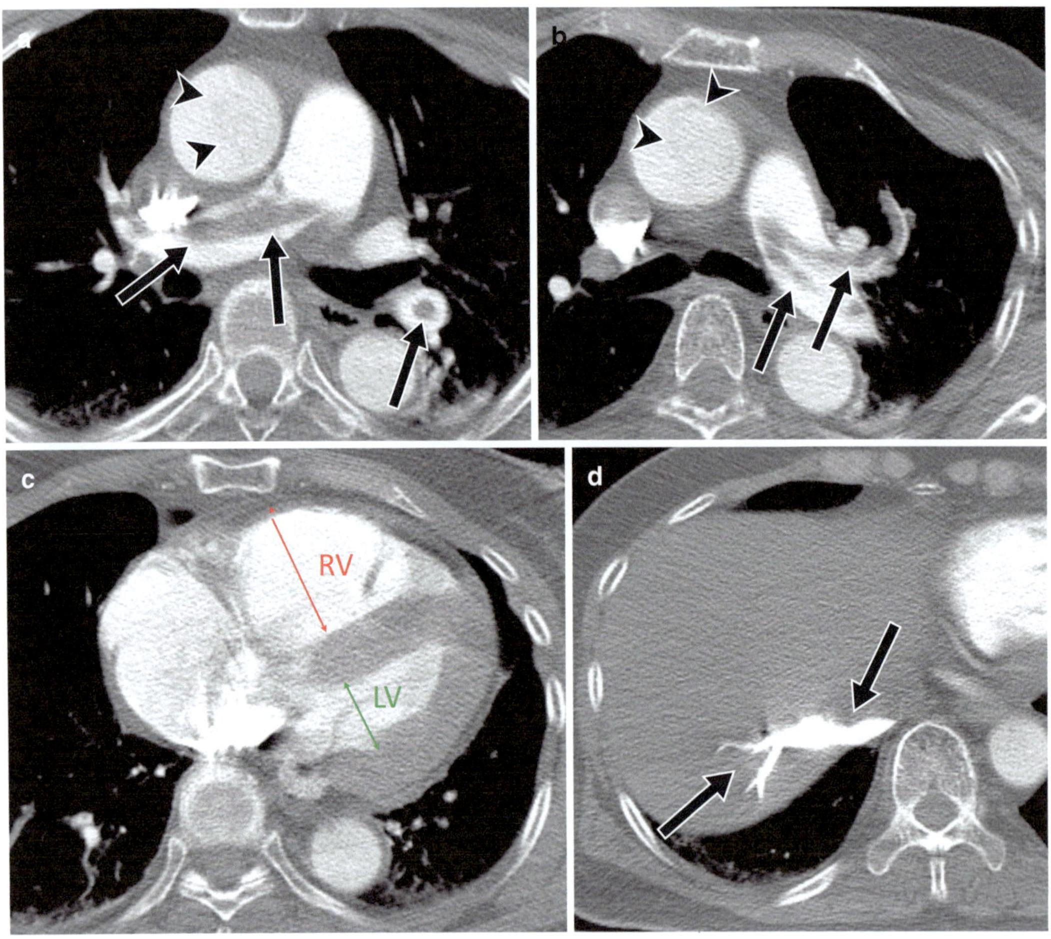

Fig. 10.6 Acute pulmonary thromboembolism with hemodynamic instability. (**a**, **b**) There are acute pulmonary thromboembolisms in the bilateral pulmonary main and lobar pulmonary arteries (arrows). There is also an intimal flap in the ascending aorta (arrowheads) due to aortic dissection. (**c**) In addition, there is right ventricle enlargement with interventricular septal straightening. The diameters of the right and left ventricles were measured at the largest points between the inner margins of the interventricular septum and the free wall. (**d**) There is contrast reflux into the inferior vena cava (arrows) due to right ventricle failure

low-risk PE [16]. This was applied as a guide for early therapeutic decisions (anticoagulation plus reperfusion treatment vs. anticoagulation alone) in a large randomized controlled trial of PE patients presenting without hemodynamic instability [19]. In this trial, fibrinolytic therapy prevented hemodynamic decompensation but increased the risk of major hemorrhage and stroke in patients with intermediate-risk PE.

Several CT pulmonary angiography parameters may be used to stratify risk in patients with PE: RV/LV diameter ratio, RV/LV volume ratio, RA/LA volume ratio, and contrast reflux into the inferior vena cava (Fig. 10.6). Generally, RV/LV ratios ≥1.0 on CT angiography indicate poor prognosis [16]. A meta-analysis of 49 studies investigating 13,162 patients with PE showed that an increased RV/LV ratio of ≥1.0 on CT was associated with a 2.5-fold increased risk for all-cause mortality (odds ratio [OR] 2.5, 95% CI 1.8–3.5) and with a fivefold increased risk for PE-related mortality (OR 5.0, 95% CI 2.7–9.2) [20]. Although mild RV dilation (RV/LV slightly above 0.9) on CT is a frequent finding (seen in >50% of hemodynamically stable PE patients) [21], increasing RV/LV diameter ratios are associated with rising prognostic specificity [22, 23], even in patients considered to be at low risk [21]. CT may provide further prognostic information based on volumetric analysis of the heart chambers [24–26] and assessment of contrast reflux into the inferior vena cava [20, 27, 28]. In a retrospective study that assessed the prognostic significance of clot volume, greater clot volume was associated with a higher incidence of right heart dilatation but was not significantly associated with patient mortality [29].

10.2.1.3 Subsegmental Pulmonary Arteries

Overdiagnosis of pulmonary embolism is an issue in the modern CT era [10]. The diagnostic value and clinical significance of isolated subsegmental contrast-filling defects

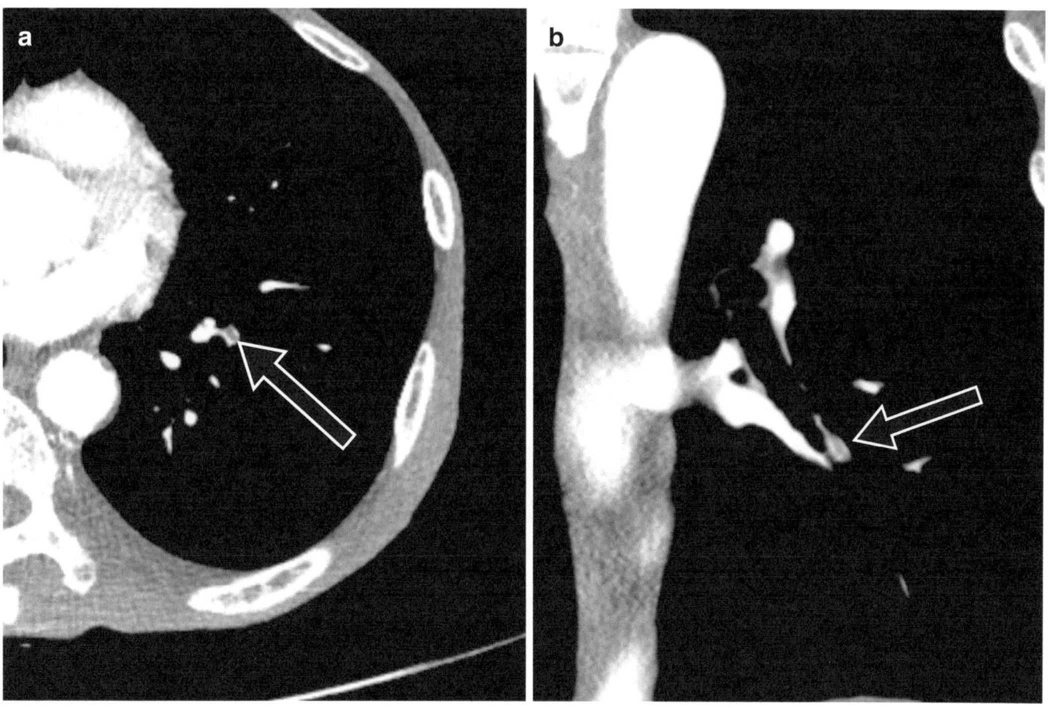

Fig. 10.7 Subsegmental pulmonary thromboembolism. (**a**, **b**) Chest CT shows pulmonary thromboembolism (arrow) in the left lower lobe subsegmental pulmonary artery

(Fig. 10.7) remain controversial. No robust data exist to indicate whether it is best to treat incidental PE with anticoagulants vs. close observation [16].

10.2.2 Iodine Maps from Dual-Energy CT or Subtraction CT

Iodine maps can be used to visualize blood perfusion abnormalities caused by acute or chronic PE [30–33] (Fig. 10.8). Iodine maps can be generated with dual-energy CT or subtraction CT. In a recent study of 1144 consecutive dual-energy CT examinations, dual-energy CT iodine maps showed a small incremental benefit for the detection of occlusive segmental and subsegmental pulmonary emboli [34]: 2.3% of the examinations ended in diagnosis of a new PE using iodine maps, resulting in a new diagnosis of PE in 1.1% of the patients. In another recent study, the addition of iodine maps also resulted in a small improvement in diagnostic performance beyond that obtained with CT angiography alone. This improvement in performance was due to an increase in specificity (subtraction CT, 100%; dual-energy CT, 95%; CT angiography alone, 94%; $P < 0.001$), while sensitivity was not higher for subtraction CT (83%) or dual-energy CT (85%) when compared with CT angiography alone (80%) ($P = 0.31$) [35].

10.2.3 Non-contrast CT

Although non-contrast chest CT is not a valid diagnostic modality for the detection of PE, recent studies showed that some centrally located embolisms may be recognizable even on non-contrast CT [36–39]. The incidental detection of a PE on non-contrast CT could be beneficial because patients with PE may not undergo contrast-enhanced CT as the symptoms of PE can be non-specific. The reported sensitivity (50–65%) and specificity (49–98.6%) are not very high [40, 41] but recognition of a hyperdense thrombus sometimes allows the diagnosis of acute PE in patients who underwent unenhanced chest CT for other suspected conditions [41] (Fig. 10.9).

10.3 Non-thrombotic Pulmonary Embolism

Non-thrombotic pulmonary embolism is much less common than thrombotic pulmonary embolism. Non-thrombotic pulmonary embolism is defined as embolization in the pulmonary circulation caused by a wide range of substances of endogenous and exogenous biological and non-biological origin and foreign bodies [42].

In addition to obstruction of the pulmonary vasculature, non-thrombotic pulmonary embolism

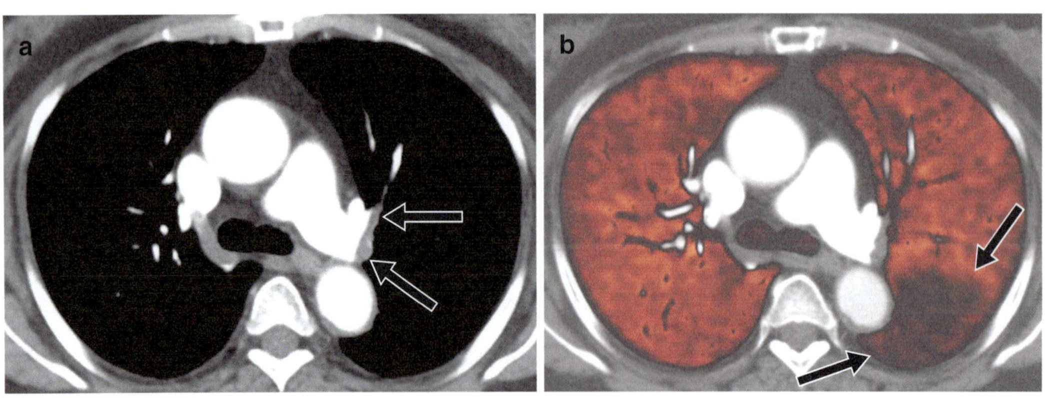

Fig. 10.8 Pulmonary thromboembolism on dual-energy CT. (**a**) CT pulmonary angiography shows a filling defect in the left distal main pulmonary artery (arrows), suggestive of thromboembolism. (**b**) Iodine perfusion map shows blood perfusion to the lung. There is a wedge-shaped perfusion defect in the left upper lobe (arrows)

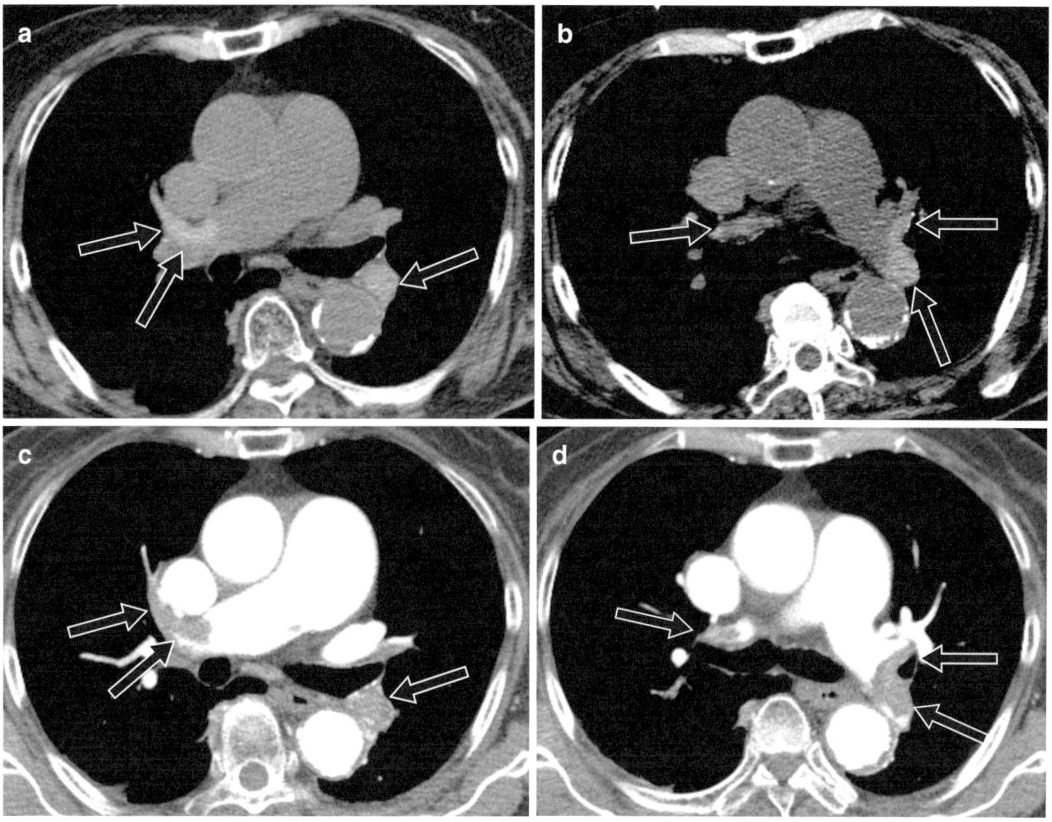

Fig. 10.9 Pulmonary thromboembolism on non-contrast CT. (**a**, **b**) Non-contrast CT shows high-attenuating filling lesions in the bilateral main and lobar pulmonary arteries (arrows). (**c**, **d**) Contrast-enhanced chest CT confirms bilateral acute pulmonary thromboembolism (arrows)

may be associated with an inflammatory cascade that deteriorates vascular, pulmonary, and cardiac function. The symptoms are similar to those of thrombotic PE and include dyspnea, tachycardia, chest pain, cough, and occasionally hemoptysis, cyanosis, and syncope. Diagnosis of non-thrombotic PE can be challenging. D-dimers are non-diagnostic because coagulation and fibrinolytic pathways are not activated. Small particles (micro-emboli) are not detectable on CT images.

10.3.1 Septic Embolism

Septic pulmonary embolism is caused by a thrombus that contains bacteria, fungi, or parasites [43]. These thrombi may lead to infarction and metastatic abscess [44]. Septic embolism occurs in patients with right-sided endocarditis [45], septic thrombophlebitis, infected central venous catheters or pacemaker wires [44], and intravenous drug use [43].

Radiographs show bilateral, peripheral lung nodules of varying size that tend to form cavities with moderately thick, irregular walls [44]. On serial radiographs, the lung nodules tend to develop and increase in size rapidly within several days. CT imaging features include patchy air space lesions like nonspecific bronchopneumonia and multiple subpleural round or wedge-shaped nodules of varying sizes. These nodules tend to be more numerous in the lower lobes and frequently form cavities [42] (Fig. 10.10). Septic embolism is often complicated by empyema [46, 47]. In many cases, a vessel can be seen leading directly to the nodules (feeding vessel sign [47]),

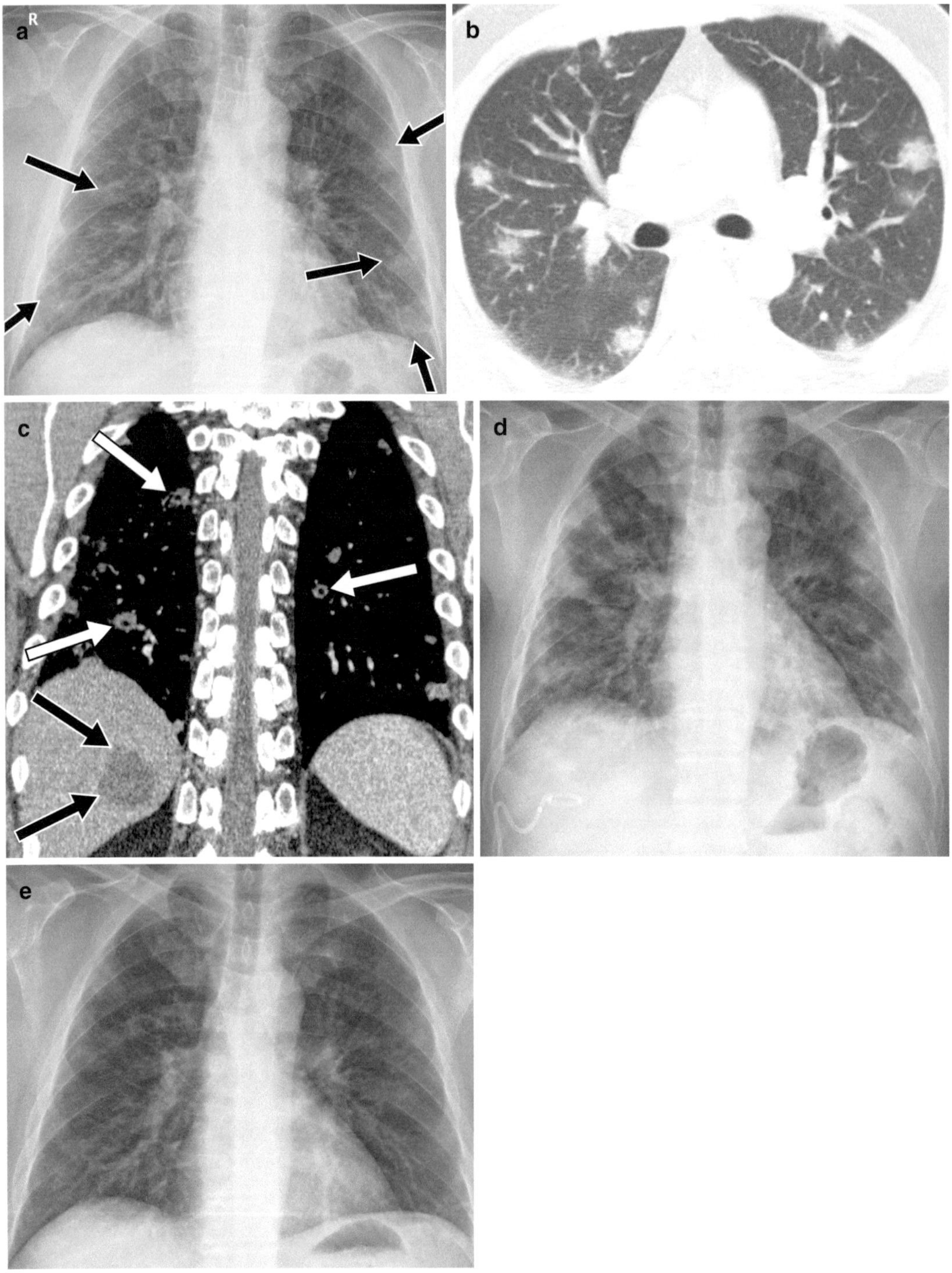

Fig. 10.10 Septic pneumonia. (**a**) Chest radiograph shows bilateral small nodular lesions in both lungs (arrows). (**b**) Chest CT shows bilateral ill-defined nodules in both lungs, which are distributed peripherally. (**c**) Cavitation is present inside some of the nodules (white arrows). There is also a hepatic abscess (black arrow). (**d**) Chest radiograph performed 3 days later shows an increase in the extent of the nodules and consolidations. (**e**) Follow-up chest radiograph performed 1 month later shows that most of the lesions disappeared

although this sign is not specific for septic pneumonia. There is no filling defect in the pulmonary arteries on CT and the condition is not associated with pulmonary hypertension. In the appropriate clinical context, diagnosis is based on identifying the source of septic emboli, positive blood culture tests, and chest radiograph or CT findings.

10.3.2 Fat Embolism

Fat embolism can occur in patients with pelvic or long bone fractures; those undergoing endomedullary nailing or placement of knee and hip prostheses; during lipid and propofol infusion, intraosseous infusion, or bone marrow harvest; in patients with pancreatitis; or after liposuction. The mechanisms of pulmonary involvement are twofold: (1) production of free fatty acid, which initiates a toxic reaction in the endothelium and (2) mechanical obstruction by fat globules and aggregates of red blood cells and platelets [14].

The classical triad of fat embolization consists of altered mental status, respiratory distress, and petechial rash; these symptoms typically appear 12–24 h after a traumatic event. Fat globules can be found in the blood, urine, sputum, bronchoalveolar lavage, and cerebrospinal fluid [48]. In most cases, fat embolisms in a pulmonary artery manifest as microembolisms. Imaging findings resemble those of acute respiratory distress syndrome and consist of widespread homogeneous and heterogeneous areas of increased opacity (Fig. 10.11) [49]. The time lapse between the traumatic event and presence of radiographic abnormalities is usually 1–2 days, which allows differentiation from traumatic contusion [50]. Small, ill-defined centrilobular, and subpleural

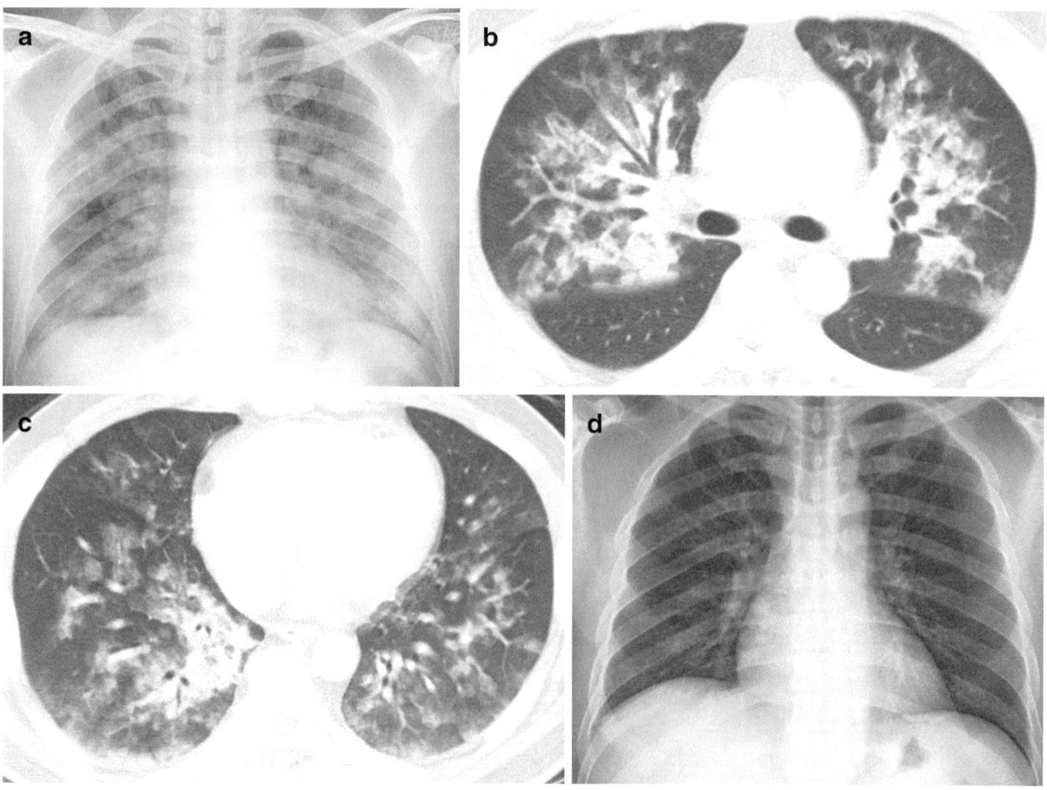

Fig. 10.11 Fat embolism in a patient who received fat implantation operation. (**a**) Chest radiograph shows multifocal increased opacities in bilateral lungs. (**b**, **c**) Chest CT shows multiple consolidations and ground-glass opacities in both lungs. Considering the patient's clinical history and imaging findings, the most probable diagnosis is fat embolism. (**d**) One week later, the lung opacities disappeared following conservative treatment

nodules can be seen, presumably representing alveolar edema, micro-hemorrhage, and an inflammatory response secondary to ischemia [51]. Normal heart size and absence of pleural effusion allow differentiation from cardiogenic pulmonary edema [46].

10.3.3 Air Embolism

Air embolization is often an iatrogenic complication which can occur following interventional procedures, surgery, or manipulation of central venous and hemodialysis catheters [52]. Most iatrogenic venous air embolisms that are related to intravenous contrast media/fluid injection involve a few milliliters of air and are asymptomatic. The lethal volume of injected air in humans is estimated to range from 300 to 500 mL injected at a rate of 100 mL/s [14, 46, 53]. If air enters the venous circulation, it passes through the right side of the heart and into the pulmonary arteries. Small air bubbles are absorbed by the pulmonary circulation and have few consequences or symptoms [54]. Moderately sized air bubbles, however, may cause pulmonary vascular damage leading to pulmonary hypertension and pulmonary edema [55]. A large bolus of air in the venous system cannot be absorbed and causes obstruction of the RV outflow tract [56]. When an air embolism enters the left side of the heart and arterial circulation, it may have fatal consequences when it proceeds to the cerebral and coronary circulations [56]. On chest CT, air bubbles may be seen in the systemic veins, right side of the heart, or main pulmonary arteries [42]. When arterial air embolization occurs, air bubbles and brain infarction may be visualized on brain CT or MRI (Figs. 10.12 and 10.13).

10.3.4 Tumor Embolism

Pulmonary intravascular tumor emboli are seen in ≤26% of autopsies of patients with solid malignancies, although the diagnosis is rarely made before death [57]. Common extrapulmonary malignancies that cause pulmonary tumor emboli include hepatocellular carcinoma, breast, renal, stomach, and prostate carcinoma, and choriocarcinoma [58]. On CT, a vascular tree-in-bud appearance is seen when the tumor cells fill in the centrilobular arteries (Fig. 10.14). When the tumor cells are located in more proximal pulmonary arteries, intravascular filling defects within the pulmonary arteries can be directly visualized (Fig. 10.14). Although it is not always possible to distinguish between intravascular tumor embo-

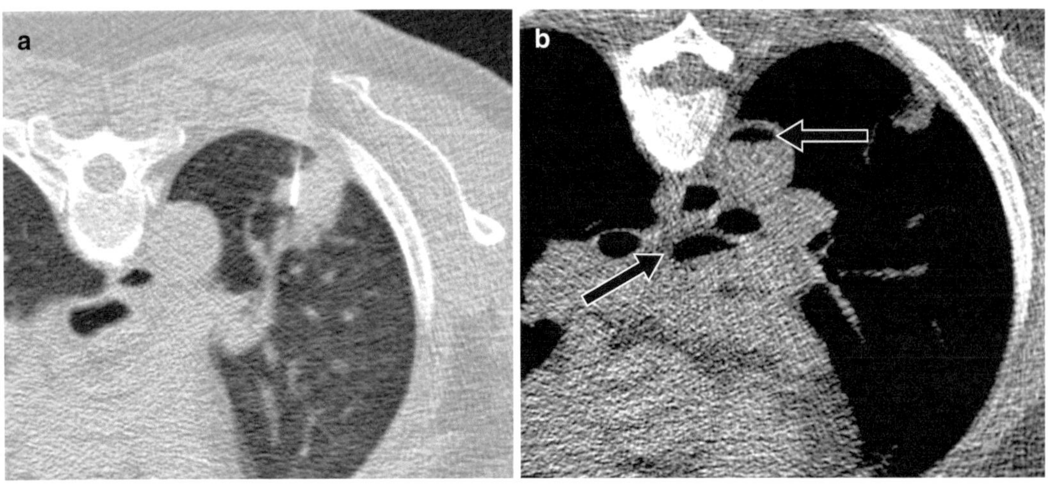

Fig. 10.12 Air embolism after percutaneous transthoracic needle lung biopsy. (**a**) CT-guided percutaneous transthoracic needle lung biopsy was performed. (**b**) Post-biopsy CT images show newly formed air bubbles in the aorta and pulmonary vein (arrows)

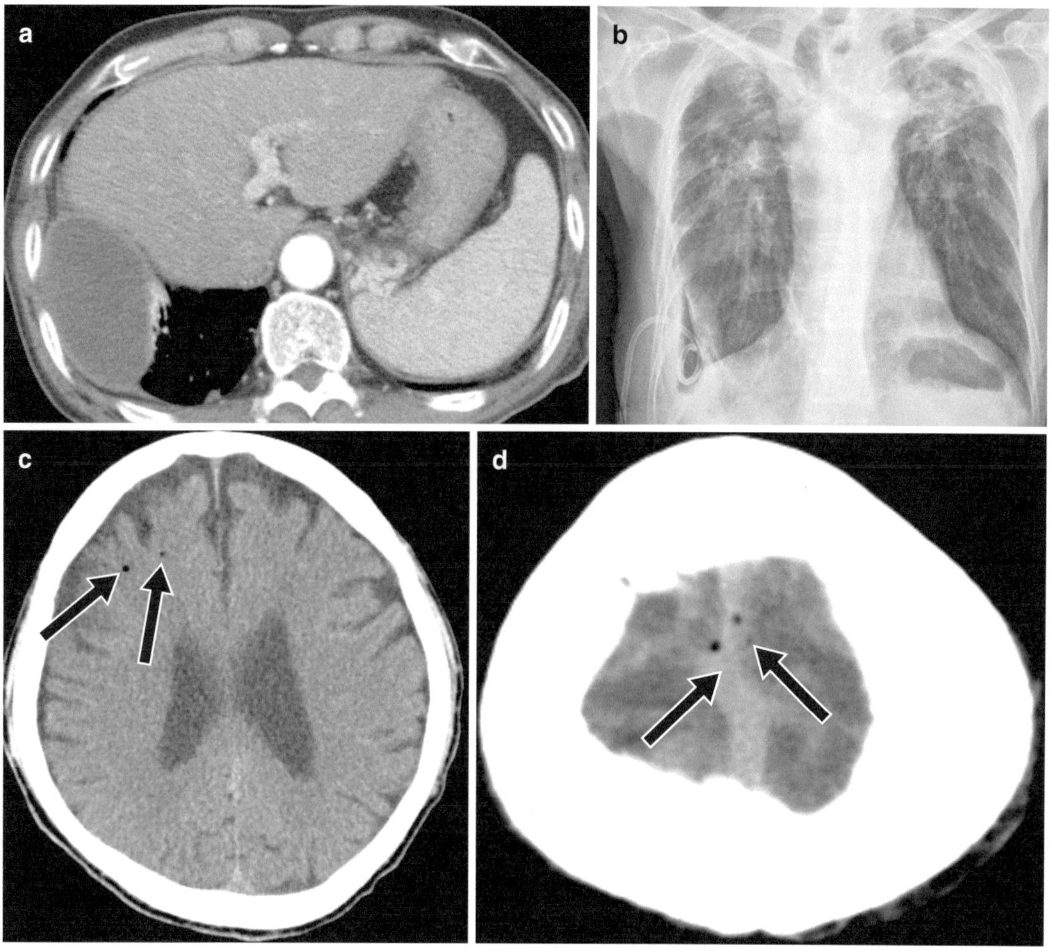

Fig. 10.13 Air embolism after pleural fibrinolysis. (**a**) Chest CT shows right loculated pleural effusion. (**b**) A chest pigtail catheter was inserted and pleural fibrinolysis was performed. After injection of the fibrinolytic agent, the patient complained of arm weakness. (**c**, **d**) Brain CT shows multiple air densities in the right fronto-parietal lobe and superior sagittal sinus, representing the air embolism

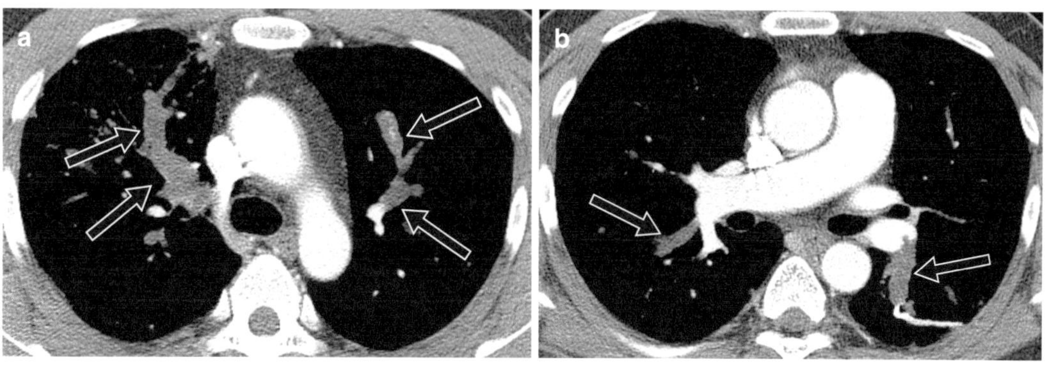

Fig. 10.14 Intravascular tumor embolism from chondrosarcoma. (**a**, **b**) There are multiple filling defects inside both pulmonary arteries (arrows). Note that the diameters of the pulmonary arteries are increased and some of the filling defects show mild contrast enhancement. (**c**, **d**) There are also nodular and branching opacities (arrows), which is the vascular tree-in-bud sign. These reflect intravascular tumor embolisms in the centrilobular arteries

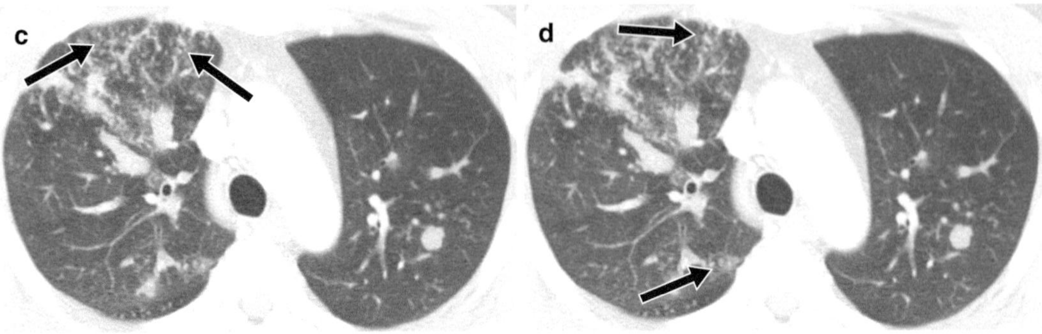

Fig. 10.14 (continued)

lism and pulmonary thromboembolism, intravascular tumor embolism may show mild contrast enhancement, a more pronounced increase in the diameter of the affected pulmonary artery, gradual increase in size on serial CT, vascular tree-in-bud sign, and increased fluorodeoxyglucose uptake on positron emission tomography. Treatment should target the underlying malignant disease. Anticoagulant treatment is often prescribed in this context because tumor embolism and thromboembolism are difficult to differentiate.

Pulmonary tumor thrombotic microangiopathy (PTTM) is a distinct but rare form of tumor embolism that has an extremely poor prognosis. It was first described by von Herbay et al. in 1990 [59] and is being increasingly recognized as a serious complication of advanced cancers. Clinically, it is characterized by acute dyspnea and pulmonary hypertension, which almost invariably progresses to right heart strain and cardiorespiratory arrest in hours to days.

Pathologically, it is characterized by widespread microscopic (usually non-occlusive) small tumor emboli in the pulmonary arterioles. It can be distinguished from conventional tumor emboli by the histopathological finding of diffuse intimal myofibroblast proliferation in small pulmonary arteries [59, 60]. Eventually, stenosis and/or occlusion occur, and an increase in pulmonary vascular resistance results in pulmonary hypertension and disseminated intravascular coagulation [61]. Conventional tumor embolism involves vascular obstruction by tumor emboli but intimal proliferation is not observed.

PTTM most commonly arises from gastric adenocarcinomas (around 60%), often those of the signet ring cell subtype. PTTM has also been reported in patients with lung, breast, colon, pancreas, prostate, gallbladder, liver, and bladder cancers [59, 62, 63]. More than 90% of cases are adenocarcinomas.

PTTM does not manifest as a filling defect in the pulmonary artery on CT, as the tumor emboli are microscopic. The radiological findings on CT are diffuse centrilobular nodular opacities in a tree-in-bud pattern throughout the bilateral lungs. The differential diagnosis for these diffuse centrilobular nodular opacities includes various diseases, but in PTTM, there are additional signs of right ventricle strain and pulmonary hypertension (Fig. 10.15). Positron emission tomography may show multifocal abnormal fluorodeoxyglucose uptake in both lungs [64]. Unfortunately, few patients survive beyond the initial acute phase and little is known regarding the optimal therapeutic strategy for treatment of PTTM.

10.4 Summary

CT pulmonary angiography is the method of choice for visualizing the pulmonary vasculature in patients with suspected PE. Thus, the ability to accurately diagnose PE on CT is crucial. Both false-positive and false-negative results are harmful to patients. Based on CT findings, it is possible to differentiate between acute and chronic PE.

The severity of PE is stratified into high-risk/massive (PE causing hemodynamic compromise), intermediate-risk/submassive (no hemodynamic

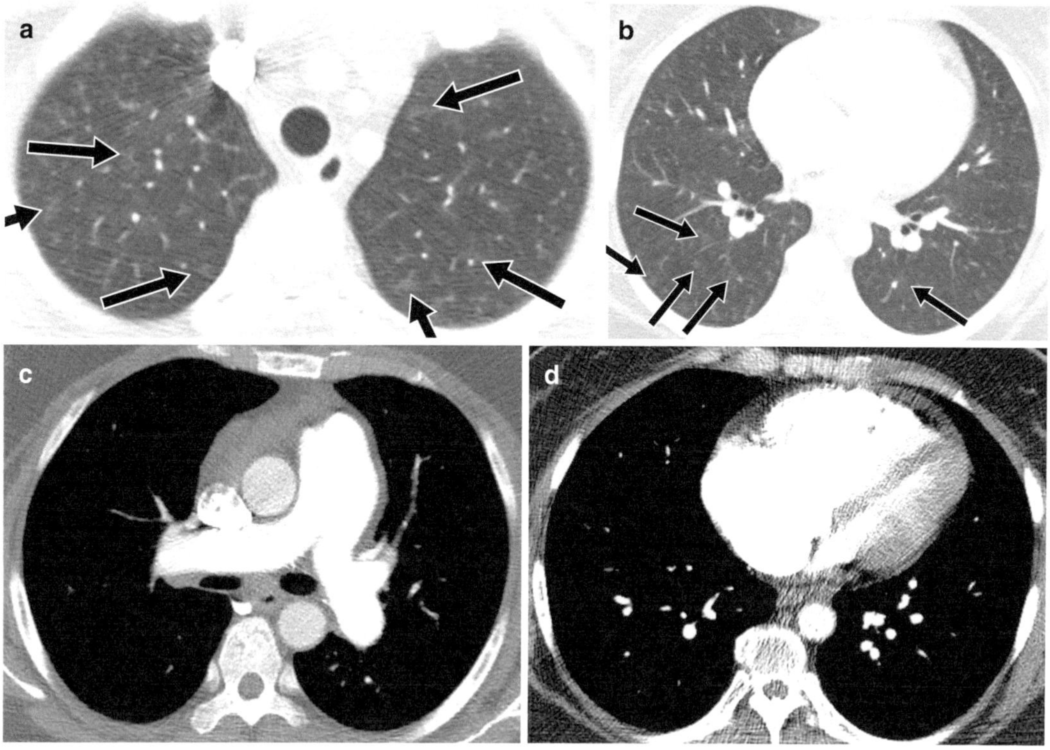

Fig. 10.15 Pulmonary tumor thrombotic microangiopathy in a 37-year-old woman who presented with dyspnea. This patient had underlying advanced gastric cancer. (**a**, **b**) Multifocal, centrilobular ground-glass opacity nodules (arrows) are present in both lungs. (**c**) There is dilatation of the pulmonary trunk but no filling defect in the pulmonary arteries. (**d**) There is also severe dilatation of the right ventricle, suggestive of right ventricle strain

instability, PE causing right ventricular [RV] dysfunction demonstrated by echocardiography, CT, or elevated cardiac biomarkers), and low-risk/non-massive (PE without evidence of RV dysfunction or hemodynamic compromise). Thus, it is important to mention whether there are imaging findings suggestive of right ventricle dysfunction (RV/LV ratios ≥1.0, contrast reflux into the inferior vena cava) on CT in patients with PE.

Representative types of non-thrombotic PE include septic pneumonia, fat embolism, air embolism, and tumor embolism. Of these, pulmonary tumor thrombotic microangiopathy (PTTM) has an extremely poor prognosis. In patients with PTTM, CT shows diffuse centrilobular nodular opacities in a tree-in-bud pattern throughout the bilateral lungs. Importantly, there are additional signs of right ventricle strain and pulmonary hypertension.

Key Points

- *Acute* versus *chronic PE*
- Acute PE: (1) Increased diameter of the pulmonary artery; (2) eccentric filling defects form acute angles with respect to the vessel wall; (3) presence of pulmonary infarction.
- Chronic PE: (1) Decreased diameter of the pulmonary artery, (2) intimal irregularities, bands and webs, and abrupt vessel narrowing; (3) obtuse angles with the vessel wall; (4) calcification; and (5) a mosaic perfusion pattern in the lung parenchyma.
- Pulmonary infarction manifests as wedge-shaped peripheral consolidation or ground-glass opacity with central lucency on CT.
- The presence of right ventricle dysfunction (RV/LV ratios ≥1.0, contrast reflux into the inferior vena cava) should be evaluated on CT in patients with PE.

References

1. Turetz M, Sideris AT, Friedman OA, Triphathi N, Horowitz JM. Epidemiology, pathophysiology, and natural history of pulmonary embolism. Semin Intervent Radiol. 2018;35(2):92–8. https://doi.org/10.1055/s-0038-1642036.
2. Calder KK, Herbert M, Henderson SO. The mortality of untreated pulmonary embolism in emergency department patients. Ann Emerg Med. 2005;45(3):302–10. https://doi.org/10.1016/j.annemergmed.2004.10.001.
3. Pena E, Dennie C. Acute and chronic pulmonary embolism: an in-depth review for radiologists through the use of frequently asked questions. Semin Ultrasound CT MR. 2012;33(6):500–21. https://doi.org/10.1053/j.sult.2012.06.001.
4. Wiener RS, Schwartz LM, Woloshin S. When a test is too good: how CT pulmonary angiograms find pulmonary emboli that do not need to be found. BMJ. 2013;347:f3368. https://doi.org/10.1136/bmj.f3368.
5. Wiener RS, Schwartz LM, Woloshin S. Time trends in pulmonary embolism in the United States: evidence of overdiagnosis. Arch Intern Med. 2011;171(9):831–7. https://doi.org/10.1001/archinternmed.2011.178.
6. Stein PD, Fowler SE, Goodman LR, et al. Multidetector computed tomography for acute pulmonary embolism. N Engl J Med. 2006;354(22):2317–27. https://doi.org/10.1056/NEJMoa052367.
7. Quiroz R, Kucher N, Zou KH, et al. Clinical validity of a negative computed tomography scan in patients with suspected pulmonary embolism: a systematic review. JAMA. 2005;293(16):2012–7. https://doi.org/10.1001/jama.293.16.2012.
8. van Belle A, Büller HR, Huisman MV, et al. Effectiveness of managing suspected pulmonary embolism using an algorithm combining clinical probability, D-dimer testing and computed tomography. JAMA. 2006;295(2):172–9. https://doi.org/10.1001/jama.295.2.172.
9. Wittram C, Kalra MK, Maher MM, Greenfield A, McLoud TC, Shepard JA. Acute and chronic pulmonary emboli: angiography-CT correlation. AJR Am J Roentgenol. 2006;186(6 Suppl 2):S421–9. https://doi.org/10.2214/ajr.04.1955.
10. Yazdani M, Lau CT, Lempel JK, et al. Historical evolution of imaging techniques for the evaluation of pulmonary embolism. Radiographics. 2015;35(4):1245–62. https://doi.org/10.1148/rg.2015140280.
11. He H, Stein MW, Zalta B, Haramati LB. Pulmonary infarction: spectrum of findings on multidetector helical CT. J Thorac Imaging. 2006;21(1):1–7. https://doi.org/10.1097/01.rti.0000187433.06762.fb.
12. Revel MP, Triki R, Chatellier G, et al. Is it possible to recognize pulmonary infarction on multisection CT images? Radiology. 2007;244(3):875–82. https://doi.org/10.1148/radiol.2443060846.
13. Schwickert HC, Schweden F, Schild HH, et al. Pulmonary arteries and lung parenchyma in chronic pulmonary embolism: preoperative and postoperative CT findings. Radiology. 1994;191(2):351–7. https://doi.org/10.1148/radiology.191.2.8153305.
14. Han D, Lee KS, Franquet T, et al. Thrombotic and nonthrombotic pulmonary arterial embolism: spectrum of imaging findings. Radiographics. 2003;23(6):1521–39. https://doi.org/10.1148/rg.1103035043.
15. King MA, Ysrael M, Bergin CJ. Chronic thromboembolic pulmonary hypertension: CT findings. AJR Am J Roentgenol. 1998;170(4):955–60. https://doi.org/10.2214/ajr.170.4.9530043.
16. Konstantinides SV, Meyer G, Becattini C, et al. ESC guidelines for the diagnosis and management of acute pulmonary embolism developed in collaboration with the European Respiratory Society (ERS): the task force for the diagnosis and management of acute pulmonary embolism of the European Society of Cardiology (ESC). Eur Respir J. 2019;54(3) https://doi.org/10.1183/13993003.01647-2019.
17. Jaff MR, McMurtry MS, Archer SL, et al. Management of massive and submassive pulmonary embolism, iliofemoral deep vein thrombosis, and chronic thromboembolic pulmonary hypertension: a scientific statement from the American Heart Association. Circulation. 2011;123(16):1788–830. https://doi.org/10.1161/CIR.0b013e318214914f.
18. Harjola VP, Mebazaa A, Čelutkienė J, et al. Contemporary management of acute right ventricular failure: a statement from the heart failure association and the working group on pulmonary circulation and right ventricular function of the European Society of Cardiology. Eur J Heart Fail. 2016;18(3):226–41. https://doi.org/10.1002/ejhf.478.
19. Meyer G, Vicaut E, Danays T, et al. Fibrinolysis for patients with intermediate-risk pulmonary embolism. N Engl J Med. 2014;370(15):1402–11. https://doi.org/10.1056/NEJMoa1302097.
20. Meinel FG, Nance JW Jr, Schoepf UJ, et al. Predictive value of computed tomography in acute pulmonary embolism: systematic review and meta-analysis. Am J Med. 2015;128(7):747–759.e742. https://doi.org/10.1016/j.amjmed.2015.01.023.
21. Côté B, Jiménez D, Planquette B, et al. Prognostic value of right ventricular dilatation in patients with low-risk pulmonary embolism. Eur Respir J. 2017;50(6) https://doi.org/10.1183/13993003.01611-2017.
22. George E, Kumamaru KK, Ghosh N, et al. Computed tomography and echocardiography in patients with acute pulmonary embolism: part 2: prognostic value. J Thorac Imaging. 2014;29(1):W7–12. https://doi.org/10.1097/rti.0000000000000048.
23. Etesamifard N, Shirani S, Jenab Y, Lotfi-Tokaldany M, Pourjafari M, Jalali A. Role of clinical and pulmonary computed tomography angiographic parameters in the prediction of short- and long-term mortality in patients with pulmonary embolism. Intern Emerg Med. 2016;11(3):405–13. https://doi.org/10.1007/s11739-015-1376-4.
24. Aviram G, Soikher E, Bendet A, et al. Prediction of mortality in pulmonary embolism based on left atrial

volume measured on CT pulmonary angiography. Chest. 2016;149(3):667–75. https://doi.org/10.1378/chest.15-0666.

25. Aviram G, Sirota-Cohen C, Steinvil A, et al. Automated volumetric analysis of four cardiac chambers in pulmonary embolism: a novel technology for fast risk stratification. Thromb Haemost. 2012;108(2):384–93. https://doi.org/10.1160/th11-07-0452.
26. Kang DK, Thilo C, Schoepf UJ, et al. CT signs of right ventricular dysfunction: prognostic role in acute pulmonary embolism. JACC Cardiovasc Imaging. 2011;4(8):841–9. https://doi.org/10.1016/j.jcmg.2011.04.013.
27. Bach AG, Nansalmaa B, Kranz J, et al. CT pulmonary angiography findings that predict 30-day mortality in patients with acute pulmonary embolism. Eur J Radiol. 2015;84(2):332–7. https://doi.org/10.1016/j.ejrad.2014.11.023.
28. Aviram G, Cohen D, Steinvil A, et al. Significance of reflux of contrast medium into the inferior vena cava on computerized tomographic pulmonary angiogram. Am J Cardiol. 2012;109(3):432–7. https://doi.org/10.1016/j.amjcard.2011.09.033.
29. Furlan A, Aghayev A, Chang CC, et al. Short-term mortality in acute pulmonary embolism: clot burden and signs of right heart dysfunction at CT pulmonary angiography. Radiology. 2012;265(1):283–93. https://doi.org/10.1148/radiol.12110802.
30. Pontana F, Faivre JB, Remy-Jardin M, et al. Lung perfusion with dual-energy multidetector-row CT (MDCT): feasibility for the evaluation of acute pulmonary embolism in 117 consecutive patients. Acad Radiol. 2008;15(12):1494–504. https://doi.org/10.1016/j.acra.2008.05.018.
31. Zhang LJ, Chai X, Wu SY, et al. Detection of pulmonary embolism by dual energy CT: correlation with perfusion scintigraphy and histopathological findings in rabbits. Eur Radiol. 2009;19(12):2844–54. https://doi.org/10.1007/s00330-009-1518-z.
32. Zhang LJ, Zhou CS, Schoepf UJ, et al. Dual-energy CT lung ventilation/perfusion imaging for diagnosing pulmonary embolism. Eur Radiol. 2013;23(10):2666–75. https://doi.org/10.1007/s00330-013-2907-x.
33. Chae EJ, Seo JB, Jang YM, et al. Dual-energy CT for assessment of the severity of acute pulmonary embolism: pulmonary perfusion defect score compared with CT angiographic obstruction score and right ventricular/left ventricular diameter ratio. AJR Am J Roentgenol. 2010;194(3):604–10. https://doi.org/10.2214/ajr.09.2681.
34. Weidman EK, Plodkowski AJ, Halpenny DF, et al. Dual-energy CT angiography for detection of pulmonary emboli: incremental benefit of iodine maps. Radiology. 2018;289(2):546–53. https://doi.org/10.1148/radiol.2018180594.
35. Grob D, Smit E, Prince J, et al. Iodine maps from subtraction CT or dual-energy CT to detect pulmonary emboli with CT angiography: a multiple-observer study. Radiology. 2019;292(1):197–205. https://doi.org/10.1148/radiol.2019182666.
36. Tatco VR, Piedad HH. The validity of hyperdense lumen sign in non-contrast chest CT scans in the detection of pulmonary thromboembolism. Int J Cardiovasc Imaging. 2011;27(3):433–40. https://doi.org/10.1007/s10554-010-9673-5.
37. Kanne JP, Gotway MB, Thoongsuwan N, Stern EJ. Six cases of acute central pulmonary embolism revealed on unenhanced multidetector CT of the chest. AJR Am J Roentgenol. 2003;180(6):1661–4. https://doi.org/10.2214/ajr.180.6.1801661.
38. Gotway M, Webb W. Acute pulmonary embolism: visualization of high attenuation clot in the pulmonary artery on noncontrast helical chest CT. Emergency Radiol. 2000;7(2):117–9.
39. Cobelli R, Zompatori M, De Luca G, Chiari G, Bresciani P, Marcato C. Clinical usefulness of computed tomography study without contrast injection in the evaluation of acute pulmonary embolism. J Comput Assist Tomogr. 2005;29(1):6–12. https://doi.org/10.1097/01.rct.0000148274.45419.95.
40. Sun S, Semionov A, Xie X, Kosiuk J, Mesurolle B. Detection of central pulmonary embolism on non-contrast computed tomography: a case control study. Int J Cardiovasc Imaging. 2014;30(3):639–46. https://doi.org/10.1007/s10554-013-0356-x.
41. Mohamed ND, Othman MH, Hassan LS, Yousef HA. The accuracy of non-contrast chest computed tomographic scan in the detection of pulmonary thromboembolism. J Curr Med Res Pract. 2019;4(1):61–6. https://doi.org/10.4103/JCMRP.JCMRP_13_19.
42. Bach AG, Restrepo CS, Abbas J, et al. Imaging of nonthrombotic pulmonary embolism: biological materials, nonbiological materials, and foreign bodies. Eur J Radiol. 2013;82(3):e120–41. https://doi.org/10.1016/j.ejrad.2012.09.019.
43. Sakuma M, Sugimura K, Nakamura M, et al. Unusual pulmonary embolism: septic pulmonary embolism and amniotic fluid embolism. Circ J. 2007;71(5):772–5. https://doi.org/10.1253/circj.71.772.
44. Riordan T, Wilson M. Lemierre's syndrome: more than a historical curiosa. Postgrad Med J. 2004;80(944):328–34. https://doi.org/10.1136/pgmj.2003.014274.
45. Cook RJ, Ashton RW, Aughenbaugh GL, Ryu JH. Septic pulmonary embolism: presenting features and clinical course of 14 patients. Chest. 2005;128(1):162–6. https://doi.org/10.1378/chest.128.1.162.
46. Rossi SE, Goodman PC, Franquet T. Nonthrombotic pulmonary emboli. AJR Am J Roentgenol. 2000;174(6):1499–508. https://doi.org/10.2214/ajr.174.6.1741499.
47. Kuhlman JE, Fishman EK, Teigen C. Pulmonary septic emboli: diagnosis with CT. Radiology. 1990;174(1):211–3. https://doi.org/10.1148/radiology.174.1.2294550.
48. Jorens PG, Van Marck E, Snoeckx A, Parizel PM. Nonthrombotic pulmonary embolism. Eur Respir J. 2009;34(2):452–74. https://doi.org/10.1183/09031936.00141708.

49. Parisi DM, Koval K, Egol K. Fat embolism syndrome. Am J Orthop (Belle Mead, NJ). 2002;31(9):507–12.
50. Muller NL, Fraser RS, Colman NC, Pare PD. Radiologic diagnosis of diseases of the chest. 1st ed. Philadelphia: Saunders; 2001. p. 378–409.
51. Van den Brande FG, Hellemans S, De Schepper A, et al. Post-traumatic severe fat embolism syndrome with uncommon CT findings. Anaesth Intensive Care. 2006;34(1):102–6. https://doi.org/10.1177/0310057x0603400120.
52. Unal E, Balci S, Atceken Z, Akpinar E, Ariyurek OM. Nonthrombotic pulmonary artery embolism: imaging findings and review of the literature. AJR Am J Roentgenol. 2017;208(3):505–16. https://doi.org/10.2214/ajr.16.17326.
53. Orebaugh SL. Venous air embolism: clinical and experimental considerations. Crit Care Med. 1992;20(8):1169–77. https://doi.org/10.1097/00003246-199208000-00017.
54. Khan H, Zaidi A. Paradoxical air embolism following central venous catheter removal. BMJ Case Rep. 2013; https://doi.org/10.1136/bcr-2013-200630.
55. Fitchet A, Fitzpatrick AP. Central venous air embolism causing pulmonary oedema mimicking left ventricular failure. BMJ. 1998;316(7131):604–6. https://doi.org/10.1136/bmj.316.7131.604.
56. Muth CM, Shank ES. Gas embolism. N Engl J Med. 2000;342(7):476–82. https://doi.org/10.1056/nejm200002173420706.
57. Roberts KE, Hamele-Bena D, Saqi A, Stein CA, Cole RP. Pulmonary tumor embolism: a review of the literature. Am J Med. 2003;115(3):228–32. https://doi.org/10.1016/s0002-9343(03)00305-x.
58. Schriner RW, Ryu JH, Edwards WD. Microscopic pulmonary tumor embolism causing subacute cor pulmonale: a difficult antemortem diagnosis. Mayo Clin Proc. 1991;66(2):143–8. https://doi.org/10.1016/s0025-6196(12)60485-6.
59. von Herbay A, Illes A, Waldherr R, Otto HF. Pulmonary tumor thrombotic microangiopathy with pulmonary hypertension. Cancer. 1990;66(3):587–92. https://doi.org/10.1002/1097-0142(19900801)66:3<587::aid-cncr2820660330>3.0.co;2-j.
60. Sato Y, Marutsuka K, Asada Y, Yamada M, Setoguchi T, Sumiyoshi A. Pulmonary tumor thrombotic microangiopathy. Pathol Int. 1995;45(6):436–40. https://doi.org/10.1111/j.1440-1827.1995.tb03481.x.
61. Uruga H, Fujii T, Kurosaki A, et al. Pulmonary tumor thrombotic microangiopathy: a clinical analysis of 30 autopsy cases. Intern Med. 2013;52(12):1317–23. https://doi.org/10.2169/internalmedicine.52.9472.
62. Malani AK, Gupta C, Kutty AV, Betlej T. Pulmonary tumor thrombotic microangiopathy from metastatic gallbladder carcinoma: an unusual cause of severe pulmonary hypertension. Dig Dis Sci. 2007;52(2):555–7. https://doi.org/10.1007/s10620-006-9232-z.
63. Ho AL, Szulakowski P, Mohamid WH. The diagnostic challenge of pulmonary tumour thrombotic microangiopathy as a presentation for metastatic gastric cancer: a case report and review of the literature. BMC Cancer. 2015;15:450. https://doi.org/10.1186/s12885-015-1467-7.
64. Tashima Y, Abe K, Matsuo Y, et al. Pulmonary tumor thrombotic microangiopathy: FDG-PET/CT findings. Clin Nucl Med. 2009;34(3):175–7. https://doi.org/10.1097/RLU.0b013e3181966f5c.

11 Noninfectious Pulmonary Emergency

11.1 Introduction

Fever is one of the most common complaints in patients who seek help in the emergency department (ED), accounting for approximately 15% of ED visits in the elderly and 5% in adults [1]. Even though many patients who present to the ED with fever have some kind of infection as an underlying disease, fever can also have noninfectious causes. Two noninfectious conditions that elicit fever and related pulmonary abnormalities and lead to ED visits are connective tissue disease (CTD) and malignant conditions such as leukemia including capillary leak syndrome and lymphoma with bilateral lung abnormalities [2]. Other conditions that cause pulmonary emergency without infection include drug-related pneumonitis, radiation pneumonitis, cardiogenic or renal and neurogenic pulmonary edema, diffuse alveolar hemorrhage, adult respiratory distress syndrome and acute interstitial pneumonia, fat embolism, acute eosinophilic pneumonia, and organizing pneumonia. In this chapter, after dividing all conditions into those in immunocompetent and immunocompromised hosts, the imaging features of each noninfectious pulmonary emergency are described and discriminated from those of infectious diseases that lead to ED visits.

11.2 Causes of Noninfectious Pulmonary Emergency

11.2.1 Immunocompetent Individuals

Pulmonary edema is a frequent noninfectious pulmonary emergency. Heart failure, volume excess and overload, and capillary leak syndrome are related to pulmonary edema. Neurogenic pulmonary edema refers to an increase in pulmonary interstitial and alveolar fluid due to an acute central nervous system injury, which usually develops rapidly after the injury [3]. It is sometimes classified as a form of acute respiratory distress syndrome (ARDS), but the two conditions differ in their pathophysiology and prognosis.

Drug-related pneumonitis (DRP) is also a common cause of ED visits. Individuals treated with molecular targeting agents and immune checkpoint inhibitors (ICIs) occasionally experience drug-related pneumonitis. Conventional cytotoxic drugs that are given to patients with a malignancy are associated with pneumonitis. Cytotoxic antibiotics, such as bleomycin and mitomycin, are also commonly involved. Nitrosourea, methotrexate, and alkylating agents (e.g., cyclophosphamide, busulfan, and chlorambucil) are also responsible for lung toxicity.

Radiation pneumonitis is the acute manifestation of radiation-induced lung disease and is relatively common following radiotherapy of the chest wall or an intrathoracic malignancy.

T. J. Kim et al., *Emergency Chest Radiology*, https://doi.org/10.1007/978-981-33-4396-2_11

Radiation pneumonitis typically occurs between 4 and 12 weeks following completion of therapy. However, the condition may be seen as early as 1 week after therapy, particularly in patients receiving a high total dose and who received chemotherapy concurrently.

A fat embolism (FE) is a piece of intravascular fat that lodges within a blood vessel and blocks blood flow. Fat emboli commonly occur after fractures of long bones in the lower body, particularly the femur, tibia, and pelvic bones. While fat emboli are common and generally resolve on their own, they can lead to a serious condition called fat embolism syndrome (FES). FES can cause inflammation, multi-organ dysfunction, and neurological changes that can be deadly. According to research, FES can be seen in 3%–4% of those with one long-bone fracture and up to 15% of those with multiple long-bone traumas.

Diffuse alveolar hemorrhage (DAH) is a common occurrence among thrombocytopenia patients. Approximately 60% of leukemia patients have pulmonary hemorrhage at autopsy, most commonly those with platelet counts <20,000/mm^3.

Connective tissue diseases (CTDs) and pulmonary vasculitis are frequent causes of fever and lung abnormalities seen in the ED.

11.2.2 Immunocompromised Individuals

Idiopathic pneumonia syndrome (IPS) is a noninfectious pulmonary complication with diffuse lung injury that is often seen after hematopoietic stem cell transplantation (HSCT) [4]. The incidence rate of IPS after allogenic HSCT is 4%–12%; the mortality rate from IPS is quite high, at 50%–90% [5–8].

Malignancies are frequently encountered in the ED and are indicated by the combination of lung abnormalities on imaging studies and fever. Particularly in leukemia and lymphoma, lung involvement can be identified with fever.

Lung transplantation, which has a three-year overall survival rate of 50%, maybe complicated with infection, which accounts for approximately 30% of deaths in the first 3 months, and with rejection, accounting for another 30% of deaths in later stages [9]. Noninfectious pulmonary complications after lung transplantation include acute and chronic rejection and early graft dysfunction (reperfusion edema or reimplantation response) and localized complications such as airway dehiscence or stricture. The details of pulmonary complications after lung transplantation will be dealt with in Chap. 12.

Hyperleukocytosis refers to a laboratory condition variably defined as a total leukemia blood cell count greater than 50,000/μL or 100,000/μL. In contrast, leukostasis (also called symptomatic hyperleukocytosis) is a medical emergency most commonly seen in patients with acute myeloid leukemia or chronic myeloid leukemia in blast crisis. It is characterized by an extremely elevated blast cell count and symptoms of decreased tissue perfusion. Leukostasis is a pathologic diagnosis in which white cell plugs are seen in the microvasculature. Clinically, leukostasis is typically diagnosed empirically when a patient with leukemia and hyperleukocytosis presents with respiratory or neurological distress. Prompt treatment is indicated since, if left untreated, the 1-week mortality rate is approximately 20%–40% [10] (Table 11.1).

11.3 Imaging Features and Clinical or Pathologic Comparisons of Pulmonary Emergencies

11.3.1 Immunocompetent Patients

11.3.1.1 Pulmonary Edema (PE)

Increased Hydrostatic Pressure Edema

Interstitial edema occurs with an increase of 15–25 mmHg in mean transmural arterial pressure and results in the early loss of definition of subsegmental and segmental vessels, mild enlargement of the peribronchovascular spaces, the appearance of Kerley lines, and small pleural effusion (Fig. 11.1). With increases in transmural pressure of >25 mmHg, fluid influx from the extravascular compartment is at maximum and the second phase (alveolar flooding) commences,

Table 11.1 Probable causes of noninfectious pulmonary emergency in immunocompetent versus immunocompromised individuals

Immune status	Immunocompetent individuals	Immunocompromised individuals
	Pulmonary edema – Hydrostatic pressure edema (heart failure and fluid overload) – Permeability edema – Capillary leak syndrome – Neurogenic edema	Idiopathic pneumonia syndrome (IPS) Lung involvements in leukemia and lymphoma Hyperleukocytosis in leukemia (Leukostasis) Superior vena cava syndrome
	Drug-induced pneumonitis (DRP)	
	Fat embolism Radiations pneumonitis Diffuse alveolar hemorrhage (DAH) Connective tissue disease and pulmonary vasculitis	

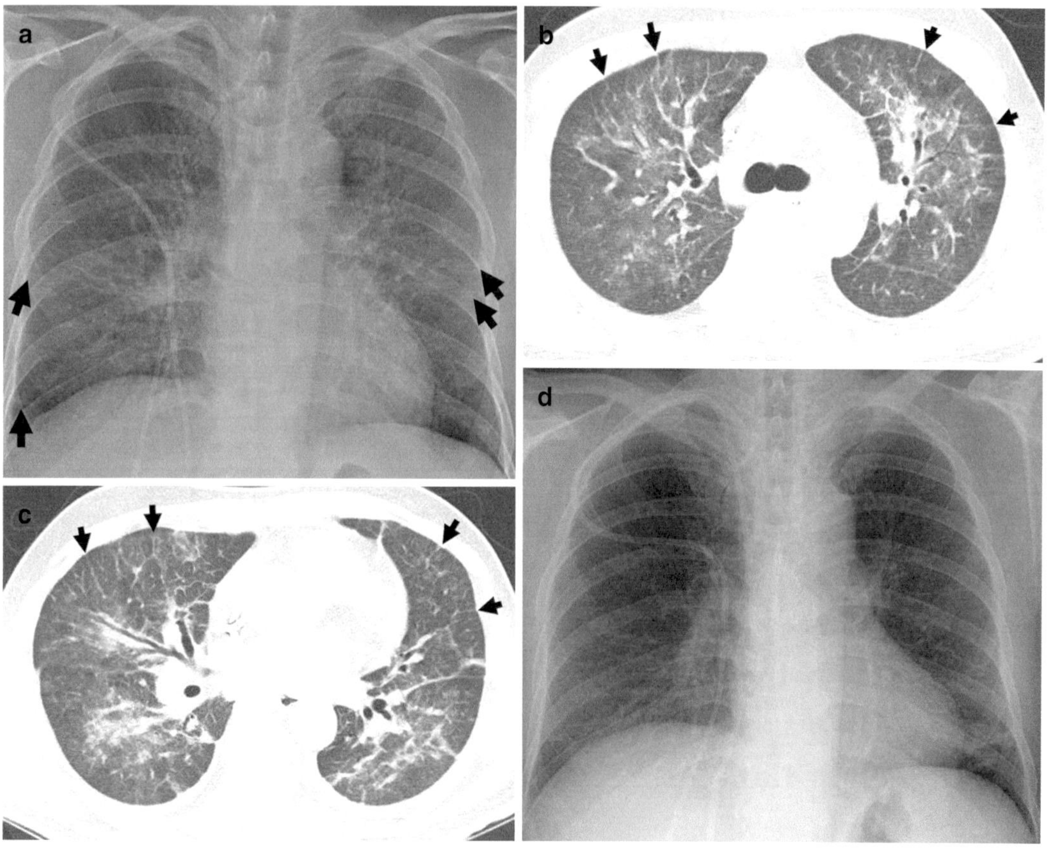

Fig. 11.1 Interstitial pulmonary edema in a 59-year-old man with mantle cell lymphoma who is about to receive chemotherapy. (**a**) Chest radiograph shows poorly defined parenchymal opacity in the parahilar areas in both lungs. Also note multiple Kerley B lines (arrows) in the peripheral portion of both lungs, particularly in the middle and lower lung zones. A central line has been inserted for chemotherapy. (**b**, **c**) Lung window images of thin-section (1.0 mm) CT scans obtained at the levels of the azygos arch (**b**) and the right middle lobar bronchus takeoff (**c**) demonstrate parenchymal opacity in the central areas of both lungs. Also note Kerley B lines (smooth thickening of the interlobular septa) (arrows). (**d**) Follow-up radiograph obtained 2 days after **a** and after diuretic therapy depicts amelioration of parenchymal opacity in both lungs

leading to a sudden extension of edema into the alveolar spaces and thus creating small nodular or acinar areas of increased opacity that may coalesce into true consolidation.

Bat wing edema is a condition in which a central, nongravitational distribution of alveolar edema is seen and the lung cortex is free of alveolar or interstitial fluid (Fig. 11.2). Bat wing edema is observed in 10% or less of cases of pulmonary edema [11]. The condition is encountered in rapidly developing pulmonary edema, such as that seen in severe cardiac failure caused by acute mitral insufficiency (e.g., papillary muscle rupture, massive myocardial infarct, and valve leaflet destruction owing to septic endocarditis) or renal failure. The condition develops rapidly and is initially observed as an alveolar opacity, with a preceding interstitial phase, typical in PE, undetected on imaging studies. The edema can be seen as an asymmetric opacity, particularly when (1) there is extensive underlying emphysema or marked lung destruction and fibrosis of the upper and middle lung zones, (2) edema is associated with mitral regurgitation (reflux stream, directed toward the

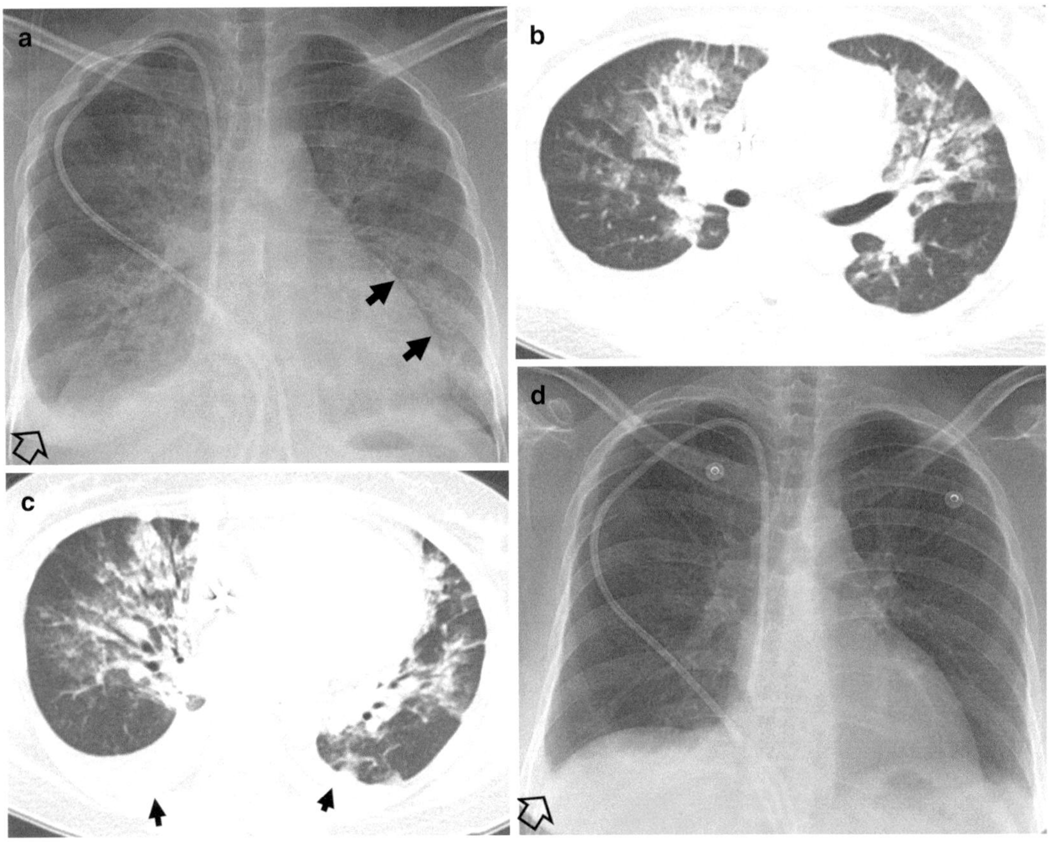

Fig. 11.2 Bat-wing pulmonary edema in acute renal injury related to hematopoietic stem cell transplantation in a 30-year-old woman with diffuse large B-cell lymphoma. (**a**) Chest radiograph shows poorly defined parenchymal opacity in the parahilar areas with sparing of the peripheral portion in both lungs. The heart is enlarged with left-side chamber enlargement (arrows) predominance. Also note right pleural effusion (open arrow). A central line has been inserted for chemotherapy for lymphoma. (**b**, **c**) Lung window images of thin-section (1.0 mm) CT scans obtained at the levels of the right bronchus intermedius (**b**) and right inferior pulmonary vein (**c**) demonstrate parenchymal opacity composed mainly of consolidation rather than ground-glass opacity in the central areas of both lungs. Again, note peripheral lung sparing. Also note bilateral pleural effusions (arrows). (**d**) Follow-up radiograph obtained 2 days after **a** and after diuretic and cardiac inotropic therapy depicts disappearance of parenchymal opacity in both lungs and decreased heart size. Right pleural effusion of small amount remains

right upper pulmonary vein) [12], and (3) the patient is in a recumbent position for a long time after prolonged surgery or immobilization.

Post-obstructive pulmonary edema occurs after relief from an upper airway obstruction and represents a pure form of hydrostatic edema [13]. It is most frequently caused by an impacted foreign body, laryngospasm, epiglottitis, or strangulation. If the obstruction occurs primarily with forced inspiration with the patient struggling to inhale and with a high negative intrathoracic pressure, the patient is in a condition of negative pleural pressure and increased venous return. With the sudden and marked decrease in the negative pleural pressure that occurs when the upper airway obstruction is cleared, a high hydrostatic pressure gradient between the intravascular and the extravascular compartments leads to a high hydrostatic pressure gradient and pulmonary edema [14, 15].

"Near drowning" is the term for survival after suffocation caused by submersion in water or other fluid. This condition is differentiated from drowning in which temporary survival ends in death within 24 h of submersion. In a near-drowning pulmonary edema, the initial condition of laryngeal spasm after the inhalation of a small amount of water results in negative pressure edema related to a prolonged episode of the Muller maneuver. Kerley's lines, peribronchial cuffing, and patchy perihilar alveolar areas of airspace consolidation are seen [16]. With appropriate therapy, these features disappear completely within 24–48 h. However, in 90% of patients, the continued hypoxia leads to cytokine release and subsequent permeability edema [16–18]. Inhaled water also has a deleterious effect on the capillary endothelium, alveolar pneumocytes, and surfactant production. These combined effects result in permeability edema with diffuse alveolar damage, atelectasis, and arteriovenous shunting, resulting in ARDS. This condition is often worsened by infection by freshwater saprophytic bacteria, further worsening alveolar damage. Imaging features are nonspecific and vary from small, ill-defined lesions to large lobar consolidation (Fig. 11.3). The volume of inhaled water, duration of the continuing hypoxia, and the nature of inhaled water (fresh versus salt water) determine the lesion size [16, 18].

Permeability Edema with Diffuse Alveolar Damage (DAD)

Adult respiratory distress syndrome (ARDS) represents the most severe form of permeability edema associated with DAD. Primary or secondary injuries to the alveolar epithelium and capillary endothelium of the lung, respectively, result from exposure of these cells to chemical agents, infectious pathogens, gastric fluid, or toxic gas, which destroy or severely damage epithelial cells. Secondary damage is associated with a systemic biochemical cascade of oxidizing agents, inflammatory mediators, and enzymes, which also harm these endothelial cells, during sepsis, pancreatitis, severe trauma, or blood transfusion [11].

ARDS encompasses three stages, with certain features that often overlap between the stages. These are the exudative, proliferative, and fibrotic stages. The early exudative stage appears with few radiologic findings; interstitial edema is observed initially, followed by perihilar areas of increased opacity. Alveolar space filling is seen as widespread areas of alveolar consolidation with air-bronchogram signs. Unlike hydrostatic edema, alveolar edema in ARDS usually has a more peripheral distribution (Fig. 11.4). The imaging features seen in cardiogenic edema, such as cardiomegaly, apical vascular redistribution, and Kerley lines, are absent. However, in ARDS, even though diffuse homogeneous parenchymal features are prominent, a gravitational gradient is easily visualized (Fig. 11.5). In other words, when the patient's position changes, CT attenuation is modified. Thus, with the patient in a prone position, the dependent opacity is seen in the anterior lungs. This confirms the idea that the homogeneous opacity in the dependent lungs includes an atelectasis component in addition to parenchymal lung injury [19]. With progression into the proliferative stage, an inhomogeneous pattern of ground-glass opacity is seen, with early modification into fibrosis. In the fibrotic stage, subpleural and intrapulmonary cystic lesions may be observed and may become the direct cause of pneumothoraces. Recurrent exudative episodes can occur during the proliferative and fibrotic stages and may be the cause of imaging features common to the three stages [20]. Infrequently, in the supine position and in the

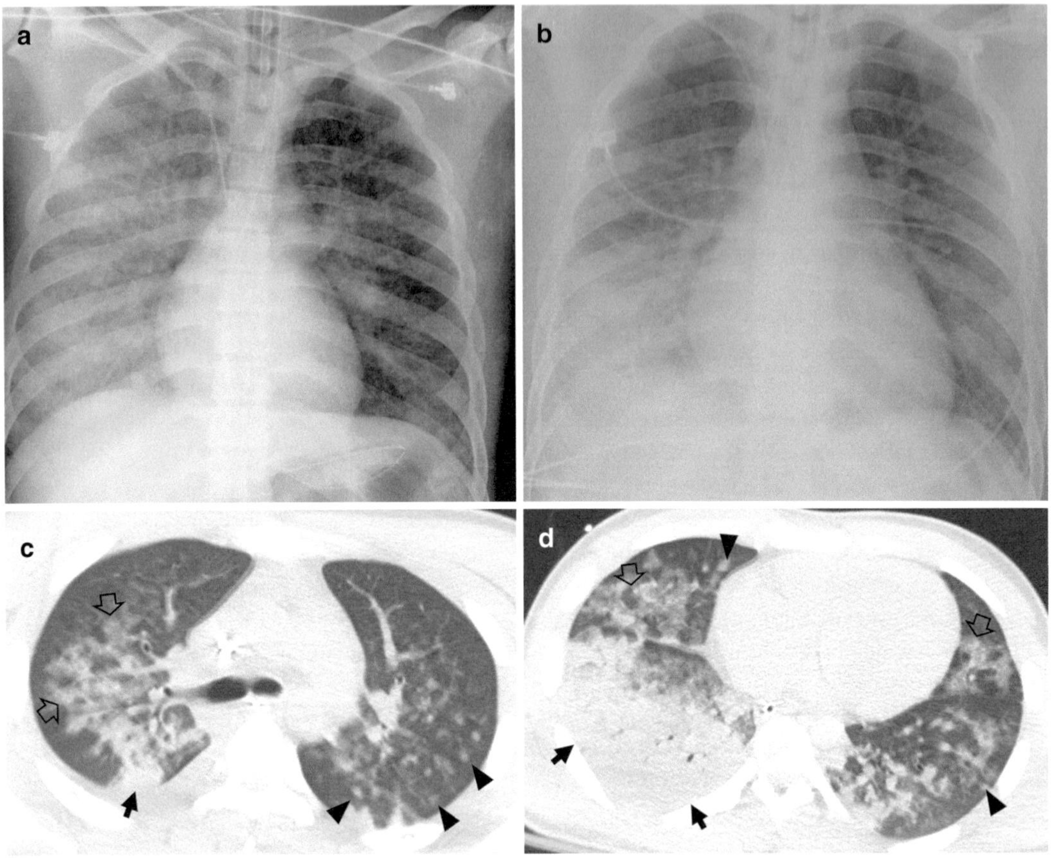

Fig. 11.3 Near drowning in a 33-year-old man who attempted suicide by jumping into a river from a high bridge. (**a**) Chest radiograph at admission to the emergency department shows parenchymal opacity in both lungs, more dense in the right lung. Also note the endotracheal intubation tube and a central line. (**b**) Follow-up radiograph taken 1 day after **a** demonstrates that opacity is localized to the middle and lower lung zones. (**c**, **d**) Lung window images of CT scans (2.5 mm section thickness) obtained at the level of the main bronchi (**c**) and cardiac ventricles (**d**) depict mixed areas of consolidation (arrows), ground-glass opacity (open arrows), and poorly defined nodules (arrowheads) in both lungs. Also note right pleural effusion. CT features are compatible with adult respiratory distress syndrome (ARDS), probably with overlapped pneumonia. The patient lived for more than 5 days (defined as near drowning)

exudative stage, anterior areas of airspace consolidation can be seen; this occurs in ~5% of ARDS cases. Such features may be caused by regional differences in the mechanically assisted ventilation process [21].

11.3.1.2 Drug-Related Pneumonitis

More than 600 drugs are known to cause pulmonary toxicity and illicit drugs are well known to result in pulmonary toxicity (drug-related pneumonitis, DRP). A list of drugs that are reported to cause DRP is available on the continually updated website PNUMOTOX online.

Increasing use of molecular targeting agents and immune-checkpoint inhibitors (ICIs) has broadened the spectrum of lung toxicity, particularly in cancer patients. The diagnosis of DRP is usually one of exclusion. Awareness of the incidence and risk factors of pneumonitis related to specific anticancer agents and ICIs is becoming increasingly important. The severity of symptoms associated with DRP may range from mild or none to life threatening with rapid progression to death.

The following diagnostic criteria for DRP are recommend [22]: (1) Newly identified pulmo-

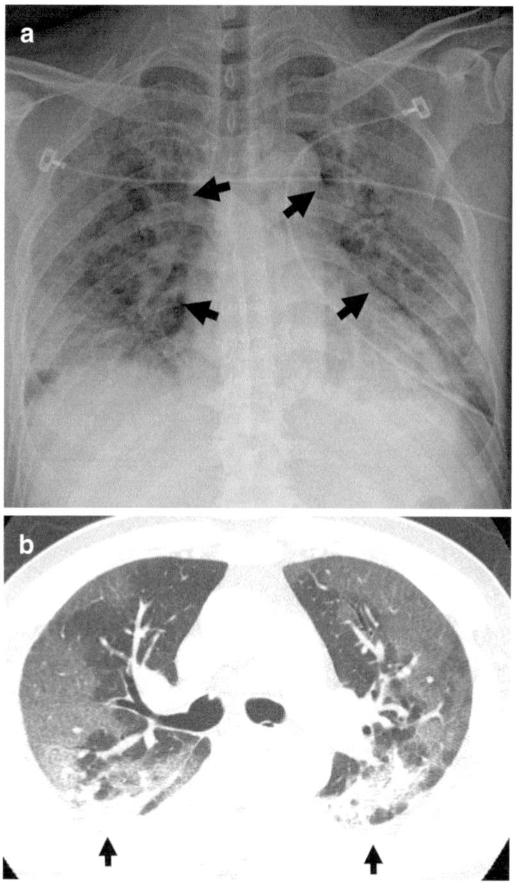

Fig. 11.4 Permeability edema in a 42-year-old man with a mercury inhalation injury. (**a**) Chest radiograph shows parenchymal opacity mainly in the peripheral portion of both lungs. Note the relative sparing (arrows) of opacity in the central portion of the lungs. (**b**) Lung window image of a thin-section (1.0 mm) CT scan obtained at the level of the right upper lobar bronchus demonstrates parenchymal opacity composed of ground-glass opacity and consolidation in the peripheral portion of both lungs. Also note small bilateral pleural effusions (arrows)

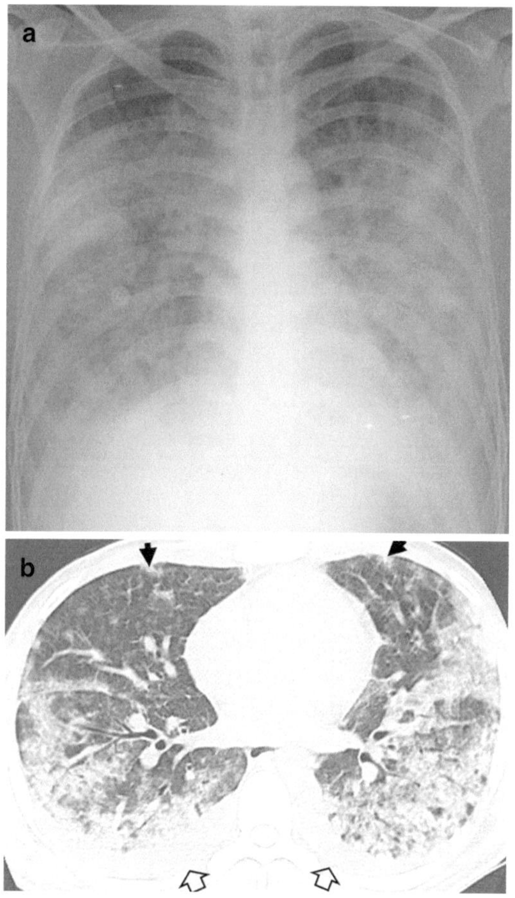

Fig. 11.5 Diffuse alveolar damage (adult respiratory distress syndrome) in both lungs in a 20-year-old man with cytomegalovirus pneumonia. The patient received hematopoietic stem cell transplantation. (**a**) Chest radiograph shows parenchymal opacity in both lungs with sparing of the upper lung zones. (**b**) Lung window image of a thin-section (1.0 mm) CT scan obtained at the level of the right inferior pulmonary vein demonstrates parenchymal opacity in both lungs with predominantly dependent lung involvement (gravitational gradient). Also note areas (arrows) of acinus-sized opacity in the anterior lungs. Again note substantial bilateral pleural effusions (open arrows)

nary parenchymal opacities, commonly in a bilateral non-segmental distribution; (2) Temporal association of presentation with initiation of a systemic therapeutic agent; and (3) Exclusion of other possible causes.

The CT features of DRP associated with systemic therapeutic agents should be assessed in consideration of the distribution of lung parenchymal abnormalities (the pattern approach). The patterns include subacute or chronic (nonspecific interstitial pneumonia) and acute (diffuse alveolar damage) interstitial pneumonia, organizing pneumonia (Fig. 11.6), hypersensitivity pneumonitis (Fig. 11.7), simple pulmonary eosinophilia, and transient asymptomatic pulmonary opacity [23, 24]. One chemotherapy agent can be associated with multiple radiologic patterns. The pattern, distribution, and extent of CT abnormalities are of limited prognostic value. However, patients showing organizing pneumonia, hypersensitivity pneumonitis, or simple pulmonary eosinophilia patterns show improvement on follow-up studies, whereas those with fibrotic nonspecific interstitial pneumonia or diffuse alveolar damage patterns do not [24]. It should be noted, however, that CT and histologic patterns coincide in only half of DRP patients [24] (Fig. 11.7). It should also be noted that the CT pattern in context reflects the extent and distribution of lung abnormalities and helps predict upcoming changes in prognosis.

Management of a patient with suspected DRP generally consists of drug discontinuation, glucocorticoid therapy, or both, along with supportive measures including supplemental oxygen as needed.

11.3.1.3 Fat Embolism Syndrome

Fat embolism (FE) represents the presence of fat droplets in the systemic circulation, which may be detected in the blood and urine of nearly all patients with long bone fractures. Fat embolism

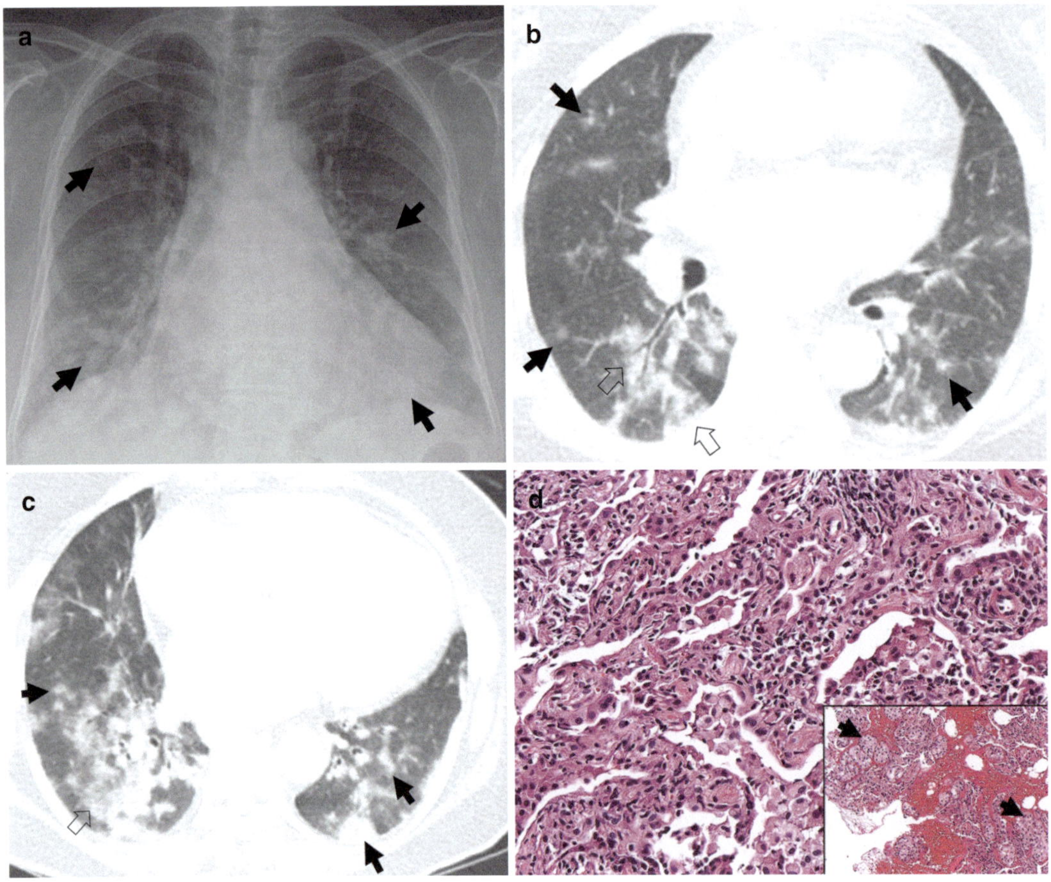

Fig. 11.6 Drug-related pneumonitis (Amiodarone) in a 64-year-old woman with atrial fibrillation and aortic stenosis. (**a**) Chest radiograph shows triangular cardiomegaly. Also note the poorly defined lung nodules (arrows) in both lungs. (**b**, **c**) Lung window images of thin-section (1.0 mm) CT scans obtained at the levels of the right bronchus intermedius (**b**) and right inferior pulmonary vein (**c**) demonstrate poorly defined nodules (arrows) and parenchymal opacity (open arrows) in both lungs, distributed along the bronchovascular bundles and subpleural lungs. This distribution of lung lesions is compatible with the organizing pneumonia pattern of interstitial lung disease. (**d**) Histopathologic specimen obtained with a transbronchial lung biopsy from the right lower lobe discloses interstitial fibrous thickening and vacuolated macrophages (arrows in Inset) in alveolar spaces, features compatible with amiodarone toxicity

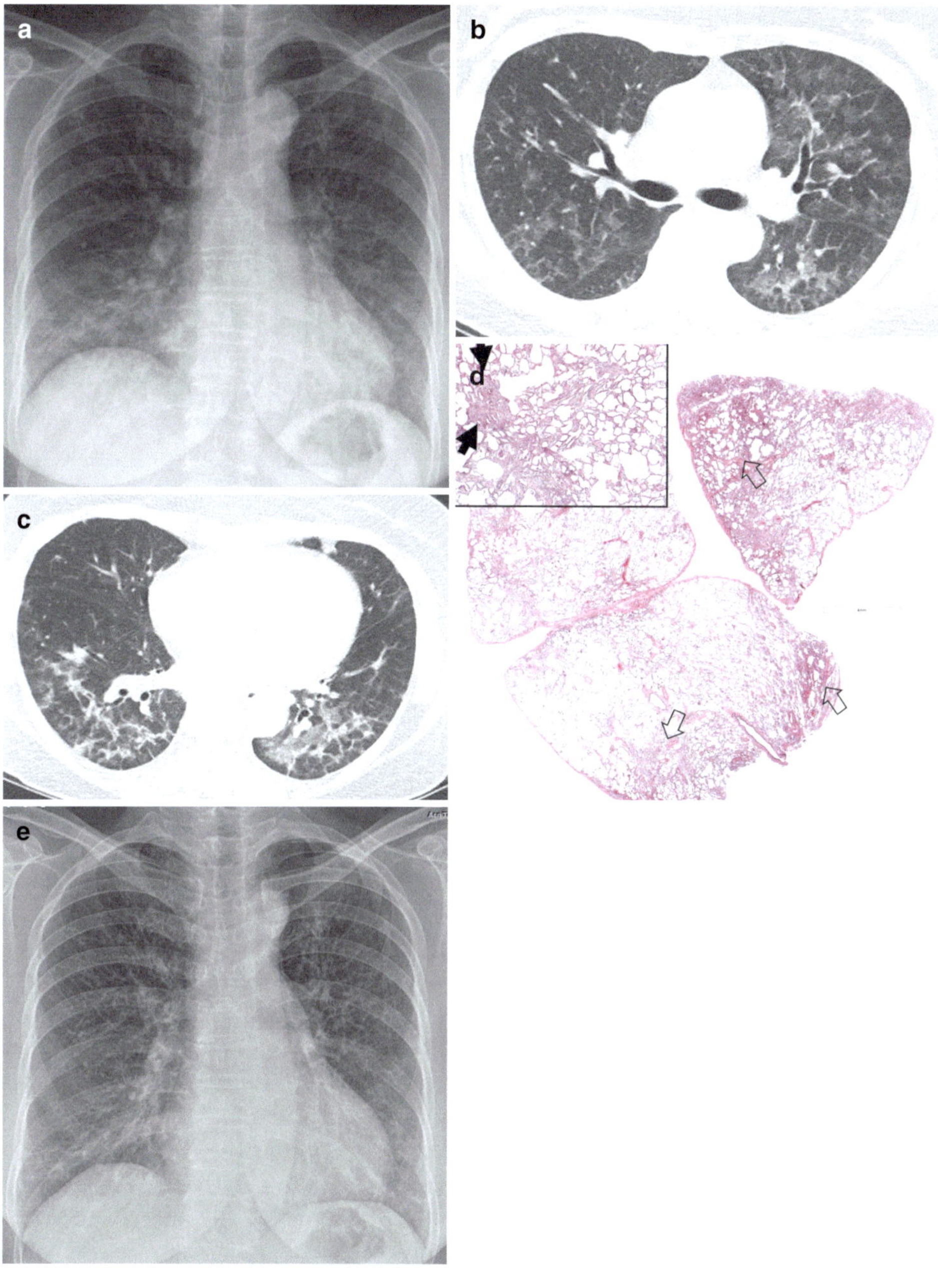

Fig. 11.7 Drug-related pneumonitis (methotrexate) in a 64-year-old woman with orbital IgG4-related disease. (**a**) Chest radiograph shows scattered poorly defined nodules in the upper lung zones and poorly defined opacity in the lower lung zones, bilaterally. (**b**, **c**) Lung window images of thin-section (1.0 mm) CT scans obtained at the levels of the right upper lobar bronchus (**b**) and right inferior pulmonary vein (**c**) demonstrate widely distributed parenchymal ground-glass opacity in both lungs and several areas of poorly defined ground-glass nodules (arrows) in the bilateral anterior lungs. This distribution of lung lesions is compatible with the subacute hypersensitivity pneumonia pattern. (**d**) Histopathologic specimens obtained from a surgical lung biopsy of the left upper lobe disclose overlapping features of organizing pneumonia (arrow in Inset) and nonspecific interstitial pneumonia (open arrows). (**e**) Follow-up radiograph obtained 5 months after **a** and after cessation of amiodarone depicts a markedly decreased extent of lung lesions

syndrome (FES), by contrast, is a clinical diagnosis requiring the presence of at least one major (hypoxia of <60 mmHg of O_2, confusion, and petechial rash) and four minor criteria (pyrexia of >39 °C, tachycardia of >120 beats per minute, retinal changes of petechia, anuria or oliguria, anemia indicated by a decrease in Hg of 20%, thrombocytopenia indicated by a decrease in platelet count of 50%, high ESR of >71 mm per hour, and fat macroglobulinemia) [25].

FES presents in a subacute manner with symptoms peaking at 48–72 h after long bone injury or long bone surgery. In fulminant FES, severe respiratory distress develops in the first 12 h after long bone surgery, probably related to the high burden and larger size of emboli resulting in acute pulmonary hypertension and right heart failure. High pulmonary arterial pressure displaces fat droplets across the pulmonary capillary bed, shunting them into the systemic circulation, leading to cerebral fat embolism and manifesting as confusion and loss of consciousness. The importance of a patent foramen ovale in contributing to the development and severity of cerebral fat embolism is controversial. Risk factors for severe FES include high-velocity trauma, surgical delay of >10 h, fixation of multiple fractures during the same procedure, fixation of pathologic fractures, and presence of a contused lung (the non-contused lung receives more fat emboli because of physiologic shunting) [26]. The pathogenesis of fat embolism syndrome is not completely understood. One theory proposes that neutral triglycerides are transported to the lung and converted to free fatty acids that elicit a toxic reaction in the capillary endothelium [27, 28]. This injury is compounded by the accumulation of inflammatory cells, especially neutrophils, which cause further damage to the vasculature. It should also be recognized that pulmonary oil embolism can occur after transcatheter oily chemoembolization of hepatocellular carcinoma. In this condition, respiratory symptoms of cough, hemoptysis, and dyspnea develop 2–5 days after an embolic procedure and the radiographic findings consist of diffuse bilateral pulmonary parenchymal opacity. The symptoms, arterial hypoxemia, and chest radiographic abnormalities completely clear 10–28 days after chemoembolization in the patients who survive. One in six patients die 10 days after chemoembolization owing to respiratory arrest with the progression of pulmonary opacity [29] (Fig. 11.8).

Bilateral diffuse or patchy opacity areas are seen on chest radiographs. However, these findings are nonspecific. Therefore, chest radiography is primarily useful in monitoring disease evolution. The opacity resolves in 50% of patients within 1 week and usually resolves in all patients within 2 weeks. CT findings (Fig. 11.8) include patchy ground-glass opacity or consolidation and small centrilobular nodules. The parenchymal opacity lesions appear as crazy-paving features with distinct demarcation (with areas of lobular sparing) between the affected and the normal lung [30]. Small nodules 10 mm or less in diameter are also seen, typically in the centrilobular regions of subpleural lungs and in the upper lung zones. The pathogenic mechanism of nodule formation has not been clearly described, but pulmonary edema, hemorrhage, or atelectasis may be the related and underlying pathophysiology [31, 32]. The appearance of parenchymal opacity of crazy-paving and centrilobular nodules 24–72 h after trauma may help differentiate FES from pulmonary contusion, pulmonary edema, aspiration pneumonia, and infectious pneumonia.

Management remains predominantly supportive care, and the benefit of medical therapy such as corticosteroids or heparin remains unclear.

11.3.1.4 Radiation Pneumonitis

Patients undergoing thoracic radiation therapy are at risk of radiation pneumonitis. Classic findings of radiation pneumonitis include the following: (1) Onset of symptoms typically within 3–12 weeks of completion of radiotherapy; (2) Symptoms of low-grade fever, shortness of breath, nonproductive cough, or malaise; (3) Laboratory studies suggestive of acute inflammation may be present, with modest increases in white blood cell count, C-reactive protein, or erythrocyte sedimentation rate; and (4) Imaging findings suggestive of pneumonitis within the treatment field [33].

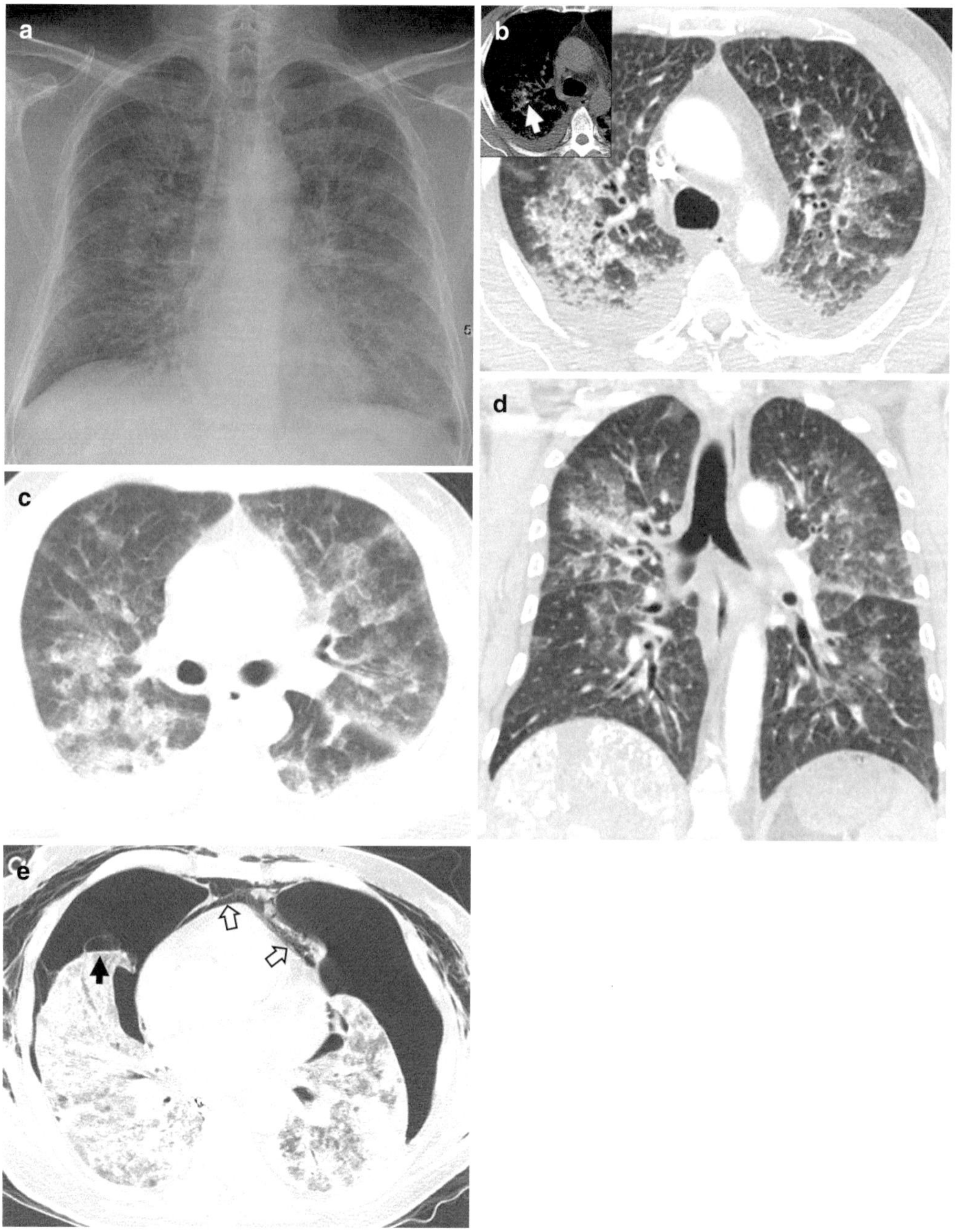

Fig. 11.8 Fat embolism appearing as adult respiratory distress syndrome 1 day after trans-arterial chemoembolization (TACE, with a mixture of Adriamycin and Lipiodol) for hepatocellular carcinoma in a 63-year-old man. (**a**) Chest radiograph shows parenchymal opacity of variable density in both lungs. The apical portion of both lungs is spared. (**b**, **c**) Lung window images of CT scans (2.5 mm) obtained at the levels of the azygos arch (**b**) and right bronchus intermedius (**c**) demonstrate widely spread parenchymal heterogeneous opacity in both lungs. Also note bilateral pleural effusion. Inset in **b** Lipiodol (arrow) is present in branch vessels of the pulmonary artery in the right upper lobe. (**d**) Coronal reformation image (2.0 mm section thickness) depicts parenchymal opacity mainly in the central portion of both lungs. (**e**) Lung window image of a CT scan obtained at the left atrial level 3 weeks after **a** discloses the fibroproliferative stage of adult respiratory distress syndrome with diffuse parenchymal opacity in both lungs. Note pneumothorax, pneumomediastinum (open arrows), and subcutaneous emphysema in both hemi-thoraces. Also note the bulla in the right anterior lung (arrow). The patient died 1 week after this CT scan was taken

Radiation pneumonitis can be graded with several methods; the following is the Common Toxicity Criteria for Adverse Events (Version 4.0) [34]: Grade 1 = Asymptomatic, radiographic findings only; Grade 2 = Symptomatic, but not interfering with activities of daily living; Grade 3 = Symptomatic and interfering with activities of daily living, oxygen indicated; Grade 4 = Life threatening, ventilator support is indicated; and Grade 5 = Death.

Before the mid-1990s, an extended-field technique was used and large areas of normal tissue were targeted, so treatment was associated with increased rates of secondary cancer and cardiac sequelae [35]. Today, patients are commonly treated with intensity-modulated radiation therapy (IMRT) using an involved-site technique that spares significant amounts of normal tissue [36]. A recent study of patients with Hodgkin and non-Hodgkin lymphoma treated with IMRT found that 14% of patients developed radiation pneumonitis (grades 1–3). Interestingly, the rates of pneumonitis appear much lower for patients undergoing treatment with stereotactic body radiation therapy (SBRT) for definitive management of lung cancer [37]. Although surgery remains the mainstay of treatment of early-stage non-small cell lung cancer, SBRT is commonly used for definitive management of patients with early-stage lung cancer who are unable or unwilling to undergo surgery. Lung SBRT consists of the delivery of high doses of radiation, typically in the range of 10 to 18 Gy per fraction, for a total of 3 to 5 fractions. The primary reason for the lower rates of pneumonitis may be related to the reduced treatment volumes as well as potential underlying differences in radiobiologic interactions with high dose-per-fraction radiation.

Radiation pneumonitis is diagnosed based on the features of classic symptoms, timing, and history of radiation therapy, appropriate imaging findings, and exclusion of alternative causes such as infection, cardiogenic edema, pulmonary embolism, drug-related pneumonitis, and other causes. Ruling out alternative diagnoses can be difficult. According to one study, assigning a diagnosis of radiation pneumonitis was challenging in 28% of patients owing to confounding medical conditions [38].

All patients undergoing radiotherapy directed at the lungs are expected to develop some degree of radiographic changes. However, the radiographic changes may not correlate with clinical symptoms or signs [39]. The classic portal-line effect that does not conform to normal lung anatomy is no longer seen very often due to modern radiation therapy techniques that use multiple beam angles. Chest CT (Fig. 11.9) usually shows evidence of patchy consolidation roughly within the high-dose radiation field and similarly does not conform to normal lobar anatomy [40]. Occasionally, progression outside of the field may be seen for reasons that are unclear but may relate to a progressive immunologic response [41, 42]. Organizing pneumonia (Fig. 11.9) is occasionally seen after high-dose radiation. It is characterized by lung opacity outside the treatment area and does not result in pulmonary fibrosis [43].

Transbronchial lung biopsy can be performed to rule out alternative causes such as tumor spread and infection. Tissue sampling may be inadequate to make a diagnosis of radiation pneumonitis. Empirical treatment with antibiotics and corticosteroids can be given, with monitoring of clinical response.

Angiotensin converting enzyme inhibitor (ACE-I) use during radiation therapy has been reported to reduce the incidence of symptomatic pneumonitis; the mechanism is not exactly known, but may include mitigation of radiation-induced endothelial cell injury or suppression of pro-inflammatory mediators [44, 45].

11.3.1.5 Diffuse Alveolar Hemorrhage

Diffuse alveolar hemorrhage (DAH) is a clinicopathologic syndrome involving accumulation of intra-alveolar red blood corpuscles (RBCs) originating from alveolar capillaries. All causes of DAH have the common denominator of an injury to the alveolar capillary microcirculation. The clinical syndrome includes hemoptysis, anemia, diffuse radiographic pulmonary opacity, and hypoxic respiratory failure.

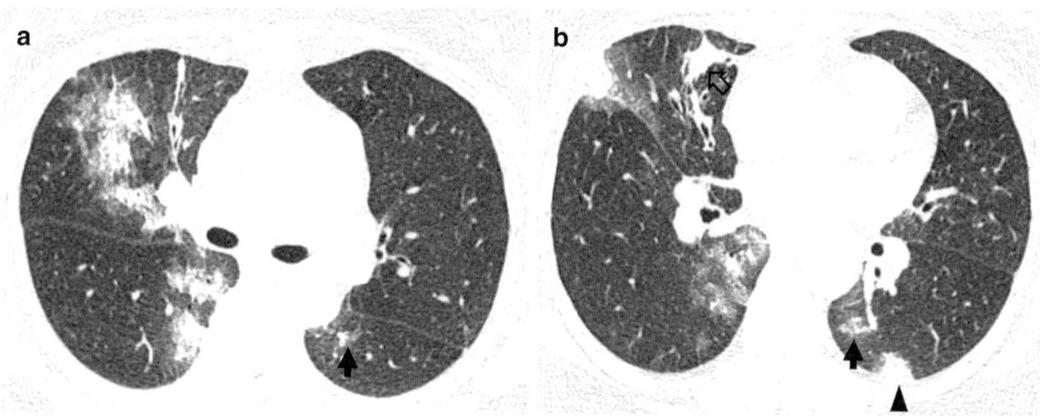

Fig. 11.9 Radiation pneumonitis in a 51-year-old woman with squamous cell carcinoma in the right middle lobe. (**a**) Lung window image of a CT scan (2.5 mm section thickness) obtained at the level of the main bronchi shows parenchymal consolidation or nodules in the right upper and lower lobes and in the superior segment (arrows) of the left lower lobe along the radiation portal. (**b**) A CT scan obtained at the level of the right inferior pulmonary vein demonstrates areas of parenchymal opacity or nodules in the right middle and lower lobes and in the superior segment (arrows) of the left lower lobe along the radiation portal. Also note area of presumed organizing pneumonia (arrowhead) in the left lower lobe away from the radiation pneumonitis. The remnants of the primary tumor (open arrow) can be seen in the right middle lobe

The most common underlying histology of DAH is a type of small vessel vasculitis know as pulmonary capillaritis which is usually seen with seropositive systemic vasculitides, or a connective tissue disorder, bland pulmonary hemorrhage, and diffuse alveolar damage due to a number of injuries including drug-induced injury (Fig. 11.10), coagulation disorders, and infections. Bronchoalveolar lavage confirms the clinical diagnosis of DAH. Surgical lung biopsy may be needed to confirm the underlying histology [46].

The radiographic features of DAH consist of patchy, bilateral air-space opacities. DAH is usually seen with extensive bilateral airspace consolidation and GGO, but maybe more prominent in the perihilar areas and in the middle and lower lung zones, sparing the lung apices and costophrenic angles [47, 48]. The most common CT features of DAH are bilateral GGOs and consolidation. The lesions are diffuse in the upper and lower lobes in approximately 75% of patients and are localized to the lower part of the lungs in the remaining 25% of patients [47, 48]. Typically, the halo sign is seen with parenchymal nodules or masses and consolidation on CT scans, representing the hemorrhagic nature of these parenchymal lesions [49]. Smooth interlobular septal thickening becomes superimposed on areas of GGO (a crazy-paving appearance) within 2–3 days. These findings may show improvement in the course of hemorrhage resorption. Additionally, ill-defined centrilobular nodules may be present, reflecting intra-alveolar accumulation of pulmonary macrophages. The nodules are uniform in size (1–3 mm in diameter) and are diffusely distributed with no zonal predominance [47, 50]. A small amount of pleural effusion may occur, but is uncommon. The airspace lesions histopathologically correlate with pulmonary hemorrhage, both with or without capillaritis [48]. Typical MR features attributable to paramagnetic properties of hemosiderin in DAH are expected, with diffusely increased signal intensity on T1-weighted MR images and markedly reduced signal intensity on T2-weighted MR images [51]. Pulmonary interstitial fibrosis, probably associated with recurrent hemorrhage, has occasionally been reported in pulmonary vasculitis and DAH [52]. CT findings in this group of patients may simulate idiopathic pulmonary fibrosis or nonspecific interstitial pneumonitis because honeycombing, reticulation, and traction bronchiectasis may occur [52].

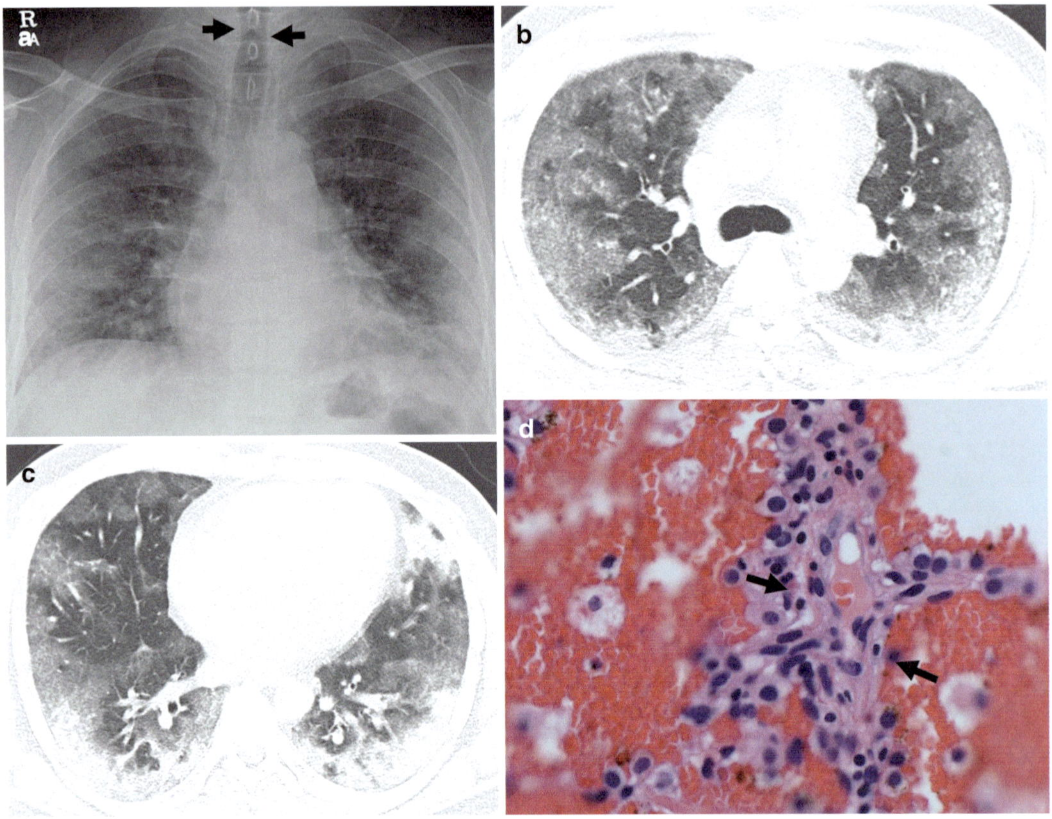

Fig. 11.10 Propylthiouracil (PTU)-associated pulmonary vasculitis manifesting as diffuse alveolar hemorrhage in a 27-year-old man. (**a**) Chest radiograph shows diffuse parenchymal opacity in both lungs. Tracheal air column shows mild hour-glass narrowing (arrows) at the thoracic inlet level, suggesting bilaterally enlarged thyroid glands. (**b**, **c**) Lung window images of CT scans (2.50 mm section thickness) obtained at the levels of the azygos arch (**b**) and right inferior pulmonary vein (**c**) depict parenchymal opacity in both lungs, mainly in the peripheral portion. (**d**) A high-magnification image of a pathologic specimen discloses focal capillaritis with neutrophil infiltration (arrows). Reprint with permission from Chung MP et al. Radiology 2010;255:322–341

11.3.1.6 Connective Tissue Diseases (CTDs) and Pulmonary Vasculitis

In systemic lupus erythematosus (SLE), lung involvement occurs in 97.8% (89 of 90) of patients at autopsy. The most common findings are pleuritis (78%), bacterial infection (58%), primary and secondary alveolar hemorrhage (26%), small airway disease (21%), opportunistic infection (14%), pulmonary thromboembolism (8%), and acute lupus pneumonitis (1–4%). Acute lupus pneumonitis is characterized pathologically by alveolar wall damage and necrosis leading to inflammatory cell infiltration, hemorrhage, edema, and hyaline membrane formation. Large vessel vasculitis has rarely been detected. Thrombi in small vessels, associated with interstitial pneumonitis, are well-documented, although this finding is an unusual feature of acute lupus pneumonitis [53]. The condition, although rare in incidence, is one of the most severe complications of SLE. Patients present with fever, cough, pleurisy, dyspnea, hypoxia, and sometimes hemoptysis. Acute lupus pneumonia usually occurs during the period of acute exacerbation of the disease with multisystem involvement such as nephritis, serositis, and arthritis. Most patients with the disease are anti-dsDNA antibody positive. Chest imaging demonstrates diffuse, bilateral alveolar lung

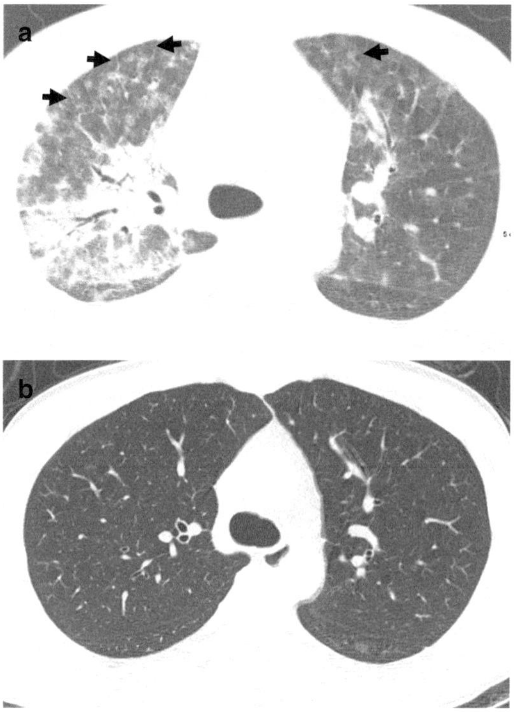

Fig. 11.11 Acute lupus pneumonitis in a 30-year-old man with systemic lupus erythematosus. (**a**) Lung window image of a thin-section (1.5 mm section thickness) CT scan obtained at the level of the azygos arch shows extensive parenchymal opacity of mixed consolidation and ground-glass opacity in both lungs. Also note smooth interlobular septal thickening (arrows) in the anterior lungs. Pathologic specimens obtained from a transbronchial lung biopsy (not shown here) demonstrated inflammatory cell infiltration in alveolar walls, a few hemosiderin-laden macrophages in alveolar spaces, and features of vasculitis (capillaritis) composed mainly of neutrophils. Those findings were compatible with the histologic diagnosis of acute lupus pneumonitis. Reprint with permission from Kim JS et al. J Comput Assist Tomogr 2000;24:9–18. (**b**) Follow-up CT scan obtained 6 months after A demonstrates that the lung lesions disappeared almost completely

lesions (Fig. 11.11). It can be difficult to discriminate SLE from DAH. BAL fluid analysis is helpful in finding other causes of acute deterioration, such as DAH or infection. It is reported that eosinophilic or neutrophilic lavage fluid is predictive of a worse prognosis compared with lymphocytic fluid.

In ANCA (antineutrophil cytoplasmic antibody)-associated pulmonary vasculitis, DAH with capillaritis or lung involvement (neutrophilic granulomas in granulomatosis with polyangiitis [GPA]) could lead to an ED visit. The most common radiographic finding in GPA is lung nodules or consolidation with cavitation (Fig. 11.12). Less frequent radiographic findings consist of nodule(s) without cavitation, increased bronchovascular lines involving the lung parenchyma, mediastinal or hilar lymph node enlargement, and pleural effusion [47]. The most common pattern on CT images at initial presentation is the presence of nodules or masses. The nodules or masses are multiple in 85% of patients, bilateral in 67% of patients, subpleural in 89% of patients, and peribronchovascular in 41% of patients based on the distribution seen on CT images. Bronchial wall thickening in the segmental or subsegmental bronchi is seen in approximately 70% of patients. The large airways are also abnormal in 30% of patients. The subglottic trachea is the site of predilection and its involvement may eventually lead to subglottic stenosis to such a degree that it necessitates tracheostomy. Another common manifestation is airspace consolidation and GGO, which is seen in 25%–50% of cases. These opacities are random or patchy in distribution and are taken to represent DAH caused by necrotizing capillaritis (please refer to DAH, above) [54].

11.3.2 Immunocompromised Patients

11.3.2.1 Idiopathic Pneumonia Syndrome

Idiopathic pneumonia syndrome (IPS) is an acute lung dysfunction of noninfectious etiology and a severe complication following hematopoietic stem cell transplantation (HSCT) [55]. IPS was conceptualized as noninfectious acute lung injury presumably caused by toxicity from pretransplantation chemotherapy, total body irradiation, and immunologic effects including graft-versus-host disease (GVHD). IPS occurs in approximately 5%–25% of allogeneic bone marrow transplant recipients [56].

The diagnostic criteria for IPS, according to the American Thoracic Society (ATS), include

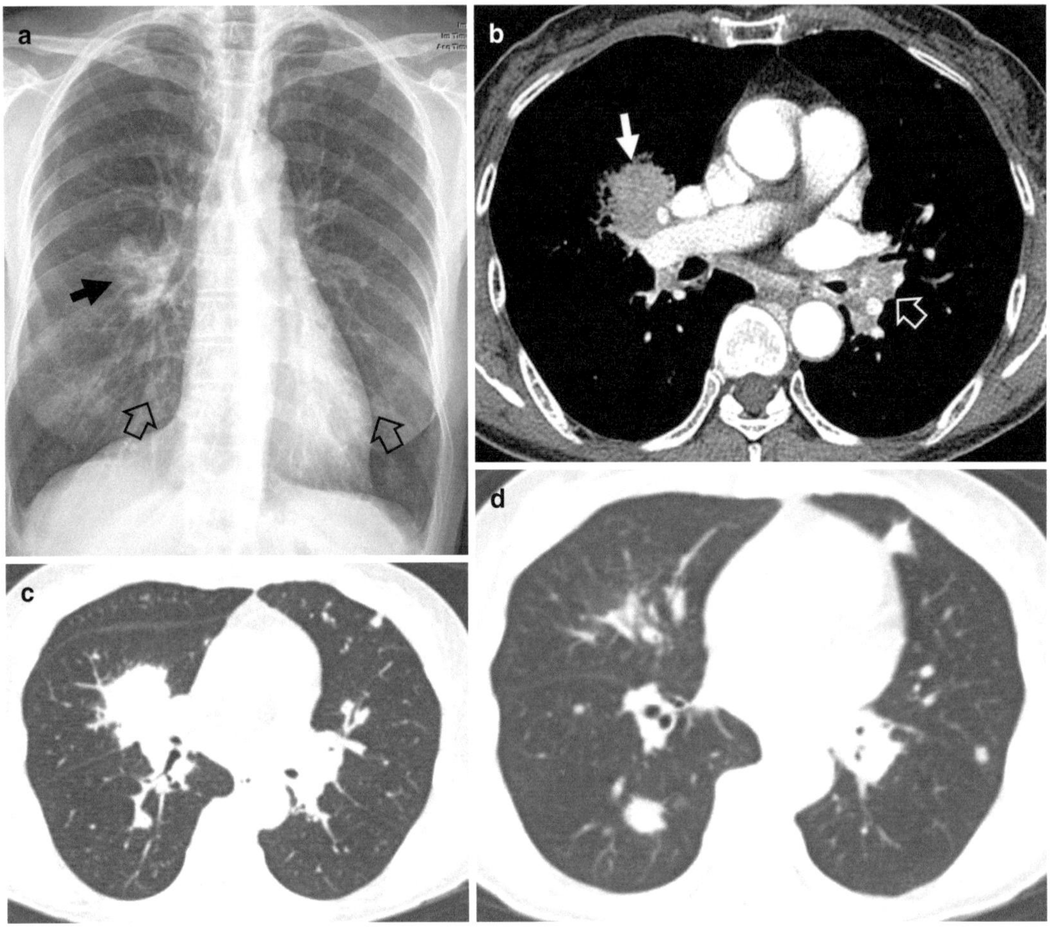

Fig. 11.12 Granulomatosis and polyangiitis (GPA, formerly Wegener's granulomatosis) in a 60-year-old woman. (**a**) Chest radiograph shows a large mass (arrow) in the right parahilar area. Also note the smaller nodules in the lower lung zones (open arrows). (**b**) Mediastinal window image of a CT scan (2.5 mm section thickness) obtained at the level of the bronchus intermedius demonstrates a mass (arrow) in the right middle lobe and enlarged lymph nodes (open arrow) in the left hilum. (**c**, **d**) Lung window images obtained at the levels of the lower lobar bronchi (**c**) and right inferior pulmonary vein (**d**) depict a large mass in the right middle lobe and multiple smaller nodules in the remaining lungs

two major requirements [4]: (1) Widespread alveolar injury with symptoms and signs of pneumonia and (2) Absence of not only active lower respiratory tract infection but also cardiac dysfunction, acute renal failure, and iatrogenic fluid overload. In the original diagnostic criteria, in order to exclude the presence of lower respiratory tract infection, conventional or shell viral culture, direct immunofluorescent antibody testing, and pathological examination were used. However, new diagnostic methods, such as testing for the biomarker galactomannan for *Aspergillus* and multiplex polymerase chain reaction (PCR) for respiratory viruses, are increasingly being used [4]. Moreover, new pathogens, especially viruses such as human metapneumovirus (HMPV) or novel coronaviruses (CoVs), have been discovered by the use of emerging technologies such as metagenomic next generation sequencing (NGS) [57, 58]. Seo and colleagues demonstrated that approximately half of patients with IPS hosted pathogens detectable with bronchoalveolar lavage (BAL) [59]. It is the very bottom, for diagnosing IPS, to exclude infectious diseases using the various above-mentioned techniques.

CT findings in IPS may be classified into three categories and are heterogeneous according to the primarily targeted lung structures; the categories are as follows: (1) Associated with pulmonary parenchyma as a target and include acute interstitial pneumonia or diffuse alveolar damage and eosinophilic pneumonia (EP); (2) Associated with vascular endothelium as a target and include non-cardiogenic capillary leak syndrome, DAH, and transfusion-related acute lung injury; and (3) Associated with airway epithelium as a target and include organizing pneumonia (OP) and bronchiolitis obliterans (BO) (Fig. 11.13) [60].

11.3.2.2 Lymphomatous and Leukemic Lung Involvement

Patients with leukemia or lymphoma may have several different pulmonary complications during the course of their illness, including pulmonary infection, drug-related pneumonitis, and diffuse alveolar hemorrhage. In addition to such complications, a substantial number of patients in autopsy series have demonstrated leukemic or lymphomatous lung infiltration (up to 64% of such cases) [61, 62]. In particular, adult T-cell lymphoma and leukemia, acute myeloid leukemia, and intravascular lymphomatosis (IVL) are the conditions in which diffuse lung involvement

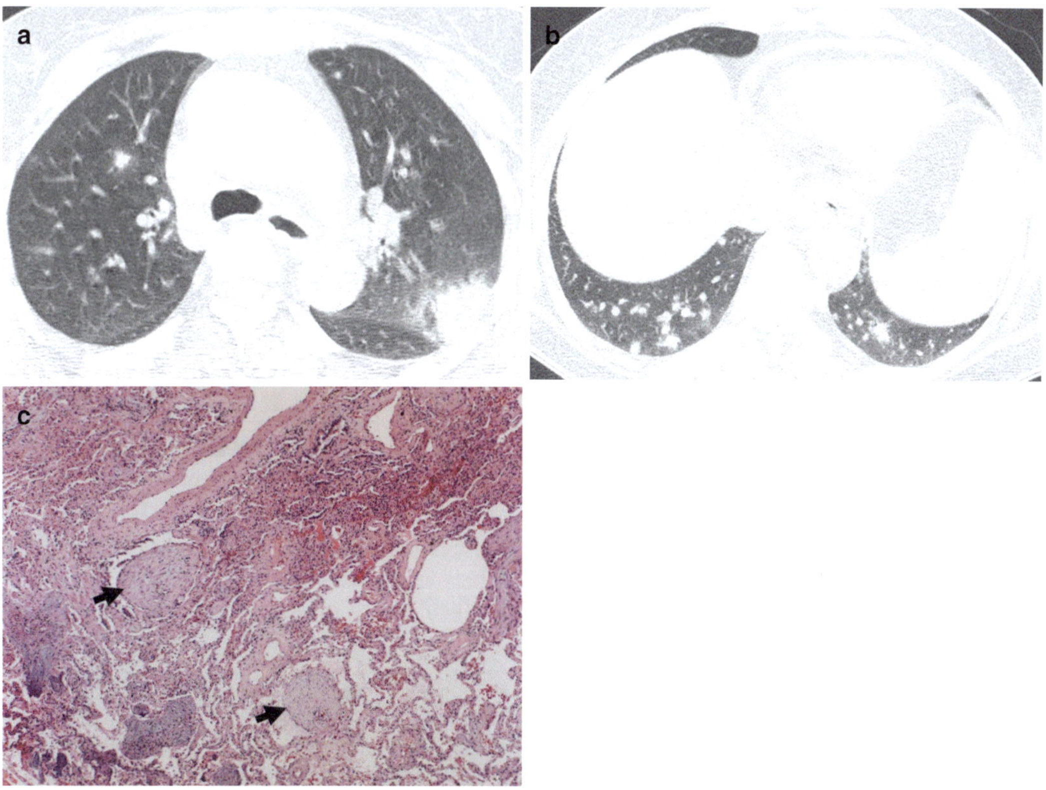

Fig. 11.13 Idiopathic pneumonia syndrome appearing as organizing pneumonia pattern in a 53-year-old who underwent hematopoietic stem-cell transplantation. (**a**, **b**) Lung window images of thin-section (1.0 mm section thickness) CT scans obtained at the levels of the azygos arch (**a**) and liver dome (**b**) show multiple variable-sized nodules in both lungs. The initial diagnosis of the nodules was invasive pulmonary aspergillosis. (**c**) A high-magnification image of a pathologic specimen obtained from a nodule in the left upper lobe discloses intra-alveolar granulation plugs (arrows) and interstitial inflammatory cell infiltration, compatible with organizing pneumonia. No fungal organism was found

are frequent and emergency clinical and imaging conditions are frequently encountered.

Leukemic Pulmonary Infiltration

According to a study [63] that compared CT and pathologic findings of leukemic lung involvement, acute myeloid leukemia accounted for 6 of 11 patients (the others were adult T-cell leukemia in three, plasma cell leukemia in one, and chronic myelomonocytic leukemia in one patient). The most frequent CT findings were thickening of bronchovascular bundles (82%) and non-lobular or nonsegmental ground-glass opacity (91%). Those CT findings represented leukemic cell infiltration around the pulmonary arteries, bronchi, or bronchioles (bronchovascular bundle thickening on CT) and leukemic cell infiltration within alveolar spaces, septa adjacent to the pulmonary arteries or bronchi, and to the areas of hemorrhage, edema, or diffuse alveolar damage (the ground-glass opacity).

Adult T-Cell Leukemia and Lymphoma

Human T-lymphotropic virus type I, which is most prevalent in southwestern Japan and the Caribbean basin, is associated with adult T-cell leukemia or lymphoma [64]. After a long latency period of 10–30 years, human T-lymphotropic virus type 1 causes the development of adult T-cell leukemia and lymphoma. The cumulative lifetime risk for an individual to develop adult T-cell leukemia and lymphoma is estimated to be between 0.5% and 5% [65, 66].

Common clinical manifestations of adult T-cell leukemia or lymphoma include lymphadenopathy (characteristically sparing the neck and mediastinal nodes), skin infiltration, hepatosplenomegaly, bone infiltration, general malaise, and gastrointestinal symptoms. Leukemic cell lung infiltration occurs in 54% of adult T-cell leukemia or lymphoma patients [67] (Fig. 11.14).

CT findings in patients with adult T-cell leukemia or lymphoma are mainly comprised of ground-glass opacity, centrilobular nodules, and thickening of the bronchovascular bundles in the peripheral lungs. Histologically, these CT findings correspond with atypical lymphocyte infiltration along the interstitium and the alveolar spaces [66].

Intravascular Lymphomatosis

Intravascular lymphomatosis (IVL) is a rare disease characterized by the proliferation of neoplastic lymphoid cells, mostly of B-cell origin, in the vascular lumina [68]. Patients who receive a diagnosis of IVL in Western countries display a tendency for central nervous system and skin involvement, whereas those diagnosed in Asian countries are more likely to demonstrate hemophagocytic syndrome, bone marrow involvement, fever, hepatosplenomegaly, and thrombocytopenia [69].

The clinical manifestations of IVL are nonspecific but most commonly include fever of unknown origin, weight loss, night sweats, dementia, and cutaneous nodules or plaques [70]. When the lungs are involved, patients experience shortness of breath, hypoxemia, and, rarely, pulmonary hypertension, and the disease may simulate various lung diseases, particularly diffuse interstitial lung disease or a subacute or chronic infectious condition [70, 71]. Moreover, owing to the rarity of this condition, ready diagnosis of the disease is difficult, and lung lesions in patients with IVL are often detected only at autopsy [72, 73].

Pulmonary IVL appears as bilateral GGO on CT images, with increased fluorodeoxyglucose uptake on PET/CT images. GGO on CT images correlates with the area of expanded alveolar septae because of distended vessels filled with neoplastic lymphoid cells [69] (Fig. 11.15).

Lymphomatous Involvement of the Lungs

Lymphoma more frequently involves the lungs in secondary or recurrent disease rather than as a primary manifestation, particularly in Hodgkin lymphoma (HL). The frequency of pulmonary involvement has changed over time due to an improvement in the survival rate resulting from aggressive lymphoma therapy [74, 75].

Pulmonary involvement is identified more often in HL than in non-Hodgkin lymphoma (NHL). Pulmonary parenchymal involvement may present with various patterns. The most common feature of pulmonary involvement is a direct extension from the hilar or mediastinal nodes toward the lungs; however, recurrences in the lungs may be seen without associated

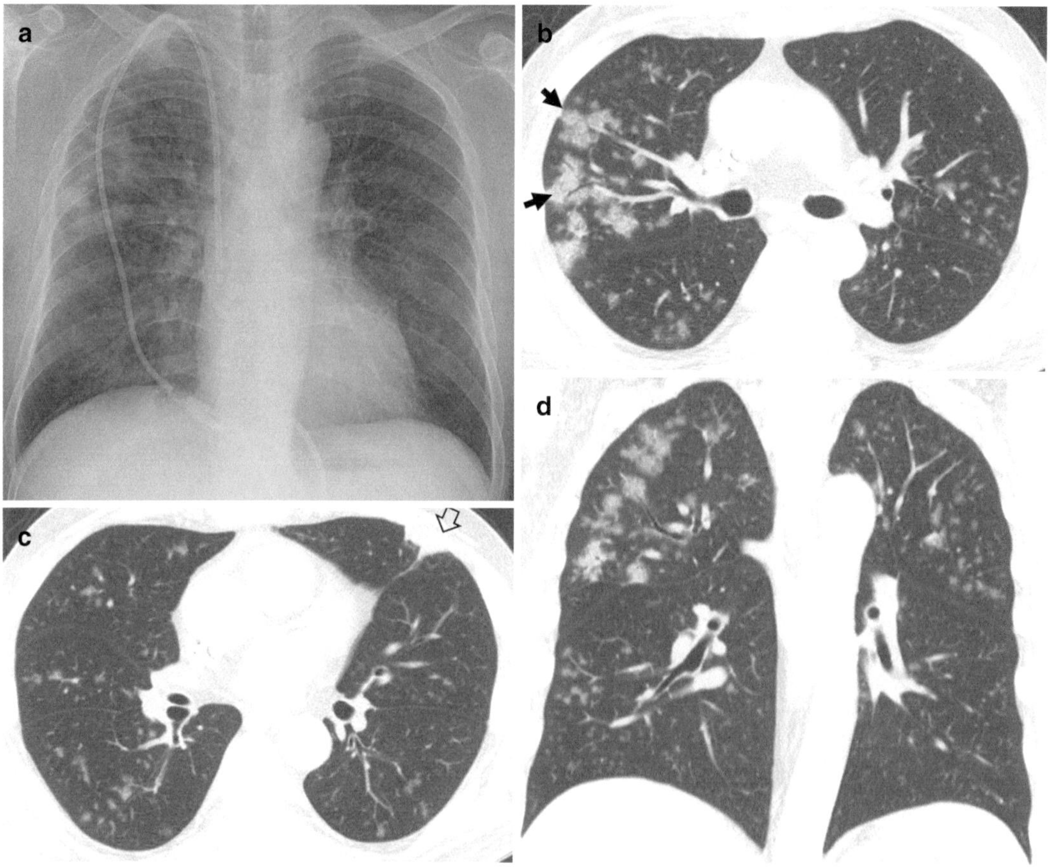

Fig. 11.14 Leukemic involvement of the lungs in a 48-year-old prolymphocytic leukemia patient. (**a**) Chest radiograph shows multiple poorly defined nodules in the right upper lung zone and smaller and more discrete nodules in the left lung. A central line is inserted. (**b**, **c**) Lung window images of thin-section (1.0 mm section thickness) CT scans obtained at the levels of the right upper lobar bronchus and left lower lobar bronchus demonstrate areas of poorly defined parenchymal opacity with a crazy-paving appearance (arrows in **b**) in the right upper lobe and smaller and more discrete nodules in the remaining lungs. Also note the triangular area (open arrow in **c**) of consolidation in the left upper lobe. (**d**) Coronal reformation image depicts crazy-paving opacity in the right upper lobe and small nodular lesions in both lungs. A pathologic specimen (not shown here) disclosed minimal infiltration of T-cell prolymphocytic leukemic cells in alveolar walls and a nodular pattern of fibrous alveolar exudates and mild mononuclear inflammatory cell collection

lymphadenopathy. Other appearances include pulmonary nodules (with or without cavitation) (Fig. 11.16), lobar or segmental consolidation with internal CT air-bronchogram signs representing peribronchial tumor infiltration without destruction of bronchial walls, reticular pattern with bronchovascular bundle and interlobular septal thickening, disseminated small nodules, cavitating masses, endobronchial lesion per se, and atelectasis or obstructive pneumonia secondary to endobronchial or nodal obstruction. When these findings are seen in a patient with newly diagnosed lymphoma, pulmonary involvement should be considered. In treated patients, however, it is often difficult to differentiate between pulmonary involvement and other benign conditions such as infection, radiation pneumonia, or drug-related pneumonitis. It is important to determine whether a tumor originated from the lung parenchyma (primary pulmonary lymphoma), originated in nodal tissue and spread to the adjacent lung, or originated in nodal tissue and hematogenously spread to extranodal sites [74, 75].

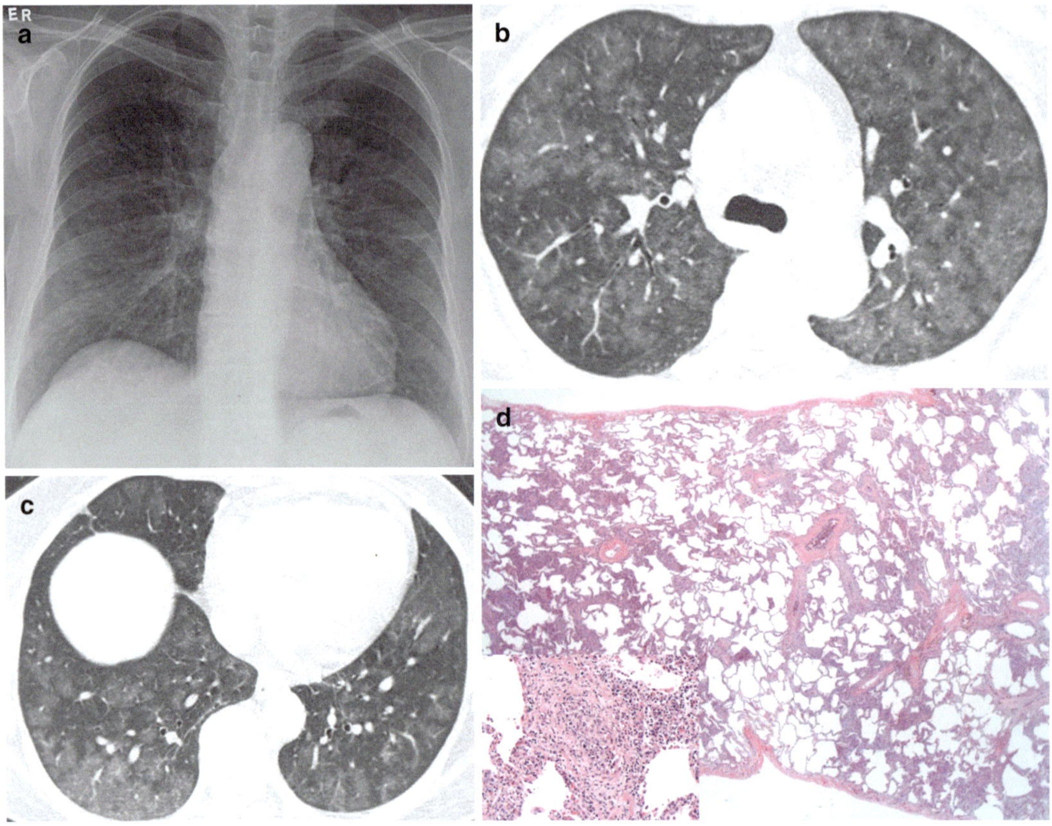

Fig. 11.15 Intravascular lymphomatosis (IVL) in a 66-year-old woman complaining of dyspnea. (**a**) Chest radiograph shows diffuse small nodular and mixed mild reticular lesions in both lungs. (**b**, **c**) Lung window images of CT scans (2.5 mm section thickness) obtained at the levels of the azygos arch (**b**) and liver dome (**c**) demonstrate patchy and wide areas of ground-glass opacity, simulating subacute hypersensitivity pneumonia (HP). (**d**) Low-magnification image of a pathologic specimen discloses features of diffuse interstitial inflammatory cell infiltration with small nodule formation and hypertrophied vessels. Inset: Accumulation of atypical large lymphocytes within alveolar capillaries

11.3.2.3 Hyperleukocytosis and Its Clinical Manifestations

Hyperleukocytosis is defined as a white blood cell count >100,000/mL in patients with acute leukemia. Risk factors for morbidity and mortality include younger age, myelomonocytic or monocytic/monoblastic morphology of leukemic cells, microgranular variant of acute promyelocytic leukemia and T-cell acute lymphocytic leukemia, and some cytogenetic abnormalities. The high number of leukocytes cause three main complications, leukocytosis, tumor lysis syndrome, and disseminated intravascular coagulation (DIC). On thoracic imaging, the leukostasis and the associated lung involvement is the most noticeable condition. Thus, we describe the imaging features of leukostasis only.

Leukostasis

Leukostasis is a clinicopathologic syndrome characterized by multi-organ failure, severe coagulopathy, tumor lysis syndrome, and metabolic abnormalities. The symptoms are usually related to the involvement of the cerebral, pulmonary, and renal microvasculature, resulting in intracranial hemorrhage, alteration of alveolar–capillary oxygen exchange until respiratory failure, and renal tubular dysfunction.

Pulmonary leukostasis is due to blast cell infiltration along the lymphatic route surrounding the

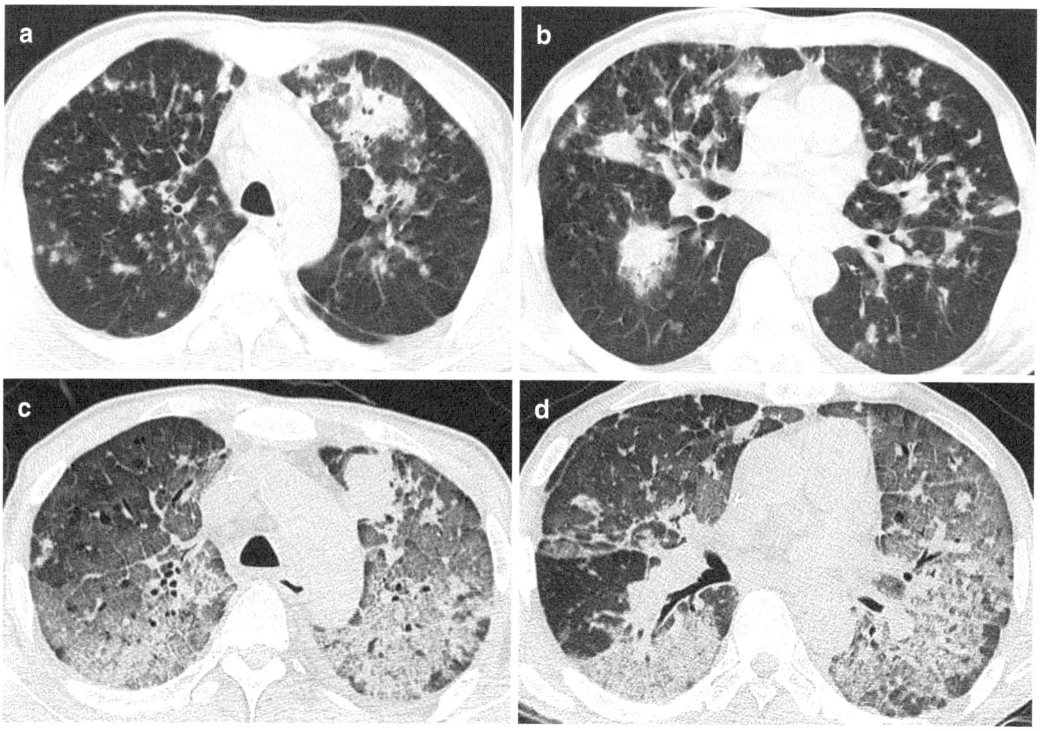

Fig. 11.16 Hodgkin lymphoma, nodular sclerosing type, and lung involvement with cytomegalovirus pneumonia. (**a**, **b**) Lung window images of thin-section (1.0 mm) CT scans, obtained at the levels of the aortic arch (**a**) and lower lobar bronchi (**b**) show multiple variable-sized nodules (representing lung involvement of Hodgkin lymphoma) in both lungs, mainly with a bronchovascular bundle distribution. (**c**, **d**) CT scans obtained at similar levels to and 2 months after **a** and **b**, respectively, demonstrate features of diffuse parenchymal opacity (compatible with cytomegalovirus pneumonia) in addition to the above-mentioned nodules in both lungs. Histopathologic specimens (not shown here) obtained on an intervening date demonstrated both Hodgkin lymphoma and intranuclear inclusion bodies in interstitial cells (cytomegalovirus pneumonia)

peribronchial and perivascular regions and within the alveolar septa or alveolar spaces. On imaging, the condition appears like a mixture of interstitial and alveolar space diseases. Because the CT findings are nonspecific for leukostasis, the combined features of CT findings, and clinical information can help to correctly diagnose the lung complications of leukostasis.

11.3.2.4 Superior Vena Cava Syndrome

Superior vena cava (SVC) syndrome results from partial or complete obstruction of the blood flow in the SVC and causes a reduction in venous return to the heart from the head, neck, and upper limbs [76–78]. Regarded as a classic oncological emergency, it is rarely immediately life-threatening [76]. Symptoms include cough, dyspnea, dysphagia, edema, and congestion in the neck, face, and upper limbs. Collateral venous circulation can cause distension of the surface veins of the thoracic cavity wall [76]. More than 50% of patients with SVC syndrome become symptomatic after receiving a diagnosis of cancer owing to severe clinical worsening of the cancer in these patients [77]. The prognosis for this syndrome depends on that of the underlying disease.

Malignant tumors such as lung cancer (particularly small cell lung cancer) (Fig. 11.17), lymphomas, and metastatic mediastinal tumors are responsible for more than 90% of SVC syndrome cases [76]. Venous thrombosis combined with the presence of a catheter within the superior vena cava is an uncommon cause of this condition in patients with cancer.

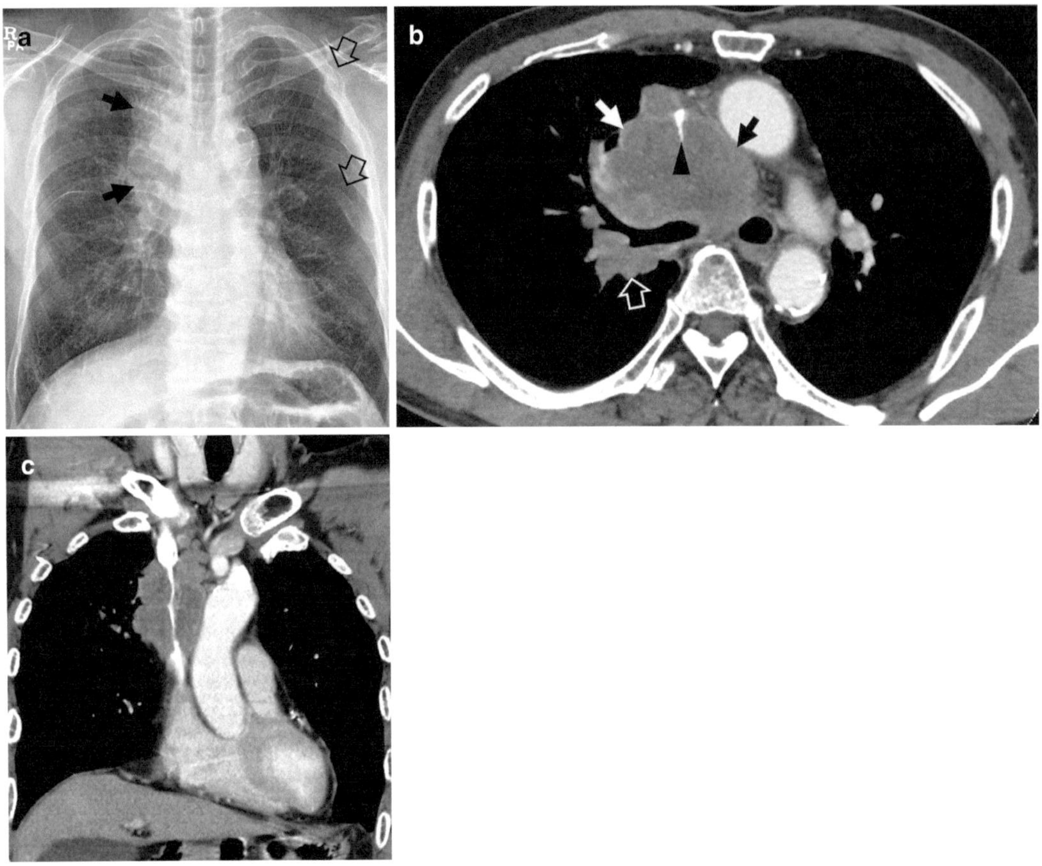

Fig. 11.17 Impending superior vena cava syndrome in a 65-year-old man with small cell lung cancer (SCLC). (**a**) Chest radiograph shows a right paratracheal mass (arrows). Also note an old rib fracture in the left hemithorax (open arrows). Interstitial markings are prominent due to pulmonary emphysema. (**b**) Mediastinal window image of a CT scan (2.5 mm section thickness) obtained at the level of the right upper lobar bronchus demonstrates a large paratracheal soft-tissue mass (arrows) and right hilar lymph node enlargement (open arrow). Also note slit-like narrowing (arrowhead) of the superior vena cava. (**c**) Coronal reformation image (2.0 mm section thickness) again depicts a narrowed segment of the superior vena cava, suggesting oncoming superior vena cava syndrome

Although superior vena cava syndrome is diagnosed clinically, CT is generally used to confirm the diagnosis via visualization of SVC luminal narrowing in association with the tumor mass or thrombosis. CT helps determine the site of obstruction and enables clinicians to differentiate extrinsic compression caused by tumor from intravascular thrombosis. CT can also provide additional information about the tumor, such as its size and relationship to other mediastinal structures (Fig. 11.17). CT should be performed with intravenous contrast medium and images acquired in the later phases to guarantee optimal contrast of the brachiocephalic veins and to avoid streak artifacts from arterial contrast [79]. If iodinated-contrast medium cannot be used, MR imaging may also be performed. Sequences with and without contrast and consequent multi-planar reconstruction assist MRI evaluation of tumor extent and compromise to the SVC and adjacent anatomical structures. Cross-sectional imaging is beneficial for therapeutic planning, especially in patients who require surgical management [80].

11.4 Summary

In order to narrow down the differential diagnoses of noninfectious emergency conditions, the authors have divided these conditions into those seen in immunocompetent and immunocompromised patients. Clinical information, including symptoms and signs and laboratory findings, appears to be very important for differential diagnosis. Fever, usually low-grade fever, can be caused by noninfectious emergency conditions. The imaging features of such conditions are usually simple: diffuse or wide patchy areas of parenchymal opacity. Nodules with poorly defined margins and of variable size may be seen as a sole manifestation or accompanied by the parenchymal opacity; they are seen in patients with DRG of organizing pneumonia or hypersensitivity pneumonia pattern and with radiation pneumonitis and organizing pneumonia pattern in immunocompetent patients. Nodules of variable size and internal necrosis are seen in patients with GPA. In immunocompromised patients, IPS can show variable patterns of lung abnormalities according to its target (lung parenchyma, endothelium, or epithelium); organizing pneumonia pattern can be the manifestation of IPS when its target is the alveolar epithelium. Leukemic and lymphomatous lung involvement also includes nodules of variable size. IVL appears as diffuse or extensive patchy areas of ground-glass opacity; small centrilobular nodules or branching nodular lesions of tree-in-bud sign may be associated or present as the lone findings.

Key Points

- The pattern approach is important in differential diagnosis. Diffuse alveolar damage pattern with diffuse or wide patchy areas of parenchymal opacity is a key feature and is seen in most diseases. In overhydration edema, parenchymal opacity is seen centrally and smooth interlobular septal thickening accompanies pleural effusion. DAH manifests as central parenchymal consolidation with subpleural sparing with or without centrilobular small nodules.
- In immunocompetent patients, nodules with poorly defined margins and of variable size may be seen as a sole manifestation or accompanied by parenchymal opacity in patients with organizing pneumonia pattern of DRG, and nodules of variable size and internal necrosis are seen in patients with GPA.
- In immunocompromised patients, IPS can appear as organizing pneumonia pattern and thus nodular lesions in both lungs, and leukemic and lymphomatous involvement of the lungs also involves nodules of variable size. IVL appears as diffuse or extensive patchy areas of ground-glass opacity. Small centrilobular nodules or branching nodular lesions of tree-in-bud sign may be associated or, rarely, be present as the lone findings.

References

1. DeWitt S, Chavez SA, Perkins J, Long B, Koyfman A. Evaluation of fever in the emergency department. Am J Emerg Med. 2017;35:1755–8.
2. Crawford SW. Noninfectious lung disease in the immunocompromised host. Respiration. 1999;66:385–95.
3. Baumann A, Audibert G, McDonnell J, Mertes PM. Neurogenic pulmonary edema. Acta Anaesthesiol Scand. 2007;51:447–55.
4. Panoskaltsis-Mortari A, Griese M, Madtes DK, et al. An official American Thoracic Society research statement: noninfectious lung injury after hematopoietic stem cell transplantation: idiopathic pneumonia syndrome. Am J Respir Crit Care Med. 2011;183:1262–79.
5. Fukuda T, Hackman RC, Guthrie KA, et al. Risks and outcomes of idiopathic pneumonia syndrome after nonmyeloablative and conventional conditioning regimens for allogeneic hematopoietic stem cell transplantation. Blood. 2003;102:2777–85.
6. Kantrow SP, Hackman RC, Boeckh M, Myerson D, Crawford SW. Idiopathic pneumonia syndrome: changing spectrum of lung injury after marrow transplantation. Transplantation. 1997;63:1079–86.
7. Yanik GA, Ho VT, Levine JE, et al. The impact of soluble tumor necrosis factor receptor etanercept on the treatment of idiopathic pneumonia syndrome after allogeneic hematopoietic stem cell transplantation. Blood. 2008;112:3073–81.
8. Solh M, Arat M, Cao Q, Majhail NS, Weisdorf D. Late-onset noninfectious pulmonary complications in adult allogeneic hematopoietic cell transplant recipients. Transplantation. 2011;91:798–803.

9. Trulock EP. Lung transplantation. Am J Respir Crit Care Med. 1997;155:789–818.
10. Porcu P, Cripe LD, Ng EW, et al. Hyperleukocytic leukemias and leukostasis: a review of pathophysiology, clinical presentation and management. Leuk Lymphoma. 2000;39:1–18.
11. Gluecker T, Capasso P, Schnyder P, et al. Clinical and radiologic features of pulmonary edema. Radiographics. 1999;19:1507–31.
12. Gurney JW, Goodman LR. Pulmonary edema localized in the right upper lobe accompanying mitral regurgitation. Radiology. 1989;171:397–9.
13. Ketai LH, Godwin JD. A new view of pulmonary edema and acute respiratory distress syndrome. J Thorac Imaging. 1998;13:147–71.
14. Cascade PN, Alexander GD, Mackie DS. Negative-pressure pulmonary edema after endotracheal intubation. Radiology. 1993;186:671–5.
15. Willms D, Shure D. Pulmonary edema due to upper airway obstruction in adults. Chest. 1988;94:1090–2.
16. Orlowski JP. Drowning, near-drowning, and ice-water submersions. Pediatr Clin N Am. 1987;34:75–92.
17. Golden FS, Tipton MJ, Scott RC. Immersion, near-drowning and drowning. Br J Anaesth. 1997;79:214–25.
18. Putman CE, Tummillo AM, Myerson DA, Myerson PJ. Drowning: another plunge. Am J Roentgenol Radium Therapy, Nucl Med. 1975;125:543–8.
19. Gattinoni L, Pelosi P, Vitale G, Pesenti A, D'Andrea L, Mascheroni D. Body position changes redistribute lung computed-tomographic density in patients with acute respiratory failure. Anesthesiology. 1991;74:15–23.
20. Morgan PW, Goodman LR. Pulmonary edema and adult respiratory distress syndrome. Radiol Clin N Am. 1991;29:943–63.
21. Kim HY, Lee KS, Kang EH, Suh GY, Kwon OJ, Chung MJ. Acute respiratory distress syndrome. Computed tomography findings and their applications to mechanical ventilation therapy. J Comput Assist Tomogr. 2004;28:686–96.
22. Camus P, Bonniaud P, Fanton A, Camus C, Baudaun N, Foucher P. Drug-induced and iatrogenic infiltrative lung disease. Clin Chest Med. 2004;25:479–519.
23. Min JH, Lee HY, Lim H, et al. Drug-induced interstitial lung disease in tyrosine kinase inhibitor therapy for non-small cell lung cancer: a review on current insight. Cancer Chemother Pharmacol. 2011;68:1099–109.
24. Cleverley JR, Screaton NJ, Hiorns MP, Flint JD, Muller NL. Drug-induced lung disease: high-resolution CT and histological findings. Clin Radiol. 2002;57:292–9.
25. Newbigin K, Souza CA, Torres C, et al. Fat embolism syndrome: state-of-the-art review focused on pulmonary imaging findings. Respir Med. 2016;113:93–100.
26. Pinney SJ, Keating JF, Meek RN. Fat embolism syndrome in isolated femoral fractures: does timing of nailing influence incidence? Injury. 1998;29:131–3.
27. Han D, Lee KS, Franquet T, et al. Thrombotic and nonthrombotic pulmonary arterial embolism: spectrum of imaging findings. Radiographics. 2003;23:1521–39.
28. Feldman F, Ellis K, Green WM. The fat embolism syndrome. Radiology. 1975;114:535–42.
29. Chung JW, Park JH, Im JG, Han JK, Han MC. Pulmonary oil embolism after transcatheter oily chemoembolization of hepatocellular carcinoma. Radiology. 1993;187:689–93.
30. Malagari K, Economopoulos N, Stoupis C, et al. High-resolution CT findings in mild pulmonary fat embolism. Chest. 2003;123:1196–201.
31. Arakawa H, Kurihara Y, Nakajima Y. Pulmonary fat embolism syndrome: CT findings in six patients. J Comput Assist Tomogr. 2000;24:24–9.
32. Heyneman LE, Muller NL. Pulmonary nodules in early fat embolism syndrome: a case report. J Thorac Imaging. 2000;15:71–4.
33. Bledsoe TJ, Nath SK, Decker RH. Radiation pneumonitis. Clin Chest Med. 2017;38:201–8.
34. NIH. Common toxicity criteria for adverse events v4.03 Available from http://evs.nci.nih.gov/ftp1/CTCAE/CTCAE_4.03_2010-06-14_QuickReference 8.5x11.pdf. Accessed 28 October 2016
35. Koh ES, Tran TH, Heydarian M, et al. A comparison of mantle versus involved-field radiotherapy for Hodgkin's lymphoma: reduction in normal tissue dose and second cancer risk. Radiat Oncol. 2007;2:13.
36. Specht L, Yahalom J, Illidge T, et al. Modern radiation therapy for Hodgkin lymphoma: field and dose guidelines from the international lymphoma radiation oncology group (ILROG). Int J Radiat Oncol Biol Phys. 2014;89:854–62.
37. Barriger RB, Forquer JA, Brabham JG, et al. A dose-volume analysis of radiation pneumonitis in non-small cell lung cancer patients treated with stereotactic body radiation therapy. Int J Radiat Oncol Biol Phys. 2012;82:457–62.
38. Kocak Z, Evans ES, Zhou SM, et al. Challenges in defining radiation pneumonitis in patients with lung cancer. Int J Radiat Oncol Biol Phys. 2005;62:635–8.
39. Faria SL, Aslani M, Tafazoli FS, Souhami L, Freeman CR. The challenge of scoring radiation-induced lung toxicity. Clin Oncol (R Coll Radiol). 2009;21:371–5.
40. Ikezoe J, Takashima S, Morimoto S, et al. CT appearance of acute radiation-induced injury in the lung. AJR Am J Roentgenol. 1988;150:765–70.
41. Arbetter KR, Prakash UB, Tazelaar HD, Douglas WW. Radiation-induced pneumonitis in the "nonirradiated" lung. Mayo Clin Proc. 1999;74:27–36.
42. Martin C, Romero S, Sanchez-Paya J, Massuti B, Arriero JM, Hernandez L. Bilateral lymphocytic alveolitis: a common reaction after unilateral thoracic irradiation. Eur Respir J. 1999;13:727–32.
43. Katayama N, Sato S, Katsui K, et al. Analysis of factors associated with radiation-induced bronchiolitis obliterans organizing pneumonia syndrome after breast-conserving therapy. Int J Radiat Oncol Biol Phys. 2009;73:1049–54.
44. Kharofa J, Cohen EP, Tomic R, Xiang Q, Gore E. Decreased risk of radiation pneumonitis with incidental concurrent use of angiotensin-converting enzyme inhibitors and thoracic radiation therapy. Int J Radiat Oncol Biol Phys. 2012;84:238–43.

45. Ward WF, Kim YT, Molteni A, Solliday NH. Radiation-induced pulmonary endothelial dysfunction in rats: modification by an inhibitor of angiotensin converting enzyme. Int J Radiat Oncol Biol Phys. 1988;15:135–40.
46. Lara AR, Schwarz MI. Diffuse alveolar hemorrhage. Chest. 2010;137:1164–71.
47. Chung MP, Yi CA, Lee HY, Han J, Lee KS. Imaging of pulmonary vasculitis. Radiology. 2010;255:322–41.
48. Primack SL, Miller RR, Muller NL. Diffuse pulmonary hemorrhage: clinical, pathologic, and imaging features. AJR Am J Roentgenol. 1995;164:295–300.
49. Primack SL, Hartman TE, Lee KS, Muller NL. Pulmonary nodules and the CT halo sign. Radiology. 1994;190:513–5.
50. Cheah FK, Sheppard MN, Hansell DM. Computed tomography of diffuse pulmonary haemorrhage with pathological correlation. Clin Radiol. 1993;48:89–93.
51. Rubin GD, Edwards DK 3rd, Reicher MA, Doemeny JM, Carson SH. Diagnosis of pulmonary hemosiderosis by MR imaging. AJR Am J Roentgenol. 1989;152:573–4.
52. Eschun GM, Mink SN, Sharma S. Pulmonary interstitial fibrosis as a presenting manifestation in perinuclear antineutrophilic cytoplasmic antibody microscopic polyangiitis. Chest. 2003;123:297–301.
53. Kim EA, Lee KS, Johkoh T, et al. Interstitial lung diseases associated with collagen vascular diseases: radiologic and histopathologic findings. Radiographics. 2002;22:S151–65.
54. Lee KS, Kim TS, Fujimoto K, et al. Thoracic manifestation of Wegener's granulomatosis: CT findings in 30 patients. Eur Radiol. 2003;13:43–51.
55. Clark JG, Hansen JA, Hertz MI, Parkman R, Jensen L, Peavy HH. NHLBI workshop summary. Idiopathic pneumonia syndrome after bone marrow transplantation. Am Rev Respir Dis. 1993;147:1601–6.
56. Cooke KR, Yanik G. Acute lung injury after allogeneic stem cell transplantation: is the lung a target of acute graft-versus-host disease? Bone Marrow Transplant. 2004;34:753–65.
57. van den Hoogen BG, de Jong JC, Groen J, et al. A newly discovered human pneumovirus isolated from young children with respiratory tract disease. Nat Med. 2001;7:719–24.
58. Zaki AM, van Boheemen S, Bestebroer TM, Osterhaus AD, Fouchier RA. Isolation of a novel coronavirus from a man with pneumonia in Saudi Arabia. N Engl J Med. 2012;367:1814–20.
59. Seo S, Renaud C, Kuypers JM, et al. Idiopathic pneumonia syndrome after hematopoietic cell transplantation: evidence of occult infectious etiologies. Blood. 2015;125:3789–97.
60. Tanaka N, Kunihiro Y, Kobayashi T, et al. High-resolution CT findings of idiopathic pneumonia syndrome after haematopoietic stem cell transplantation: based on the updated concept of idiopathic pneumonia syndrome by the American Thoracic Society in 2011. Clin Radiol. 2016;71:953–9.
61. Klatte EC, Yardley J, Smith EB, Rohn R, Campbell JA. The pulmonary manifestations and complications of leukemia. Am J Roentgenol Radium Therapy, Nucl Med. 1963;89:598–609.
62. Green RA, Nichols NJ. Pulmonary involvement in leukemia. Am Rev Respir Dis. 1959;80:833–44.
63. Tanaka N, Matsumoto T, Miura G, et al. CT findings of leukemic pulmonary infiltration with pathologic correlation. Eur Radiol. 2002;12:166–74.
64. Gibbs WN, Lofters WS, Campbell M, et al. Non-Hodgkin lymphoma in Jamaica and its relation to adult T-cell leukemia-lymphoma. Ann Intern Med. 1987;106:361–8.
65. Dixon AC, Dixon PS, Nakamura JM. Infection with the human T-lymphotropic virus type I. A review for clinicians. West J Med. 1989;151:632–7.
66. Okada F, Ando Y, Kondo Y, Matsumoto S, Maeda T, Mori H. Thoracic CT findings of adult T-cell leukemia or lymphoma. AJR Am J Roentgenol. 2004;182:761–7.
67. Sato E, Hasui K, Tokunaga M. Autopsy findings of adult T cell lymphoma-leukemia. Gann Monogr Cancer Res. 1982;28:51–64.
68. DiGiuseppe JA, Nelson WG, Seifter EJ, Boitnott JK, Mann RB. Intravascular lymphomatosis: a clinicopathologic study of 10 cases and assessment of response to chemotherapy. J Clin Oncol. 1994;12:2573–9.
69. Cha MJ, Lee KS, Hwang HS, et al. Pulmonary intravascular lymphomatosis: clinical, CT, and PET findings, correlation of CT and pathologic results, and survival outcome. Radiology. 2016;280:602–10.
70. Demirer T, Dail DH, Aboulafia DM. Four varied cases of intravascular lymphomatosis and a literature review. Cancer. 1994;73:1738–45.
71. Treves TA, Gadoth N, Blumen S, Korczyn AD. Intravascular malignant lymphomatosis: a cause of subacute dementia. Dementia. 1995;6:286–93.
72. Yamagata T, Okamoto Y, Ota K, Katayama N, Tsuda T, Yukawa S. A case of pulmonary intravascular lymphomatosis diagnosed by thoracoscopic lung biopsy. Respiration. 2003;70:414–8.
73. Jang HJ, Lee KS, Han J. Intravascular lymphomatosis of the lung: radiologic findings. J Comput Assist Tomogr. 1998;22:427–9.
74. Lewis ER, Caskey CI, Fishman EK. Lymphoma of the lung: CT findings in 31 patients. AJR Am J Roentgenol. 1991;156:711–4.
75. Bae YA, Lee KS. Cross-sectional evaluation of thoracic lymphoma. Radiol Clin N Am. 2008;46:253–64.
76. Guimaraes MD, Bitencourt AG, Marchiori E, Chojniak R, Gross JL, Kundra V. Imaging acute complications in cancer patients: what should be evaluated in the emergency setting? Cancer Imaging. 2014;14:18.
77. McCurdy MT, Shanholtz CB. Oncologic emergencies. Crit Care Med. 2012;40:2212–22.
78. Cheng S. Superior vena cava syndrome: a contemporary review of a historic disease. Cardiol Rev. 2009;17:16–23.
79. Eren S, Karaman A, Okur A. The superior vena cava syndrome caused by malignant disease. Imaging with multi-detector row CT. Eur J Radiol. 2006;59:93–103.
80. Wilson LD, Detterbeck FC, Yahalom J. Clinical practice. Superior vena cava syndrome with malignant causes. N Engl J Med. 2007;356:1862–9.

12 Postoperative Emergency

12.1 Introduction

Complications after pulmonary resection surgery differ according to the type of surgery performed and the time elapsed since surgery. Early and late complications following pneumonectomy and lobectomy or sleeve lobectomy are different. Early complications after pneumonectomy include empyema, cardiac herniation, pulmonary edema (both cardiogenic and permeability), chylothorax, hemothorax, bronchopleural fistula, wound infection, and esophagopleural fistula; the most common late complications are postpneumonectomy syndrome, recurrent tumor, and esophagopleural fistula. Early complications after lobectomy include space problems, persistent air leakage, postsurgical lobar torsion, ischemic necrotizing pneumonia, nonobstructive atelectasis, pulmonary edema, anastomotic dehiscence, hemothorax, bronchopleural fistula, wound infection, and esophagopleural fistula. Late complications include anastomotic stricture, recurrent tumor, gossypiboma, and esophagopleural fistula. Among these various complications, authors have selected empyema, cardiac herniation, permeability pulmonary edema (adult respiratory distress syndrome [ARDS]), hemothorax, and bronchopleural fistula as urgent conditions necessitating immediate intervention after pneumonectomy, and postsurgical lobar torsion, ischemic necrotizing pneumonia, ARDS, hemothorax, and bronchopleural fistula as the most urgent conditions after lobectomy [1].

Esophageal resection is a high-risk procedure associated with considerable morbidity and mortality. Significant improvements in surgical techniques and perioperative management methods have led to a decrease in both morbidity and mortality rates for esophageal resection. For example, the mortality rate dropped from 12% in the 1970s and early 1980s to 3% in the late 1980s and early 1990s [2]. A study by Swisher et al. [3] on surgery for esophageal cancer showed that the morbidity and mortality rates vary greatly depending on surgical volume, hospital size, and degree of cancer specialization. Complications after major esophageal surgery, namely surgery for esophageal cancer and esophageal stricture, are also diverse. Postoperative complications include delayed hemorrhage, anastomotic leak, mediastinitis, pulmonary complications (atelectasis, pneumonia, ARDS, and aspiration pneumonia/cellular [inflammatory] bronchiolitis), cardiac complications (arrhythmia, myocardial infarction, and pericardial tamponade), delayed gastric emptying, chylothorax, and herniation of the abdominal viscera through the esophageal hiatus. Postsurgical mediastinitis, ARDS, pneumonia, and herniation of the abdominal viscera through the esophageal hiatus are the urgent complications after major esophageal surgery [4, 5].

T. J. Kim et al., *Emergency Chest Radiology*, https://doi.org/10.1007/978-981-33-4396-2_12

Table 12.1 Postsurgical emergency complications

Surgical organs and types	Complications
Lungs or lung lobes	Postsurgical empyema, cardiac herniation, postsurgical ALI/ARDS, Hemothorax, Bronchopleural fistula, Postlobectomy lobar torsion, ischemic necrotizing pneumonia
Esophagus	Postsurgical mediastinitis, ALI/ARDS, pneumonia, herniation of abdominal viscera through esophageal hiatus
Lung transplantation	Primary graft dysfunction (transient ischemic/reperfusion injury), anastomosis dehiscence, diffuse alveolar hemorrhage

Note: *ALI* acute lung injury; *ARDS* acute (adult) respiratory distress syndrome; ALI, a common condition characterized by acute severe hypoxia encompassing a continuum of clinical and radiographic changes and affecting lungs with ARDS, of which the emergency condition represents the more severe end of the continuum

Five main kinds of complications may occur after lung transplantation; these are primary graft dysfunction, postsurgical complications, alloimmune responses, infections, and malignancy. Among postsurgical complications, anastomosis dehiscence and diffuse alveolar hemorrhage (DAH) of unknown cause may become emergent conditions.

In this chapter, the authors will discuss postsurgical empyema, cardiac herniation, postsurgical ARDS, hemothorax, bronchopleural fistula, postlobectomy lobar torsion, and ischemic necrotizing pneumonia after pneumonectomy or lobectomy. Also, the authors will elaborate on postsurgical mediastinitis, ARDS, pneumonia, and herniation of the abdominal viscera through the esophageal hiatus after major esophageal surgery. Readers are expected to encounter cases involving primary graft dysfunction and repeated diffuse alveolar hemorrhage and resultant hemochromatosis as the result of postsurgical complications (Table 12.1).

12.2 Clinical and Imaging Features of Postsurgical Complications of the Lungs or Lung Lobes

12.2.1 Postsurgical Empyema

Empyema is a serious but uncommon complication of pulmonary resection, occurring in 2–16% of patients. It is associated with a high mortality rate, which ranges widely from 16% to 71% [6]. Mortality is especially high when the empyema is associated with a large bronchopleural fistula (BPF) [7]. Postpneumonectomy empyema commonly occurs with completion pneumonectomy (i.e., pneumonectomy following previous lobectomy), right pneumonectomy, preoperative irradiation, gross contamination of the pleura, postoperative sepsis, mediastinal lymph node dissection, and a long bronchial stump and in patients requiring postoperative mechanical ventilation [6].

Empyema usually occurs in the early postoperative period but can develop months or even years after surgery. Empyema that occurs shortly after surgery is due to residual infection in the pleural cavity. Empyema may also occur secondary to BPF or an esophagopleural fistula. *Staphylococcus aureus*, *Pseudomonas aeruginosa*, *Streptococcus* species, and *Aerobacter aerogenes* are the most commonly cultured organisms in the most reported case series [8].

On chest radiography, postpneumonectomy empyema typically manifests as multiple air–fluid levels in the early postsurgical period and as mediastinal shifting away from the surgical site in the late postsurgical period. CT reveals the volume-expanding process within the postpneumonectomy space with reversal of the normal concavity of the mediastinal pleura even without mediastinal displacement (Fig. 12.1) [1].

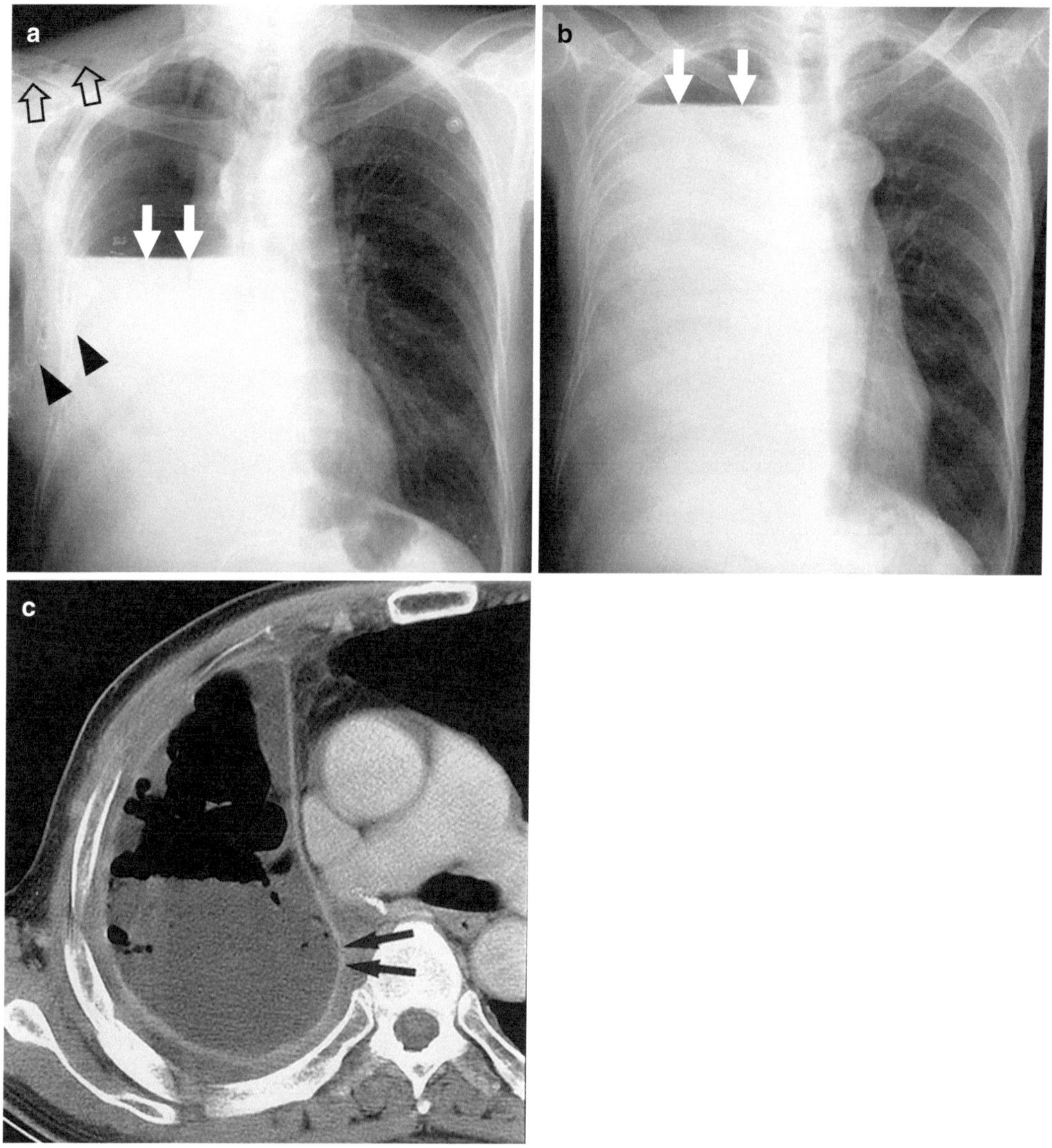

Fig. 12.1 Postpneumonectomy empyema in a 64-year-old man complaining of chest wall pain after right pneumonectomy for lung squamous cell carcinoma. (**a**) Chest radiograph obtained immediately after surgery shows an air–fluid level (arrows) in the right pneumonectomy space. Note also subcutaneous emphysema (open arrows) and surgical wires (arrowheads) in the right chest wall. (**b**) Follow-up chest radiograph obtained 63 days after (**a**) shows prominent fluid collection in the right pneumonectomy space with a persistent air–fluid level (arrows) in the right hemithorax. Also note mediastinal shifting to the left side. (**c**) Postpneumonectomy empyema in a different patient (70-year-old man) with fever, seen 5 months after right pneumonectomy for lung squamous cell carcinoma. Enhanced CT scan obtained at the right main pulmonary artery level shows hydropneumothorax with diffusely enhancing parietal pleura in the right pneumonectomy space. Note also inward convexity of the mediastinal pleura in the azygoesophageal recess (arrows), suggestive of mass effect. Cases courtesy of Kim EA et al. *Radiographics* 2002;22:67–86

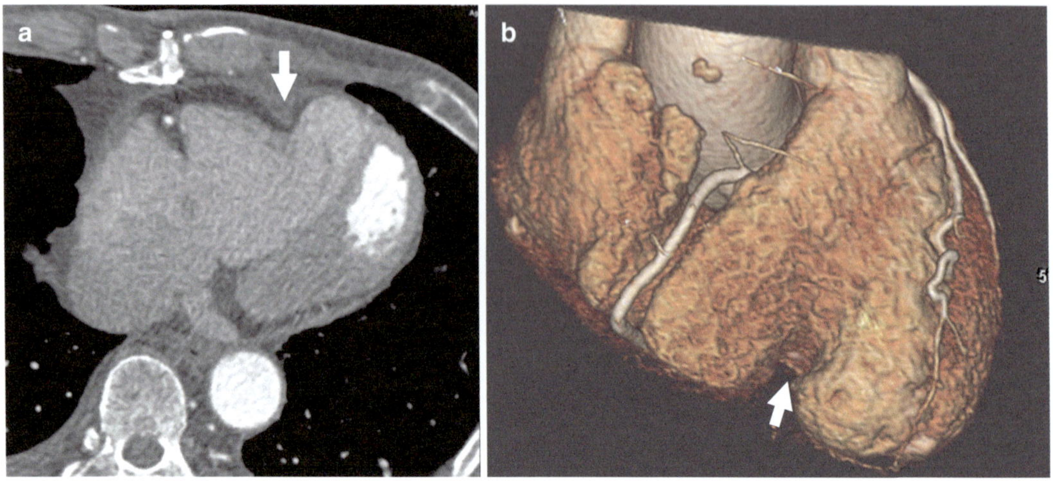

Fig. 12.2 Cardiac herniation after descending thoracic aortic aneurysm surgery in a 48-year-old man. (**a**) Transverse CT coronary angiography shows indentation of the right ventricular wall (arrow) owing to pericardial constriction. (**b**) 3D volume-rendered image also demonstrates right ventricular indentation (arrow)

12.2.2 Cardiac Herniation

Cardiac herniation with subsequent torsion is a very rare postpneumonectomy complication requiring urgent reduction. Most cases of cardiac herniation are the result of prolapse of the heart through the pericardial defect created at the time of surgery. The most common cause of cardiac herniation is an intrapericardial pneumonectomy without closure of the defect. An unusual case that occurred after lobectomy has also been reported [9]. Cardiac herniation occurs independent of the size of the pericardial defect created during surgery and shows no side predilection. It occurs most often after pneumonectomy, which creates a large dead space with negative pressure for herniation. Cardiac herniation may involve acute angulation laterally with the apex touching the lateral chest wall, or there may be lateral posterior rotation, placing the apex in the region of the posterior costophrenic sulcus [8]. Air may surround the empty pericardial space [10]. On the right side, the heart comes out of the pericardial sac and rotates in a counterclockwise manner around the axis of the vena cava, which produces superior vena cava syndrome of the upper half of the body. On the left side, the ventricles protrude through a medium-sized pericardial defect into the left pleural cavity and are strangulated by the edge of the pericardial sac [4] (Fig. 12.2).

12.2.3 Postsurgical Adult Respiratory Distress Syndrome

Adult respiratory distress syndrome is a recognized complication of lung resection surgery [11]. ARDS occurs in approximately 5% of lung or lobar resections; the reported frequency ranges from 4% to 15% [12, 13]. Although the exact definition of postpneumonectomy ARDS varies between studies [12, 13], the defining features of ARDS are common to all descriptions, such that in its most severe form, postpneumonectomy ARDS is indistinguishable from ARDS from other causes with regard to both clinical manifestations and pathologic features [1]. The mortality rate for postlobectomy ARDS has not been well defined. Estimates of mortality following the development of postpneumonectomy ARDS range between 50% and 100% [12–14].

The diagnosis of ARDS or acute lung injury is largely based on observation of the characteristic pulmonary opacity on chest radiographs and a pulmonary artery wedge pressure lower than 18 mmHg [15]. Serial chest radiographs show the

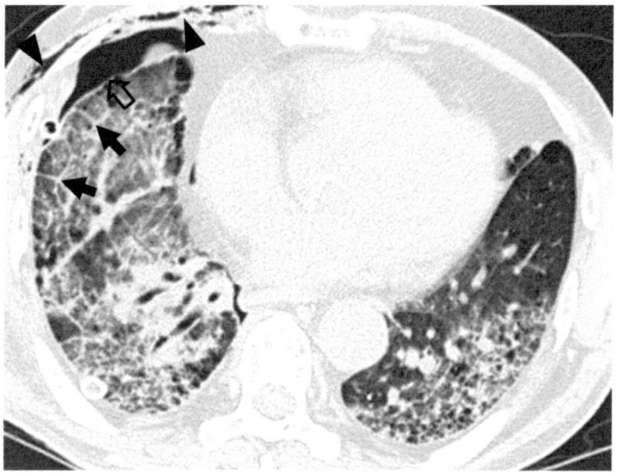

Fig. 12.3 Acute respiratory distress syndrome in a 72-year-old man after right upper lobectomy. A lung window on CT obtained at the level of the aortic valve 4 days after surgery shows parenchymal opacity in both lungs. Also note smooth interlobular septal thickening (arrows) in the right anterior lung. Right pneumothorax (open arrow) and subcutaneous emphysema (arrowheads) are associated

rapid development of diffusely increased opacity in the remaining lung (Fig. 12.3). CT depicts ground-glass opacity, increased visibility of interlobular septa, and an anteroposterior opacity gradient [16]. ARDS may also develop in combination with other postpneumonectomy complications, such as pneumonia and bronchopleural fistula with or without empyema [17].

ARDS following lobectomy is associated with asymmetric lung injury visible on CT, with the non-lobectomy-site lung more extensively involved than the remaining lobectomy-site lung/lobes. The extent of ARDS involvement in the non-lobectomy lung is more than that of compensatory hyperexpansion plus ARDS involvement of the residual lung on the operated side [16].

12.2.4 Postsurgical Hemothorax

Major hemorrhage following thoracotomy and resection is most often the result of inappropriate hemostasis of a bronchial artery or systemic vessels in the chest wall. It infrequently results from slippage of a ligature from a major pulmonary vessel or an unrecognized injury to a systemic vein. Bleeding related to a coagulation abnormality is rare. The overall mortality rate associated with uncontrolled bleeding is less than 0.1% [10]. Hemothorax often manifests as a rapidly enlarging pleural effusion. CT can demonstrate hemorrhagic pleural effusions as areas of high attenuation. CT findings in hemothorax include heterogeneous attenuation of pleural fluid, hyperattenuating areas of debris within the pleural fluid, and a fluid-hematocrit level (Fig. 12.4). As the hemorrhagic pleural effusion begins to clot, locules develop within the pleural fluid and fibrin balls emerge. These pleural pseudotumors can be distinguished from pleural-based masses by their high attenuation on unenhanced CT scans [18]. The presence of extrapleural fat within a hyperattenuated hematoma on CT helps differentiate extrapleural chest wall hematoma from hemothorax.

12.2.5 Bronchopleural Fistula

Bronchopleural fistula (BPF) remains the most dreaded complication following thoracic surgery. Its prevalence is reported to range between 2% and 13%. Reported mortality rates of BPF range from 30% to 70% [7]. The most common cause of death associated with this condition is aspiration pneumonia with subsequent ARDS. BPF is more common after right pneumonectomy than after left pneumonectomy. This is probably due to anatomic features of the right main bronchus, including its larger size, greater tendency to spring open, and less mediastinal coverage than the left main bronchus. BPF is frequently associated with postsurgical mechanical ventilation [7]. Predisposing factors include preoperative uncontrolled pleuropulmonary infection, trauma, and presurgical radiation therapy [7, 19]. BPF is the main cause of postpneumonectomy empyema.

In the immediate postsurgical period, bronchial leaks are rare and are usually due to faulty closure of the bronchus. Delayed BPF is much more common and is usually due to infection or recurrent tumor of the bronchial stump. An adequately short stump, a disease-free margin, and maintenance of bronchial vascularity by preservation of the bronchial artery or peribronchial tissue have been strongly suggested as means of avoiding avascular necrosis of the stump [7]. BPF usually develops in the bronchial stump

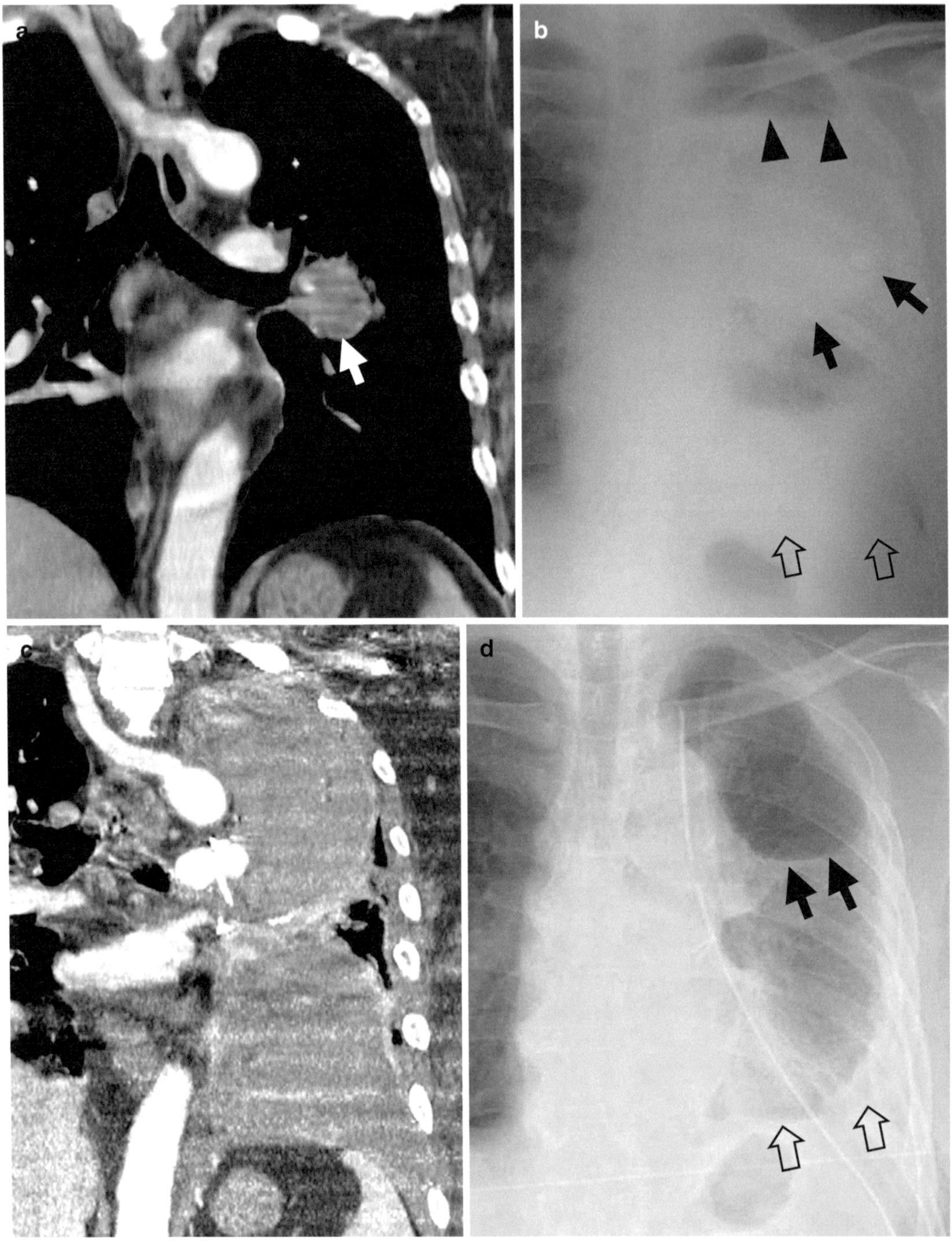

Fig. 12.4 Postsurgical hematoma in a 49-year-old man with a history of left upper lobectomy for large cell neuroendocrine carcinoma. (**a**) Coronal image of presurgical CT scan shows a 35-mm-sized mass (arrow) in the lingular segment of the left upper lobe. (**b**) Chest radiograph obtained 9 days after left upper lobectomy demonstrates mass-like opacity in the left upper (arrows) and lower (open arrows) lung zones. Also note air–blood level (arrowheads) in the apical portion. (**c**) Coronal image of a CT scan obtained on the same day as (**b**) depicts hematoma masses in the left upper and lower lung zones. (**d**) Follow-up chest radiograph obtained after completion pneumonectomy, 1.5 months after (**b**), shows hydropneumothorax in the left upper lung zone (arrows) and hemopneumothorax (open arrows) in the left lower lung zone. A chest tube has been inserted

after pneumonectomy or lobectomy and is generally diagnosed with bronchoscopy [6].

Radiologic findings in BPF consist of [1] a continuous increase in the residual intrapleural airspace, [2] the appearance of an air–fluid level, [3] changes in an already present air–fluid level, [4] development of tension pneumothorax, and [5] a drop in the air–fluid level exceeding 2 cm during the postsurgical period or reappearance of an air–fluid level in a patient who has undergone pneumonectomy [8]. Movement of the mediastinum back toward its preoperative position, a finding that suggests volume enlargement of the resected hemithorax with leaked air, may be evidence of BPF. CT is useful for the diagnosis and management of peripheral BPF. CT findings in BPF include air and fluid collections in the pleural space and the presence of a communication or tract from an airway or the lung parenchyma to the pleural space (Fig. 12.5). Direct visualization

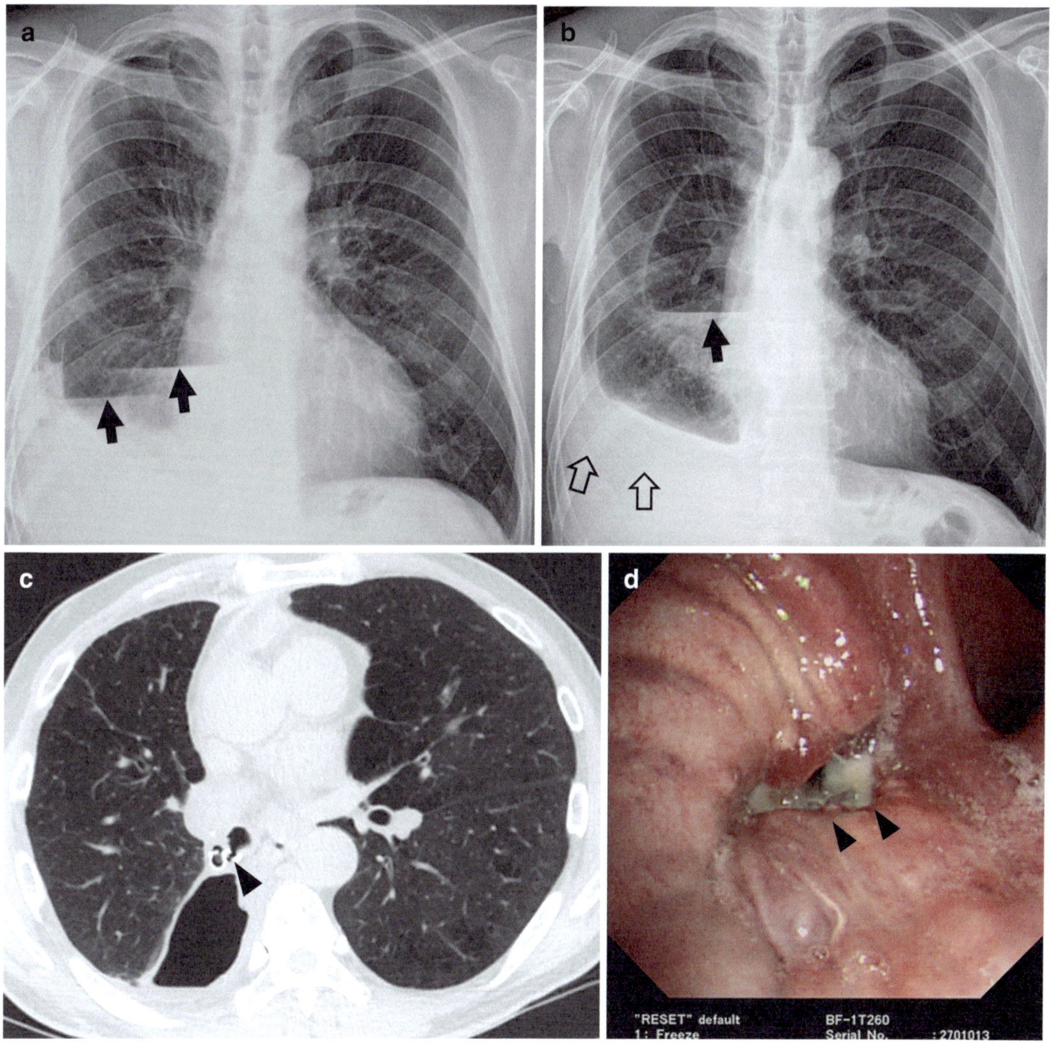

Fig. 12.5 Bronchopleural fistula after right lower lobectomy in a 54-year-old man with lung adenocarcinoma. (**a**) Chest radiograph obtained 12 days after right lower lobectomy shows multiple air–fluid levels (arrows) in the right lower lung zone. (**b**) Chest radiograph obtained 3 weeks after (**a**) demonstrates an air–fluid level (arrow) in the right lower lung zone and obliterated right costophrenic angle (open arrows). (**c**) Lung window image of a CT scan obtained at the level of the left basal trunk and at a similar time as (**b**) depicts dehiscence of the right lower lobectomy stump (arrowhead). Also note air and fluid collection in the right lower lobectomy space. (**d**) Bronchoscopy discloses an untied and opened lobectomy stump with inflammatory exudates (arrowheads)

of BPF is achieved with standard or thin-section CT in approximately 50% of patients. In the remaining patients, persistent localized air and fluid collections or a postsurgical air leak suggest the presence of BPF [20].

12.2.6 Postlobectomy Lobar Torsion

In postsurgical torsion, rapidly progressing signs and symptoms (shock, sepsis, deterioration of the patient) with resultant infarction may appear. The mortality rate is high if the torsion goes unrecognized and surgical fixation or excision of the involved lobe is delayed. The degree of rotation in pulmonary torsion is generally 180°, although occasionally, 90°or 360° torsion is recorded. Torsion of hilar structures and especially of the pulmonary veins leads to impaired circulation with reflux into the venous pathways, resulting in interstitial edema and alveolar exudation. Depending on the condition's severity, a hemorrhagic infarction may develop [21]. CT findings in lobar torsion include tapered obliteration of the proximal pulmonary artery and accompanying bronchus of the involved lobe and amorphous soft-tissue attenuation at the hilum. The torsed lobe demonstrates poorly enhancing consolidation with increased volume, ground-glass opacity, interlobular septal thickening, and intralobular linear attenuation. Neofissure following lobectomy demonstrates bulging and an unusual orientation (Figs. 12.6 and 12.7). Early recognition of postsurgical lobar torsion is vital. CT may be helpful in making an early confirmatory diagnosis.

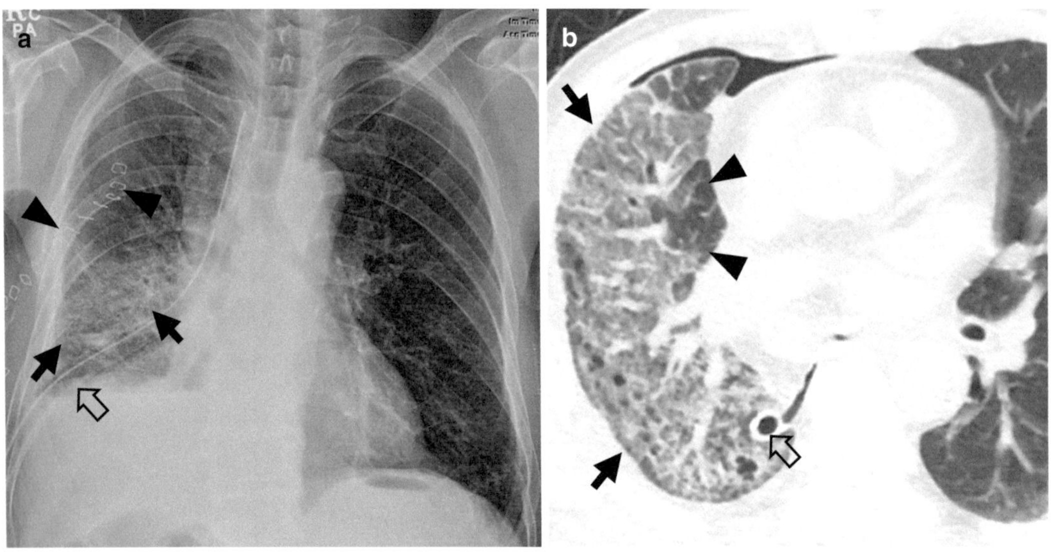

Fig. 12.6 Right middle lobe torsion after right lower lobectomy plus partial resection of the right middle lobe in a 74-year-old man with lung adenocarcinoma. (**a**) Chest radiograph obtained 18 h after surgery shows parenchymal opacity (arrows) in the right lower lung zone. Also note chest tube (open arrow) and surgical wires in the right chest wall (arrowheads). (**b**) Lung window image of a CT scan obtained at the level of the basal trunk at the same time as (**a**) demonstrates diffuse ground-glass opacity (arrows) in the remaining right middle lobe. Also note normal attenuation (arrowheads) of the bottom of the right upper lobe. A chest tube (open arrow) has been inserted. (**c**) Coronal reformatted image depicts parenchymal opacity (arrows) in the right middle lobe. A chest tube (open arrow) is seen in the right pleural space containing partial pneumothorax. (**d**) Lung window image of a CT scan obtained at the right middle lobar bronchus takeoff shows a small volume of the right middle lobe (arrows) and air–fluid level (open arrows) in the right lobectomy space, suggesting the presence of a bronchopleural fistula. (**e**) Low-magnification image of a pathologic specimen obtained after completion pneumonectomy reveals necrosis and dislocation (arrows) of cartilage in the right middle lobar bronchus. These findings are thought to be derived from torsion of the right middle lobe and resultant bronchial necrosis. (**f**) High-magnification view reveals congestion, hemorrhagic infarction, and necrotizing pneumonia (arrows) in the resected right middle lobe

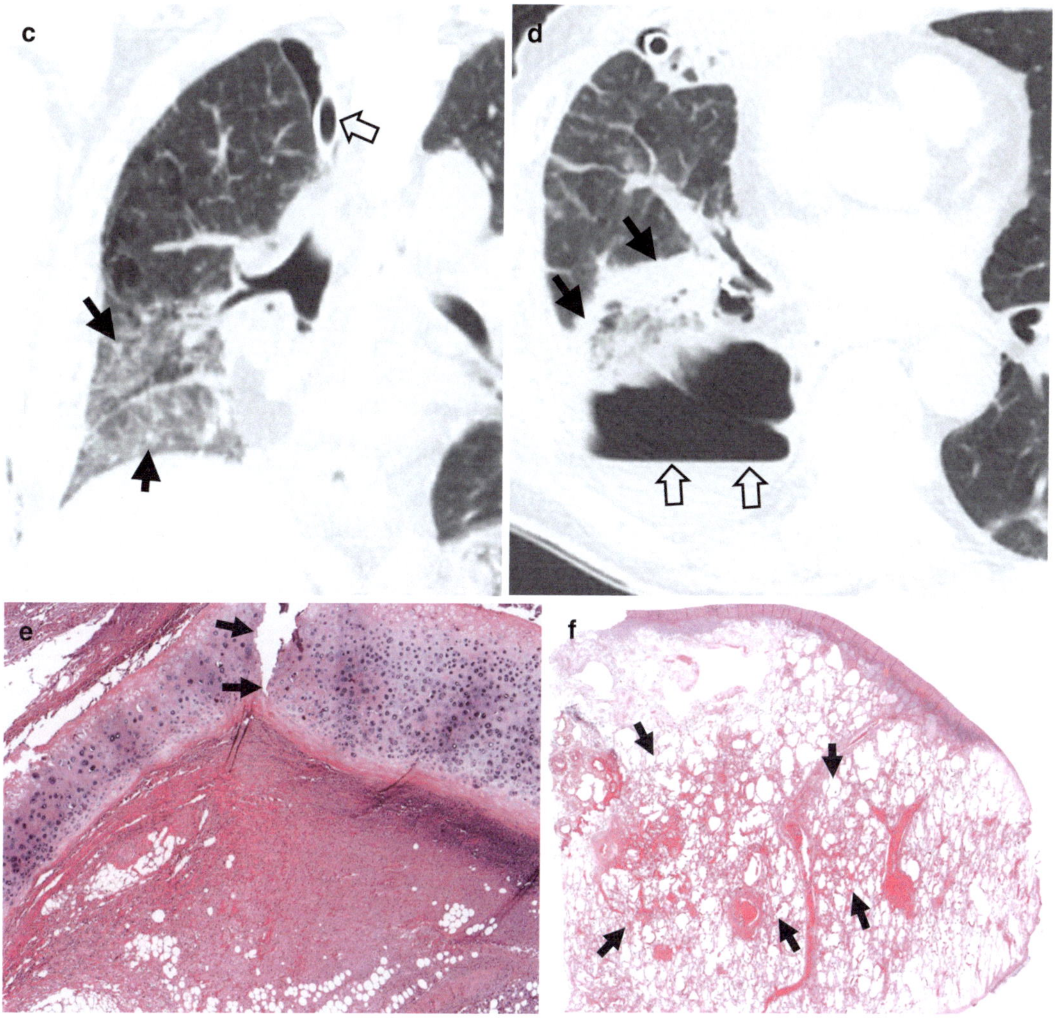

Fig. 12.6 (continued)

12.2.7 Ischemic Necrotizing Pneumonia

The reported prevalence of postthoracotomy pneumonia ranges from 2% to 22% [22]. Approximately 30% of new pulmonary infiltrates in a surgical intensive care unit are caused by a disease process other than pneumonia. Lack of radiographic evidence of pneumonia does not rule out the possibility of postsurgical pneumonia owing to the presence of a time lag between clinical presentation and radiographic manifestations. Postsurgical pneumonia is most common in patients requiring prolonged ventilator support or who have ongoing difficulty in clearing tracheobronchial secretions [8]. Postsurgical pneumonia is most often caused by aspiration of gastric secretions and bacterial colonization of the atelectatic lobe [23]. Intubation and mechanical ventilation may increase the size and prevalence of aspirations, with a concurrent increase in the development of pneumonia [24]. In hospitalized patients with colonies of highly virulent organisms, aspiration may overwhelm lung defenses, leading to the development of pneumonia.

Radiographic findings vary somewhat among the diverse species of Gram-negative bacilli.

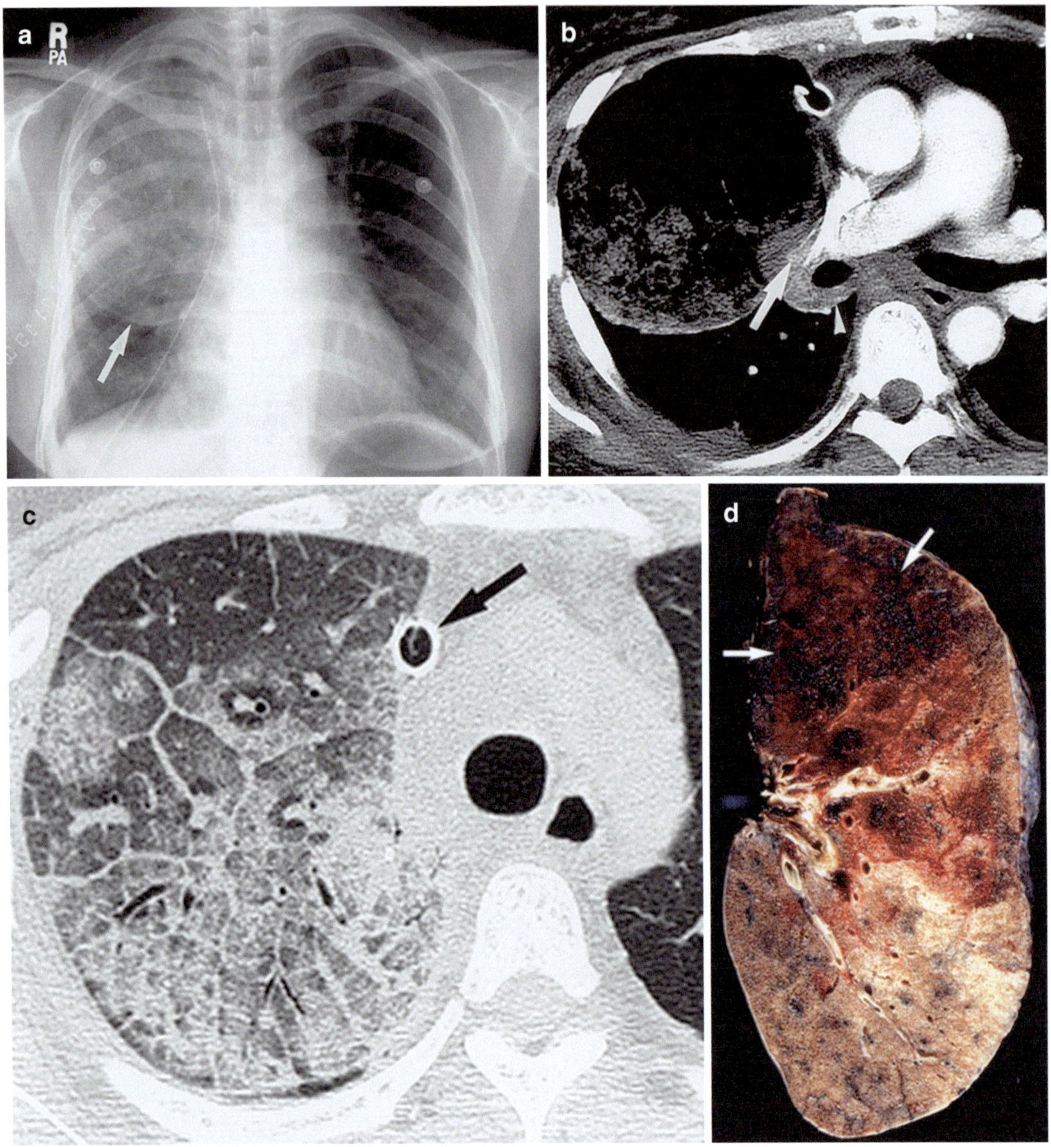

Fig. 12.7 Right upper lobe torsion in a 55-year-old woman who underwent right middle lobectomy for lung adenocarcinoma. (**a**) Chest radiograph obtained 1 day after right middle lobectomy shows rapidly developing consolidation with volume expansion in the right upper lobe. A neofissure is seen bulging downward (arrow), indicating volume increase in the right upper lobe. A chest tube is seen in the right pleural space. (**b**) Mediastinal window image of a CT scan obtained at the level of the bronchus intermedius demonstrates obstruction of the right upper lobar pulmonary artery (arrow) with surrounding soft-tissue attenuation. Also note thickening of the posterior wall of the bronchus intermedius (arrowhead). (**c**) Lung window image of a CT scan obtained at the level of the aortic arch depicts ground-glass opacity and consolidation and interlobular septal thickening with volume expansion in the right upper lobe. A chest tube (arrow) has been inserted. (**d**) Photograph of a gross pathologic specimen obtained following completion pneumonectomy discloses hemorrhagic infarction with congestion (arrows) in the right upper lobe. Cases courtesy of Kim EA et al. *Radiographics* 2002;22:67–86

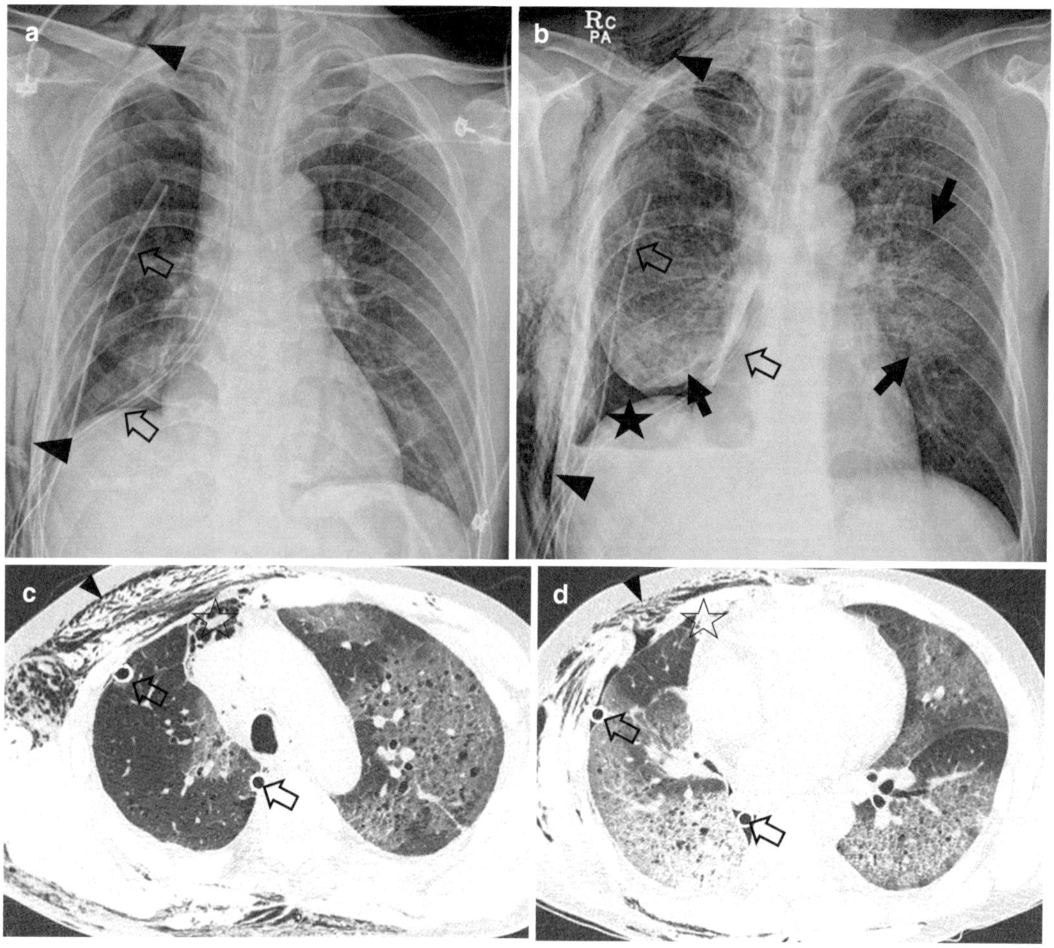

Fig. 12.8 Postsurgical pneumonia in a 60-year-old man who underwent right middle and lower bilobectomy for lung adenocarcinoma and who complained of fever and dyspnea. (**a**) Chest radiograph obtained on postsurgical day one shows two chest tubes (open arrows) in the right lobectomy space. Also note subcutaneous emphysema (arrowheads). The lungs are clear, without any parenchymal lesion. (**b**) Follow-up chest radiograph obtained 2 days after (**a**) demonstrates bilateral multifocal areas of parenchymal opacity (arrows), right hydropneumothorax (asterisk), and extensive chest wall subcutaneous emphysema (arrowheads). Chest tubes (open arrows) remain in the right pleural space. (**c**, **d**) Lung window images of CT scans obtained at the levels of the aortic arch (**c**) and left basal trunk (**d**) depict wide areas of parenchymal opacity comprised of consolidation and ground-glass opacity in both lungs. Also note chest tubes (open arrows), pneumomediastinum (asterisks), and subcutaneous emphysema (arrowheads)

Chest radiographs typically show patchy bronchopneumonic patterns. The lobar airspace consolidation pattern is much less common [25] (Fig. 12.8). A prolonged disease course or large aspirations may result in severe necrotizing bronchopneumonia.

12.3 Clinical and Imaging Features of Postsurgical Esophageal Complications

Major esophageal surgery, especially for esophageal cancer and esophageal stricture, consists of the following procedures: (1) esophageal resection through right or left thoracotomy and transhiatal blunt esophageal resection without thoracotomy; (2) securing of an esophageal substitute constructed from free revascularized whole stomach, colon, gastric tube, or jejunum; and (3) anastomosis between the remaining esophagus and the esophageal substitute. Usually, both thoracotomy and laparoscopy/laparotomy are necessary. Thus, major esophageal surgery is a lengthy procedure. The details of such surgeries are illustrated nicely in a pictorial review published by Kim et al. [4]. The following complications are urgent conditions that require prompt and appropriate intervention.

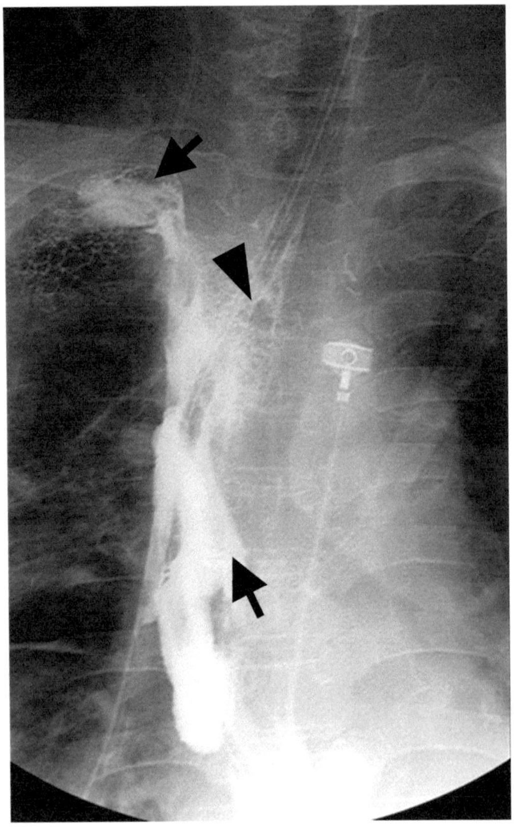

Fig. 12.9 Esophagopleural fistula after Ivor Lewis operation (separate laparotomy and right thoracotomy incision for esophagectomy and esophagogastrostomy) in a 56-year-old man with intrathoracic middle esophageal cancer. Gastrografin esophagography shows leakage of contrast dye into the pleural space (arrows) through a fistulous connection (arrowhead) between the esophagus and pleural space

12.3.1 Anastomotic Leak

Anastomotic leak is one of the major postsurgical complications following esophagectomy and is reported to occur in up to 50% of patients who undergo esophageal resection surgery [26]. Modern surgical management of intrathoracic leaks results in a mortality rate of only 3.3% and therefore, anastomotic leakage has no impact on long-term survival [27]. Anastomotic leak may occur either in the early postsurgical period (2–3 days postoperative) due to technical failure, or later (3–7 days), when it is commonly attributable to ischemic changes in the pulled-up stomach, usually at or just below the anastomosis site [5]. One-half of intrathoracic leaks are subclinical.

Such leaks can be detected with a routine contrast study, which is usually performed on postsurgical day 7. Most subclinical leaks heal without treatment. Minor leaks require conservative treatment such as antibiotics, nasogastric tube placement, or total parenteral nutrition. Larger leaks are treated in the same manner, but they often require adequate drainage of contained fluid (infected or not infected) that has collected in the vicinity of the anastomosis [28]. Intrathoracic leaks can be treated with placement of a pigtail catheter or chest tube under fluoroscopic or CT guidance. An uncontained leak, which is defined as a large leak that allows free flow of contrast material into the pleural space on esophagography (Fig. 12.9), may require surgical intervention [29]. Anastomotic leak can cause fistula formation with adjacent anatomic structures, such as airways (esophagobronchial), the pleura (esophagopleural), or the skin (esophagocutaneous fistula). Patients who develop anastomotic leaks have a higher chance of eventual stricture formation and should be considered for early esophageal dilation [5].

12.3.2 Postsurgical Mediastinitis

Mediastinitis caused by anastomotic leak is the most severe complication after esophagectomy. Mediastinitis presents as a local intrathoracic reaction or both intrathoracic and systemic extrathoracic reactions (sepsis). When the normal postsurgical course is disturbed, early diagnostic workup is needed in order to achieve successful management. Direct endoscopic surveillance of the anastomosis site should be used to verify the vitality of the anastomosed organs; if a leak is present, its size should be assessed. A wide spectrum of therapeutic options, ranging from simple drainage procedures, endoscopic interventions, and stent implantation to reoperation or discontinuity resection, are appropriate according to the location of leakage/mediastinitis and the patient's condition. The goals of treatment should be (1) immediate and sufficient drainage of the leakage and (2) prevention of further contamination via the leakage site by gastrointestinal contents. Also important in patient management is the early initiation of supportive systemic measures according to the pathophysiologic principles of sepsis [30].

12.3.3 Adult Respiratory Distress Syndrome

Acute lung injury (ALI)/ARDS is a serious complication in patients undergoing esophagectomy because the condition is associated with prolonged hospital stay and increased in-hospital mortality. Multivariate logistic regression analysis indicated that presurgical lowered FEV1/FVC, American Society of Anesthesiologists (ASA) classification, and duration of one-lung ventilation are independent risk factors for the development of ALI/ARDS after esophagectomy. Careful assessment of the patient before surgery and reduced duration of one-lung ventilation are key in preventing ALI/ARDS after esophagectomy [31].

The use of corticosteroids in patients with ALI following esophagectomy requires attention to surgical site complications and close surveillance to identify new infections [32]. As for ALI/ARDS after lung resection surgery, a diagnosis of ALI/ARDS is largely based on observation of the characteristic pulmonary opacity on chest radiographs that demonstrate rapid development of diffusely increased opacity in the lungs. CT exhibits ground-glass opacity, thickened interlobular septa, and increasing opacity from the anterior lungs to dependent lungs [15] (Fig. 12.10).

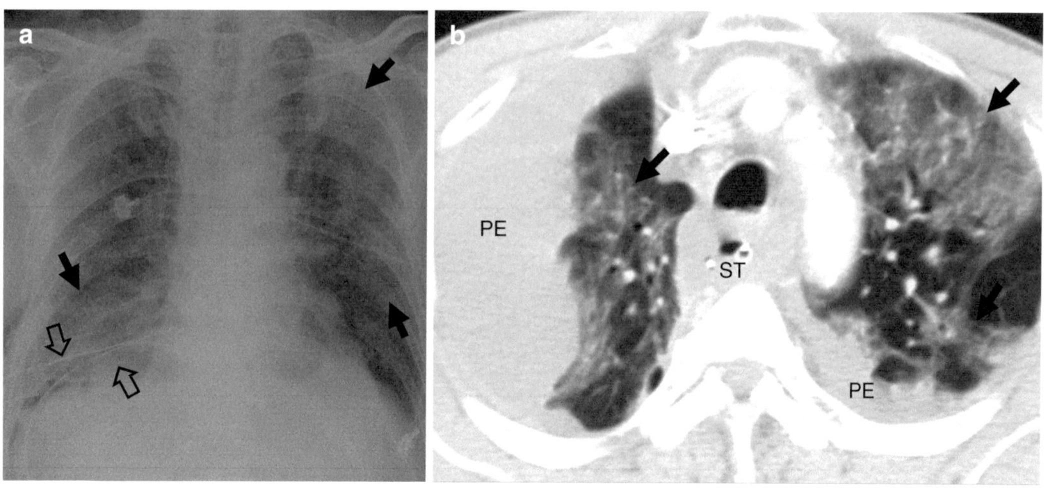

Fig. 12.10 Adult respiratory distress syndrome that developed after Ivor Lewis operation for esophageal cancer. (**a**) Chest radiograph obtained 6 days after surgery shows patchy areas of parenchymal opacity (arrows) in both lungs. Also note two chest tubes in the right pleural space (open arrows, in lower lung zone). (**b**) Lung window image of a CT scan obtained at the level of the aortic arch demonstrates patchy areas of ground-glass opacity (arrows) in both lungs. Also note bilateral pleural effusions (PE) and pulled-up stomach (ST)

12.3.4 Pneumonia

Pneumonia is the most common clinically important pulmonary complication, occurring in up to 30% of patients (15%–30%) undergoing esophageal resection surgery. The overall mortality rate of pneumonia is approximately10% [33, 34]. Decreased vital capacity is well correlated with the incidence of pulmonary complications [35].

12.3.5 Hiatal Hernia after Esophagectomy

Hiatal hernia (HH) is an infrequent but potentially life-threatening complication after esophagectomy. According to a meta-analysis, postsurgical HH occurred in 240 (3.96%) of 6058 patients who underwent esophagectomy. The pooled incidence of symptomatic HH after MIE is 4.5%, compared to a pooled incidence of 1.0% after open esophagectomy. Most importantly, surgical repair of HH is associated with a high morbidity rate (25%) [36].

12.4 Clinical and Imaging Features of Complications Related to Lung Transplantation

After lung transplantation, five types of main complications can occur: (1) primary graft dysfunction (transient ischemic/reperfusion injury during the first 3 days after surgery) (Fig. 12.11); (2) postsurgical complications; (3) allo-immune responses (acute rejection or chronic lung allograft dysfunction); (4) infections; and (5) malignancy (post-transplantation lymphoproliferative disease: PTLD) [37].

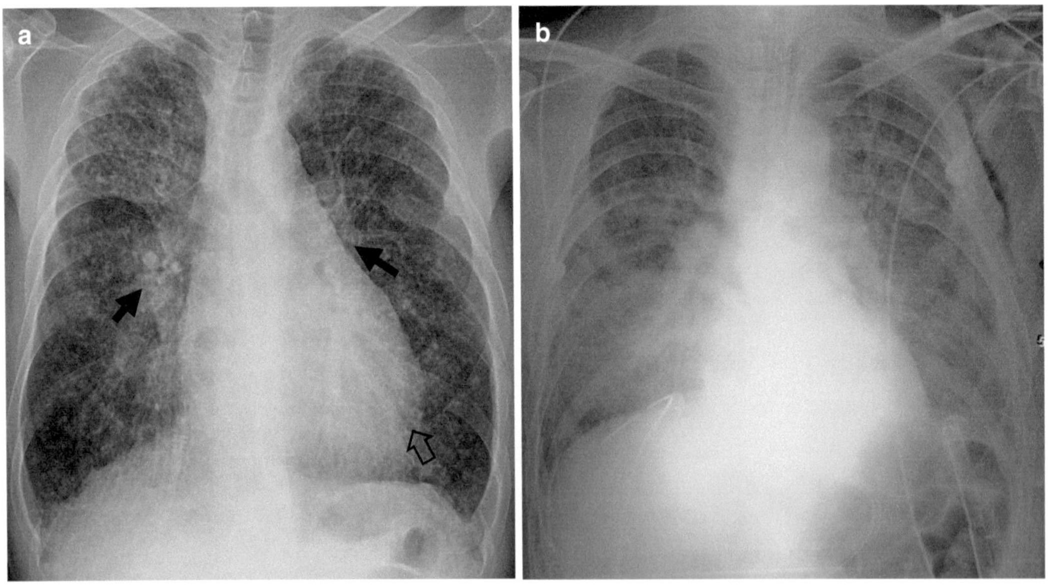

Fig. 12.11 Reperfusion edema after bilateral lung transplantation in a 44-year-old man. (**a**) Chest radiograph taken before lung transplantation shows extensive small nodular lesions in both lungs, bilateral hilar enlargement (arrows), and cardiomegaly and left apical elevation (open arrow) suggesting the presence of pulmonary hypertension and right-side chamber enlargement. The explanted lung (not shown here) demonstrated bronchiectasis, acute inflammatory bronchiolitis, and diffuse formation of micro-abscesses in both lungs. (**b**) Chest radiograph obtained 3 days after transplantation depicts extensive parenchymal opacity in both lungs. Endotracheal tube and chest tubes in the bilateral lower lung zones are located in situ. (**c**) Lung window of a CT scan obtained at the cardiac ventricular level shows gravity-dependent opacity in both lungs simulating adult respiratory distress syndrome. Opacity decreased markedly on a chest radiograph (not shown here) obtained 3 days after the current CT study

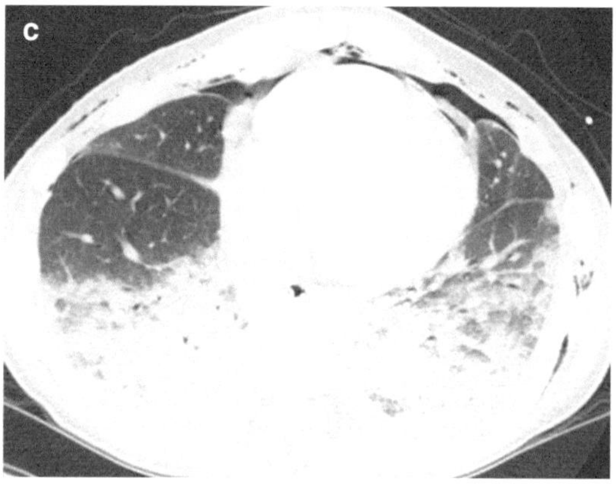

Fig. 12.11 (continued)

Postsurgical complications, as depicted on CT, include bronchial anastomosis dehiscence, bronchial stenosis and bronchomalacia, pulmonary artery stenosis, size mismatch, and repeated hemorrhage and hemosiderosis (Fig. 12.12). Similar to postsurgical emergency after lung surgery or esophageal resection surgery, bronchial anastomosis dehiscence could become an emergency post-transplantation complication.

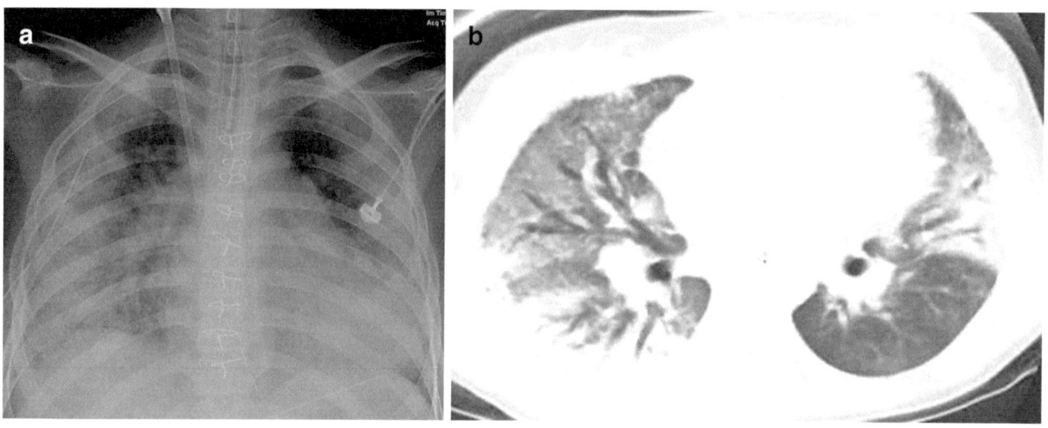

Fig. 12.12 Repeated hemorrhage and hemochromatosis after heart transplantation (for dilated cardiomyopathy) in a 13-year-old girl. The patient also underwent bilateral lung transplantation (due to recurrent infection, sepsis, and difficult weaning of extra-corporeal membrane oxygenation) following the heart transplantation. The interval between heart and lung transplantations was 9 months. (**a**) Chest radiograph obtained after heart transplantation shows extensive lung parenchymal opacity in both lungs with relative sparing of the parahilar regions, features suggestive of diffuse alveolar damage (DAD; adult respiratory distress syndrome). A heart biopsy specimen (not shown here) obtained at this time showed acute rejection. (**b**, **c**) Lung window images of CT scans obtained at the levels of the right middle lobar bronchus and (**b**) and right inferior pulmonary vein (**c**) on the same day as (**a**) demonstrate extensive parenchymal opacity in both lungs with internal CT air-bronchogram signs. A transbronchial lung biopsy specimen did not show any organismal growth. (**d**, **e**) Lung window images of CT scans obtained at similar levels as **b** and **c** 9 months afterward depict patchy areas of parenchymal opacity in both lungs and multi-loculated pneumothoraces (P) in the bilateral pleural spaces. Bilateral lung transplantation was performed after acquisition of CT images **d** and **e**. (**f**) Pathologic specimens obtained from explanted lungs disclose diffuse interstitial thickening and fibrosis with hemochromatosis. Inset: Hemosiderin-laden macrophages in the alveolar spaces (arrows) and thickened and fibrotic interstitium (arrowheads)

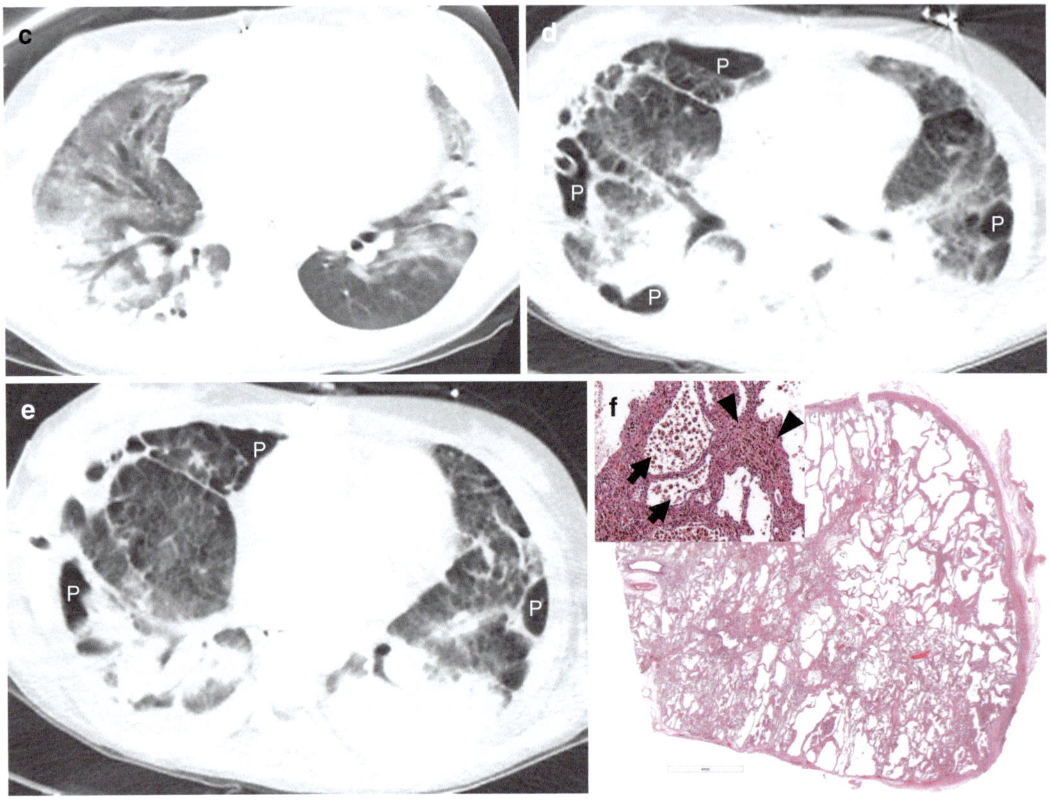

Fig. 12.12 (continued)

12.5 Summary

The radiologist plays a major role in the diagnosis of various complications following pulmonary or esophageal resection surgery and lung transplantation. The relatively low diagnostic accuracy of chest radiography may be improved by familiarity with the clinical settings in which specific complications are likely to occur. Awareness of the diverse radiographic appearances of complications following pulmonary or lung resection and lung transplantation should lead to improved early recognition of these complications, several of which may be life-threatening and require emergency management. When radiographic findings are subtle or equivocal, CT frequently allows more accurate identification of the disease process as well as prompt and appropriate intervention.

Key Points

Familiarity with surgical procedures related to lung and esophageal resection and lung transplantation appears to be the main prerequisite for understanding postsurgical urgent conditions. The most common and dreaded complication is ARDS. Chest radiograph and CT show extensive parenchymal opacity in the remaining lung or lobes in ARDS. After lobectomy, ARDS shows denser opacity within the contralateral lung than in the remaining ipsilateral lung or lobe (i.e., the non-lobectomy-site lung is more extensively involved than the remaining lobectomy-site lung/lobes). Lobar torsion is rare, but when it occurs, it causes lobar volume increase with opacity. CT helps identify unusual anatomy (distortion) of the vessels and bronchus of the corresponding lobe. Cardiac herniation is also very rare, but with recent improvements in imaging techniques (multi-planar reformation and 3D rendering), indentation of normal cardiac morphology or constriction of the pericardial anatomy may be observed on CT scans. Demonstration of BPF (central or peripheral type) and anastomotic dehiscence is also feasible with sophisticated CT rendering techniques. Various complications are expected after lung transplantation. Again, complications related to surgical technique, primary graft dysfunction, and postsurgical infection are the main urgent conditions necessitating immediate management.

References

1. Kim EA, Lee KS, Shim YM, et al. Radiographic and CT findings in complications following pulmonary resection. Radiographics. 2002;22(1):67–86. https://doi.org/10.1148/radiographics.22.1.g02ja0367.
2. Swisher SG, Hunt KK, Holmes EC, Zinner MJ, McFadden DW. Changes in the surgical management of esophageal cancer from 1970 to 1993. Am J Surg. 1995;169(6):609–14. https://doi.org/10.1016/s0002-9610(99)80231-1.
3. Swisher SG, Deford L, Merriman KW, et al. Effect of operative volume on morbidity, mortality, and hospital use after esophagectomy for cancer. J Thorac Cardiovasc Surg. 2000;119(6):1126–32. https://doi.org/10.1067/mtc.2000.105644.
4. Kim SH, Lee KS, Shim YM, Kim K, Yang PS, Kim TS. Esophageal resection: indications, techniques, and radiologic assessment. Radiographics. 2001;21(5):1119–37.; discussion 1138-1140. https://doi.org/10.1148/radiographics.21.5.g01se031119.
5. Kim TJ, Lee KH, Kim YH, et al. Postoperative imaging of esophageal cancer: what chest radiologists need to know. Radiographics. 2007;27(2):409–29. https://doi.org/10.1148/rg.272065034.
6. Wain JC. Management of late postpneumonectomy empyema and bronchopleural fistula. Chest Surg Clin N Am. 1996;6(3):529–41.
7. Wright CD, Wain JC, Mathisen DJ, Grillo HC. Postpneumonectomy bronchopleural fistula after sutured bronchial closure: incidence, risk factors, and management. J Thorac Cardiovasc Surg. 1996;112(5):1367–71. https://doi.org/10.1016/S0022-5223(96)70153-8.
8. Kirsh MM, Rotman H, Behrendt DM, Orringer MB, Sloan H. Complications of pulmonary resection. Ann Thorac Surg. 1975;20(2):215–36. https://doi.org/10.1016/s0003-4975(10)63878-7.
9. Ohri SK, Siddiqui AA, Townsend ER. Cardiac torsion after lobectomy with partial pericardectomy. Ann Thorac Surg. 1992;53(4):703–5. https://doi.org/10.1016/0003-4975(92)90341-z.
10. Goodman LR. Postoperative chest radiograph: II. Alterations after major intrathoracic surgery. AJR Am J Roentgenol. 1980;134(4):803–13. https://doi.org/10.2214/ajr.134.4.803.
11. Zeldin RA, Normandin D, Landtwing D, Peters RM. Postpneumonectomy pulmonary edema. J Thorac Cardiovasc Surg. 1984;87(3):359–65.
12. Turnage WS, Lunn JJ. Postpneumonectomy pulmonary edema. A retrospective analysis of associated variables. Chest. 1993;103(6):1646–50. https://doi.org/10.1378/chest.103.6.1646.
13. van der Werff YD, van der Houwen HK, Heijmans PJ, et al. Postpneumonectomy pulmonary edema. A retrospective analysis of incidence and possible risk factors. Chest. 1997;111(5):1278–84. https://doi.org/10.1378/chest.111.5.1278.
14. Hayes JP, Williams EA, Goldstraw P, Evans TW. Lung injury in patients following thoracotomy. Thorax. 1995;50(9):990–1. https://doi.org/10.1136/thx.50.9.990.
15. Chae EJ, Seo JB, Kim SY, et al. Radiographic and CT findings of thoracic complications after pneumonectomy. Radiographics. 2006;26(5):1449–68. https://doi.org/10.1148/rg.265055156.
16. Padley SP, Jordan SJ, Goldstraw P, Wells AU, Hansell DM. Asymmetric ARDS following pulmonary resection: CT findings initial observations. Radiology. 2002;223(2):468–73. https://doi.org/10.1148/radiol.2232010721.
17. Deb S, Fonseca P. Respiratory distress following pneumonectomy. Chest. 1999;116(5):1461–3. https://doi.org/10.1378/chest.116.5.1461.
18. Kuhlman JE, Singha NK. Complex disease of the pleural space: radiographic and CT evaluation. Radiographics. 1997;17(1):63–79. https://doi.org/10.1148/radiographics.17.1.9017800.
19. Friedman PJ, Hellekant CA. Radiologic recognition of bronchopleural fistula. Radiology. 1977;124(2):289–95. https://doi.org/10.1148/124.2.289.
20. Westcott JL, Volpe JP. Peripheral bronchopleural fistula: CT evaluation in 20 patients with pneumonia, empyema, or postoperative air leak. Radiology. 1995;196(1):175–81. https://doi.org/10.1148/radiology.196.1.7784563.
21. Berkmen YM, Yankelevitz D, Davis SD, Zanzonico P. Torsion of the upper lobe in pneumothorax. Radiology. 1989;173(2):447–9. https://doi.org/10.1148/radiology.173.2.2798876.
22. Ferdinand B, Shennib H. Postoperative pneumonia. Chest Surg Clin N Am. 1998;8(3):529–39.
23. Schweizer A, de Perrot M, Hohn L, Spiliopoulos A, Licker M. Massive contralateral pneumonia following thoracotomy for lung resection. J Clin Anesth. 1998;10(8):678–80. https://doi.org/10.1016/s0952-8180(98)00088-9.
24. DePaso WJ. Aspiration pneumonia. Clin Chest Med. 1991;12(2):269–84.
25. Franquet T, Gimenez A, Roson N, Torrubia S, Sabate JM, Perez C. Aspiration diseases: findings, pitfalls, and differential diagnosis. Radiographics.

2000;20(3):673–85. https://doi.org/10.1148/radiographics.20.3.g00ma01673.
26. Bruce J, Krukowski ZH, Al-Khairy G, Russell EM, Park KG. Systematic review of the definition and measurement of anastomotic leak after gastrointestinal surgery. Br J Surg. 2001;88(9):1157–68. https://doi.org/10.1046/j.0007-1323.2001.01829.x.
27. Martin LW, Swisher SG, Hofstetter W, et al. Intrathoracic leaks following esophagectomy are no longer associated with increased mortality. Ann Surg. 2005;242(3):392–9. https://doi.org/10.1097/01.sla.0000179645.17384.12.
28. Bains MS. Complications of abdominal right-thoracic (Ivor Lewis) esophagectomy. Chest Surg Clin N Am. 1997;7(3):587–98. discussion 598-589
29. Urschel JD. Esophagogastrostomy anastomotic leaks complicating esophagectomy: a review. Am J Surg. 1995;169(6):634–40. https://doi.org/10.1016/s0002-9610(99)80238-4.
30. Bartels H, Siewert JR. Therapy of mediastinitis in patients with esophageal cancer. Chirurg. 2008;79(1):30–7. https://doi.org/10.1007/s00104-007-1441-2.
31. Xu JX, Wang HZ, Dong J, et al. Analysis of risk factors for acute lung injury/acute respiratory distress syndrome after esophagectomy. Beijing Da Xue Xue Bao Yi Xue Ban. 2018;50(6):1057–62.
32. Choi H, Cho JH, Kim HK, et al. Prevalence and clinical course of postoperative acute lung injury after esophagectomy for esophageal cancer. J Thorac Dis. 2019;11(1):200–5. https://doi.org/10.21037/jtd.2018.12.102.
33. Millikan KW, Silverstein J, Hart V, et al. A 15-year review of esophagectomy for carcinoma of the esophagus and cardia. Arch Surg. 1995;130(6):617–24. https://doi.org/10.1001/archsurg.1995.01430060055011.
34. Shirinzadeh A, Talebi Y. Pulmonary complications due to esophagectomy. J Cardiovasc Thorac Res. 2011;3(3):93–6. https://doi.org/10.5681/jcvtr.2011.020.
35. Nagawa H, Kobori O, Muto T. Prediction of pulmonary complications after transthoracic oesophagectomy. Br J Surg. 1994;81(6):860–2. https://doi.org/10.1002/bjs.1800810622.
36. Oor JE, Wiezer MJ, Hazebroek EJ. Hiatal hernia after open versus minimally invasive esophagectomy: a systematic review and meta-analysis. Ann Surg Oncol. 2016;23(8):2690–8. https://doi.org/10.1245/s10434-016-5155-x.
37. Habre C, Soccal PM, Triponez F, et al. Radiological findings of complications after lung transplantation. Insights Imaging. 2018;9(5):709–19. https://doi.org/10.1007/s13244-018-0647-9.

13 Pleural Diseases

13.1 Introduction

Many clinical conditions encountered in an emergency department can accompany pleural abnormality. Pleural abnormality includes various disorders, from simple pleural effusion to pleural malignancy. This chapter deals with three categories of pleural conditions (pneumothorax, hemothorax, and pleural infection), as prompt and timely patient management is crucial for these cases. Chest imaging (both radiograph and CT) plays an essential role in detecting and diagnosing these pleural conditions.

13.2 Pneumothorax

Pneumothorax is defined as the presence of an air collection in the pleural space. It can be classified as spontaneous (no preceding trauma or other obvious cause) or traumatic (direct or indirect trauma) [1]. Spontaneous pneumothorax can be subclassified as primary (no underlying lung disease) or secondary (with underlying lung disease, most commonly chronic obstructive pulmonary disease). Pneumothorax is a very common condition in the trauma setting: it is present in 40 and 20%, respectively, of blunt and penetrating thoracic trauma patients [2]. It is caused by alveolar rupture due to a sudden increase in intrathoracic pressure, blunt crushing force or deceleration force to the chest, or direct penetrating injury to the pleura.

13.2.1 Imaging Findings

The initial imaging diagnosis of pneumothorax is usually made based on chest radiography (Fig. 13.1). On radiography, skin folds (Fig. 13.2), tape, gowns, vascular lines, and the medial scapular border can mimic pneumothorax. The complete absence of vascular shadows beyond the apparent visceral pleural line is a key supporting finding that is suggestive of pneumothorax [3]. Giant bullous emphysema can also mimic pneumothorax (Fig. 13.3). In addition, pneumothorax ex vacuo due to lung entrapment should be differentiated from pneumothorax due to air leakage, as pneumothorax ex vacuo usually does not require chest tube drainage (Fig. 13.4).

In supine patients, 10%–80% of pneumothoraces from blunt trauma cannot be visualized on chest radiography but can be seen on CT [4–6]. These pneumothoraces seen only on CT are called occult pneumothoraces (Fig. 13.5). Air in the pleural space accumulates nondependent area; it accumulates in the upper and lateral pleural space when patients are in an upright position. However, it moves anteriorly and medially when patients are in a supine position. As a result, a pneumothorax may be occult on chest radiographs obtained in the supine position, even though it can be seen on a chest radiograph obtained in the upright position. The presence of a pneumothorax should be suspected when the following imaging findings are seen on a supine radiograph: (a) increased lucency at the affected

T. J. Kim et al., *Emergency Chest Radiology*, https://doi.org/10.1007/978-981-33-4396-2_13

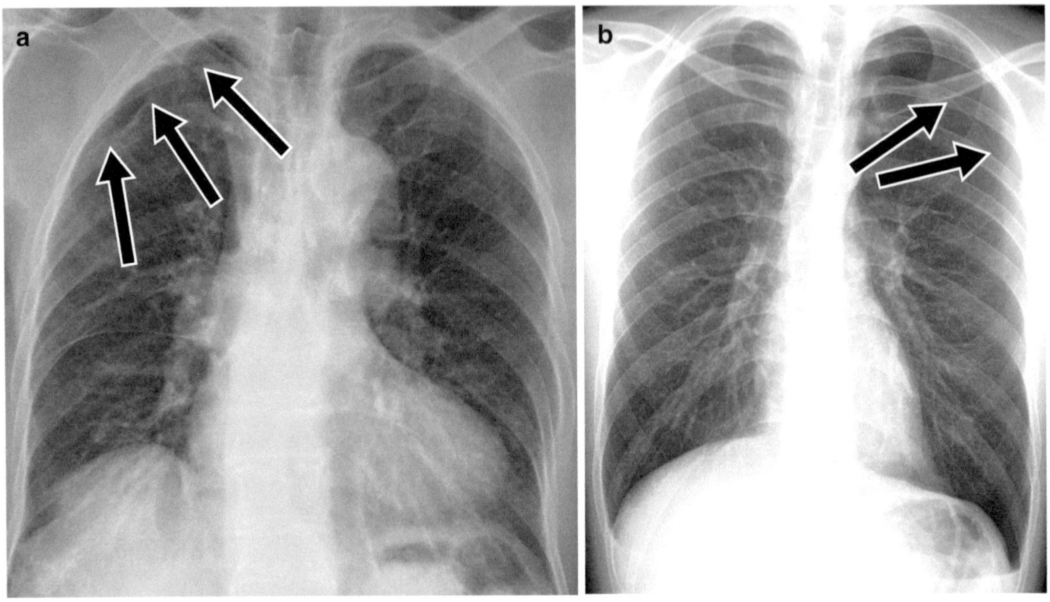

Fig. 13.1 Pneumothorax on posteroanterior chest radiograph in erect patients. (**a**, **b**) Chest radiographs demonstrate pneumothorax (**a** right; **b** left) in the upper, lateral pleural space. There is a complete absence of vascular shadows beyond the visceral pleural line (arrows)

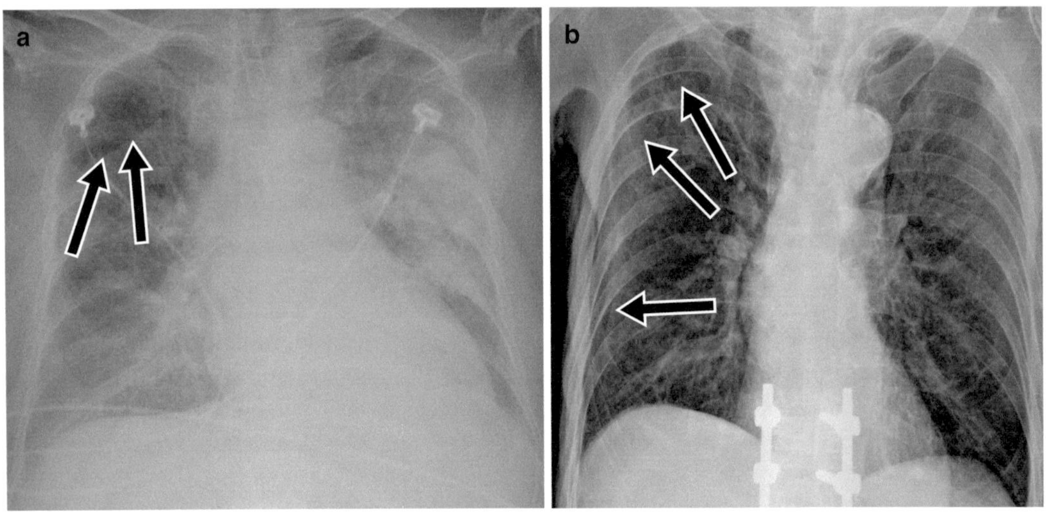

Fig. 13.2 Skin folds. (**a**, **b**) Chest radiographs show skin folds (arrows), which can mimic pneumothorax. In contrast to pneumothorax, pulmonary vascular shadows are present beyond the skin folds. In addition, the lines of skin folds are thicker and more blunt than the visceral pleural lines of pneumothorax

lung base, (b) the "deep sulcus" sign, and (c) sharp delineation of the mediastinal border (Fig. 13.6). Even a small occult pneumothorax may become clinically symptomatic when it enlarges in patients who are placed on positive mechanical ventilation or undergo general anesthesia with endotracheal tube placement.

13.2.2 Tension Pneumothorax

Tension pneumothorax is particularly lethal and has been reported in up to 5% of all major trauma patients [7, 8]. Tension pneumothorax occurs when the intrapleural pressure exceeds the atmospheric pressure throughout expiration and often

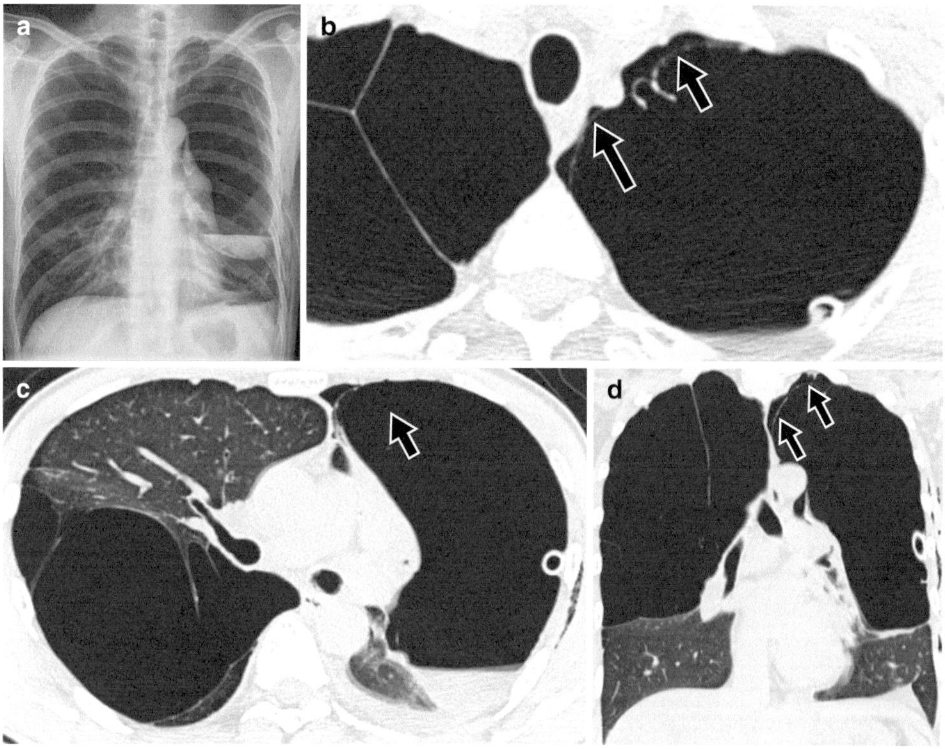

Fig. 13.3 Giant bullous emphysema. (**a**) Chest radiographs show giant bullous emphysema in a 37-year-old man. A chest tube was inserted for a giant bulla in the left lung, as it was misdiagnosed as pneumothorax. (**b–d**) Chest CT demonstrates that most air is in a large bulla in both upper lobes. There is also a small amount of pneumothorax (air external to the bulla wall). The bulla wall (arrows) is parallel to the parietal pleura

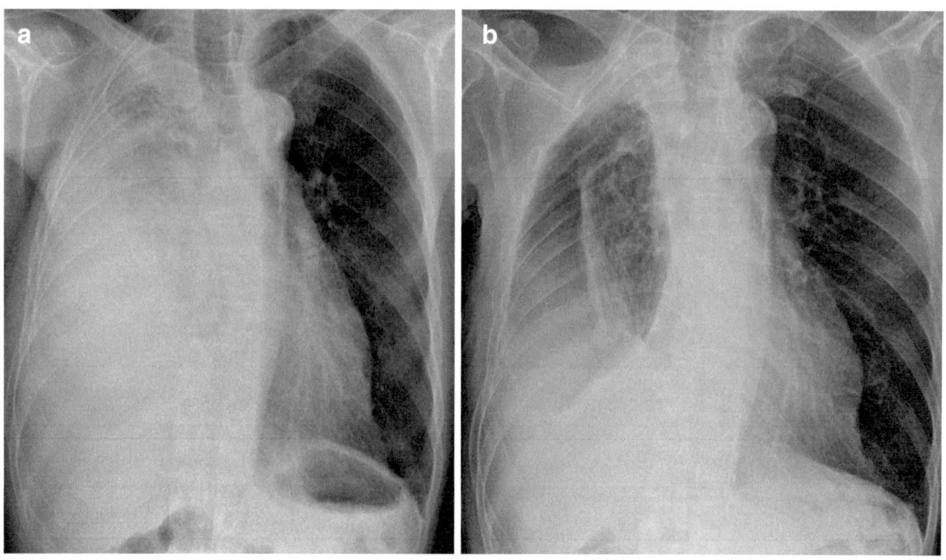

Fig. 13.4 Pneumothorax ex vacuo (unexpandable lung due to lung entrapment) in a 76-year-old man with squamous cell lung cancer with pleural seeding. (**a**) Chest radiograph shows a large amount of right pleural effusion. (**b**) Chest radiograph performed after thoracentesis shows that the amount of pleural effusion has decreased. Instead, a large amount of air is filling the right pleural space. The lung was not able to fully expand and fill the thoracic cavity owing to underlying pleural seeding

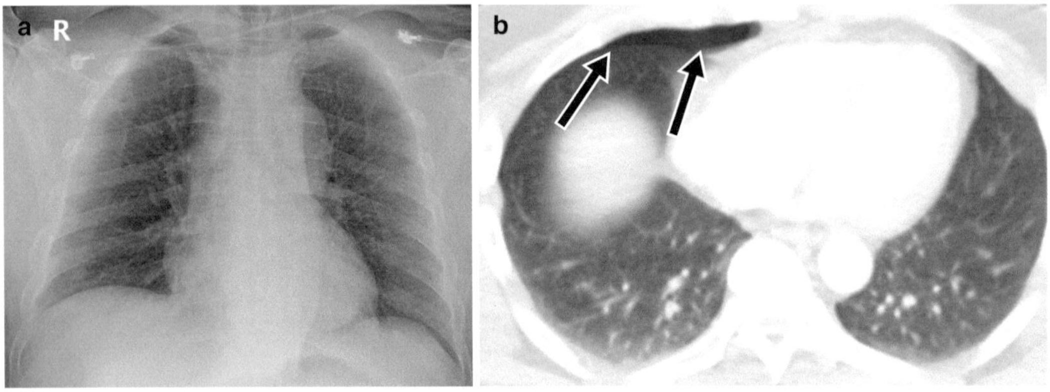

Fig. 13.5 Occult pneumothorax. (**a**) Chest radiograph shows no abnormality. (**b**) On chest CT, there is a small amount of right pneumothorax (arrows). In supine position, the air accumulates in the anterior and medial pleural space

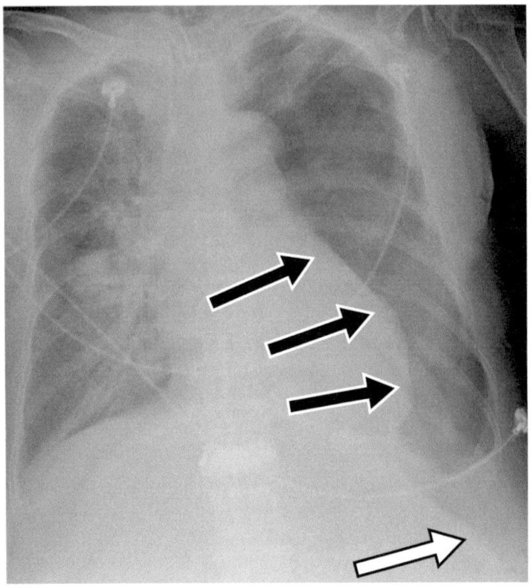

Fig. 13.6 Pneumothorax on anteroposterior chest radiograph in supine patients. In supine patients, pneumothorax manifests as increased lucency at the affected lung base, a deep sulcus (white arrow), and sharp delineation of the mediastinal border (black arrows)

during inspiration as well [9]. For a tension pneumothorax to develop, a one-way valve mechanism must be present so that more air enters the pleural space on inspiration than exits the pleural space on expiration, and thus air accumulates in the pleural space under positive pressure [9]. When tension pneumothorax develops, the increased intrathoracic pressure collapses the ipsilateral lung and prevents adequate diastolic filling of the heart. The combination of decreased cardiac output due to impaired venous return and profound hypoxia due to ventilation–perfusion mismatches leads to sudden deterioration of cardiopulmonary status [10].

Tension pneumothorax is a clinical diagnosis with a variety of definitions [8]. On imaging, tension pneumothorax may be suggested when the following signs are present in addition to the pneumothorax: (a) mediastinal shift to the contralateral side, (b) ipsilateral flattening of the heart border, (c) flattening or inversion of the ipsilateral hemidiaphragm, (d) hyperexpanded ipsilateral chest, and/or (e) increased rib separation [8, 11] (Fig. 13.7). It should be noted that mediastinal shift does not necessarily indicate a tension pneumothorax, as it may occur in both tension and simple pneumothoraces [8]. When a tension pneumothorax persists despite chest tube drainage, the possibility of major airway injury should be considered [3].

13.2.3 Treatment

Pneumothorax greater than 25% of thoracic volume typically requires tube thoracostomy drainage [12]. For less severe pneumothorax, treatment decisions should be made based on the degree of respiratory symptoms, the potential for the development of a tension pneumothorax, underlying patient condition, and other associated injuries [13]. Occult pneumothoraces, those not seen on chest radiograph, may be observed in a stable

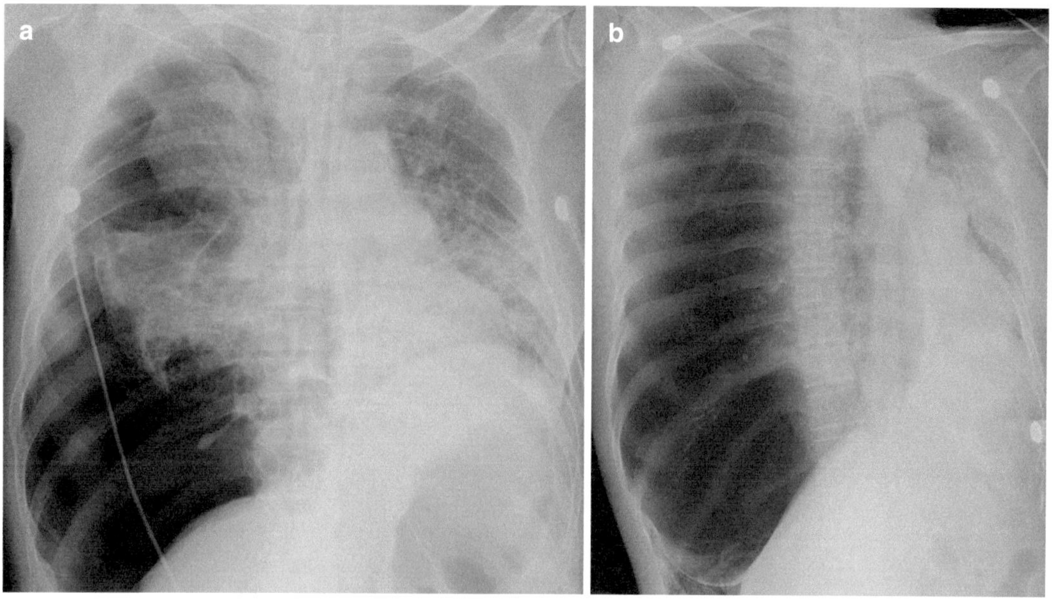

Fig. 13.7 Tension pneumothorax. (**a**, **b**) The following signs of tension pneumothorax are seen on chest radiograph: mediastinal shift to the contralateral side, ipsilateral flattening of the heart border, flattening or inversion of the ipsilateral hemidiaphragm, hyperexpanded ipsilateral chest, and increased rib separation

patient regardless of positive pressure ventilation [14]. According to the literature, only 26%–30% of patients with occult pneumothorax undergo chest tube placement [6, 15], whereas the remaining patients were successfully observed without tube thoracostomy. The average pneumothorax absorption rate when managed without tube thoracostomy has been estimated at 1.25% per day [16]. Accumulating evidence indicates that smaller pigtail catheters (14- to 16-French) are equally effective as large-bore chest tubes (28- to 40-French) and less painful [17, 18]. One rare but potentially fatal complication following pneumothorax drainage is re-expansion pulmonary edema. Re-expansion pulmonary edema may occur following pneumothorax drainage due to an increase in permeability of the alveolar–capillary membrane while the collapsed lung expands (Fig. 13.8) [19].

13.3 Hemothorax

Hemothorax is defined as the presence of blood products in the pleural space. It can be classified as traumatic, iatrogenic, or non-traumatic [20]. In the trauma setting, it may originate from a variety of thoracic injuries (e.g., involving the lung, chest wall, heart, or great vessels) or abdominal injuries (liver and splenic injuries with diaphragmatic rupture).

13.3.1 Imaging Findings

On radiography, cardio-phrenic angle blunting is seen on posteroanterior chest radiography when there is accumulation of at least 200 ml of pleural fluid. Decubitus view can demonstrate as little as 5 ml of pleural fluid [21].

The attenuation value on CT helps characterize the pleural fluid and sometimes enables differentiation of hemothorax from pleural effusion. Blood in the pleural space typically has an attenuation of 35–70 Hounsfield units (HU) [11], whereas pleural effusion typically shows attenuation of less than 15 HU. Blood can be seen in the pleural space at different degrees of coagulation, which results in a layered appearance, called the "hematocrit sign" (Fig. 13.9) [22, 23]. Liquid blood in the pleural space has a density between

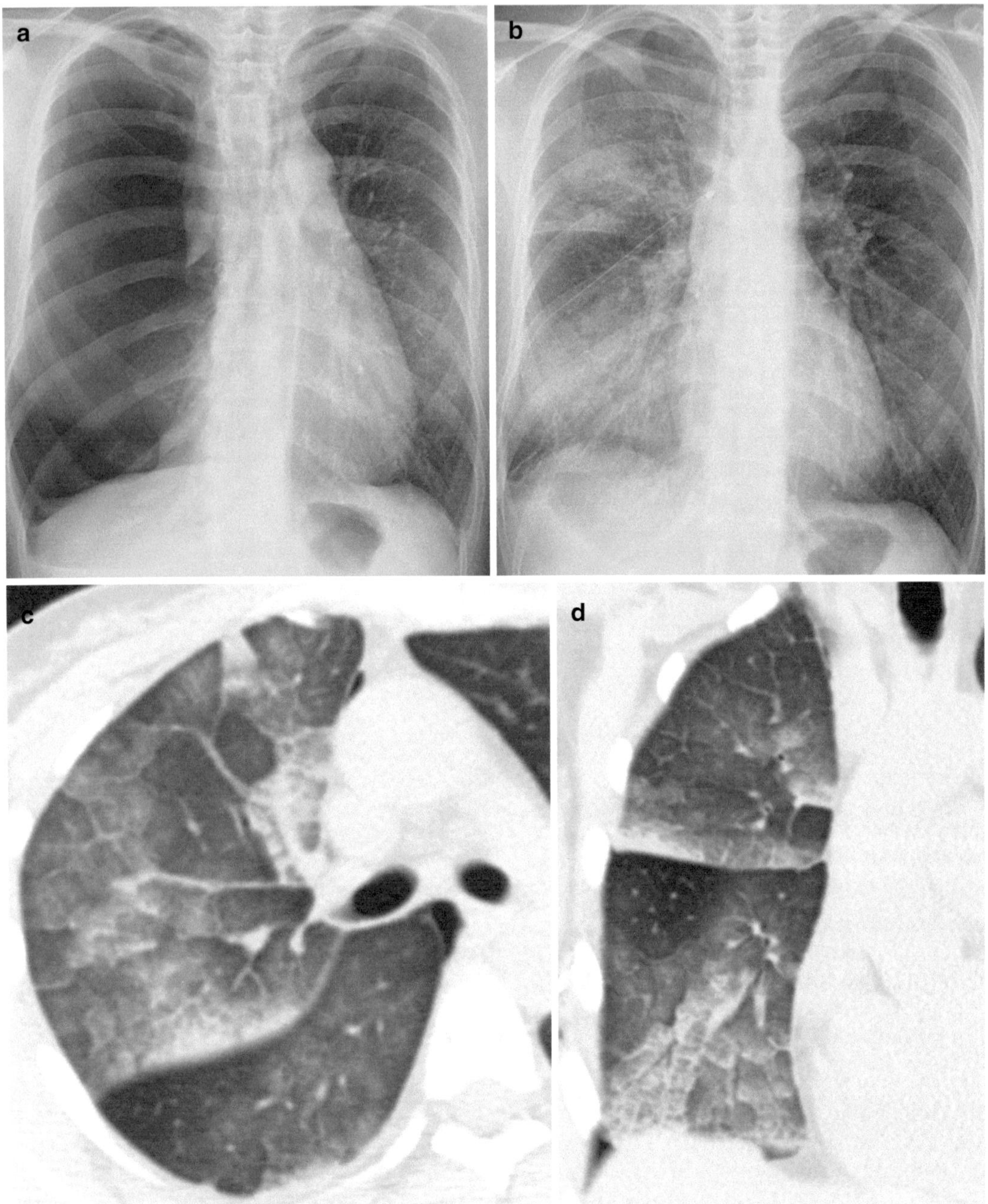

Fig. 13.8 Re-expansion pulmonary edema. (**a**) Chest radiograph shows a large amount of right pneumothorax. (**b**) After chest tube drainage, the amount of pneumothorax decreased; however, multifocal increased opacities developed in the right lung. (**c**, **d**) On chest CT, there are interlobular septal thickening and multifocal ground-glass opacities in the right lung, which suggest re-expansion pulmonary edema. (**e**) A chest radiograph taken the following day shows that the re-expansion pulmonary edema resolved

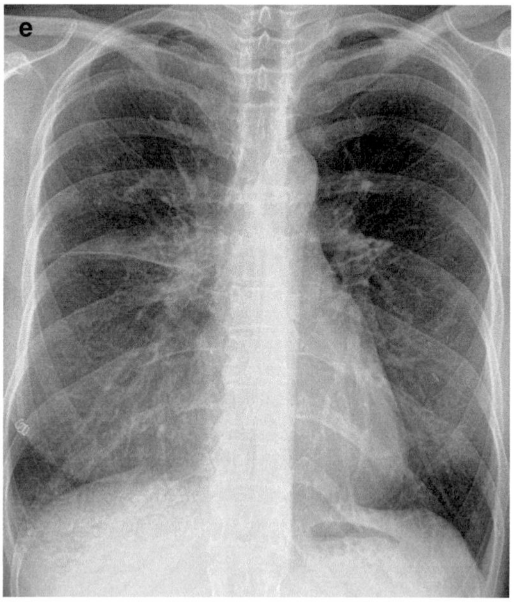

Fig. 13.8 (continued)

30 and 45 HU, whereas clotted blood becomes more dense, measuring between 50 and 90 HU [3]. The bleeding focus can occasionally be identified as contrast extravasation or pseudoaneurysm on CT (e.g., intercostal or internal mammary artery laceration).

When hemothorax is identified in the absence of trauma or an iatrogenic cause, spontaneous hemothorax may be the initial manifestation of a malignancy (Fig. 13.10). Indeed, the most common cause of nontraumatic hemothorax is malignant pleural disease [20].

13.3.2 Treatment

The initial treatment of hemothorax is tube thoracostomy. In general, hemothorax evident on supine chest radiograph should be drained imme-

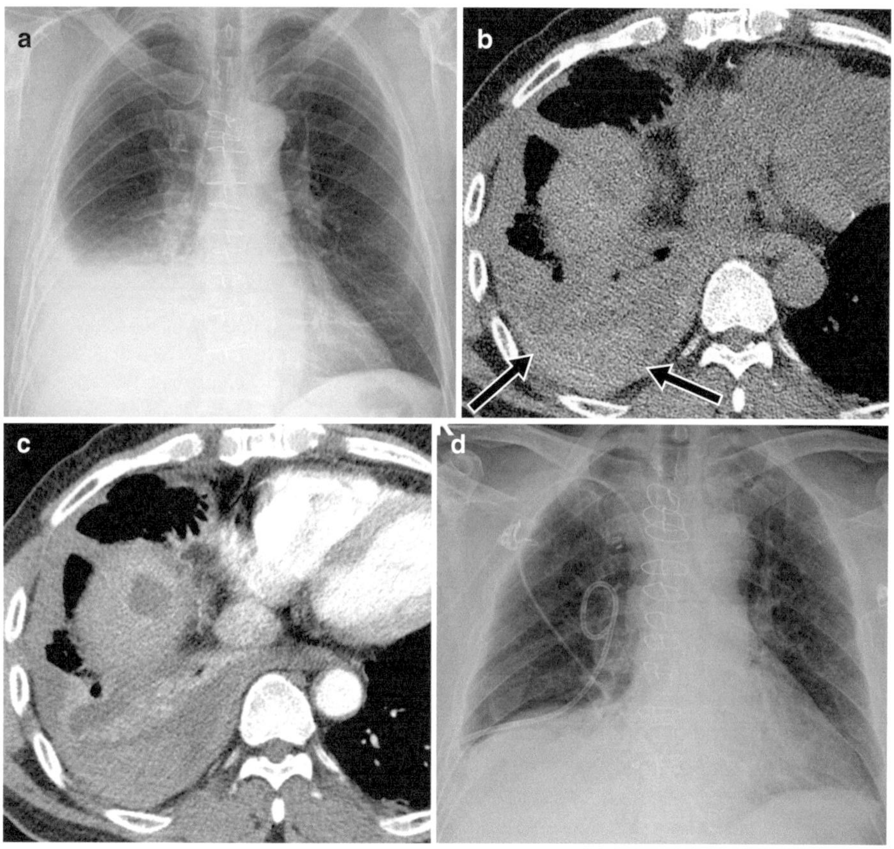

Fig. 13.9 Hemothorax that occurred after radio frequency ablation of a liver tumor. (**a**) Chest radiograph shows right pleural effusion or hemothorax. (**b**, **c**) Chest CT shows high-attenuating fluid with a layered appearance in the right pleural space (arrows), which indicates right hemothorax. (**d**) Hemothorax resolved after drainage with a pigtail catheter

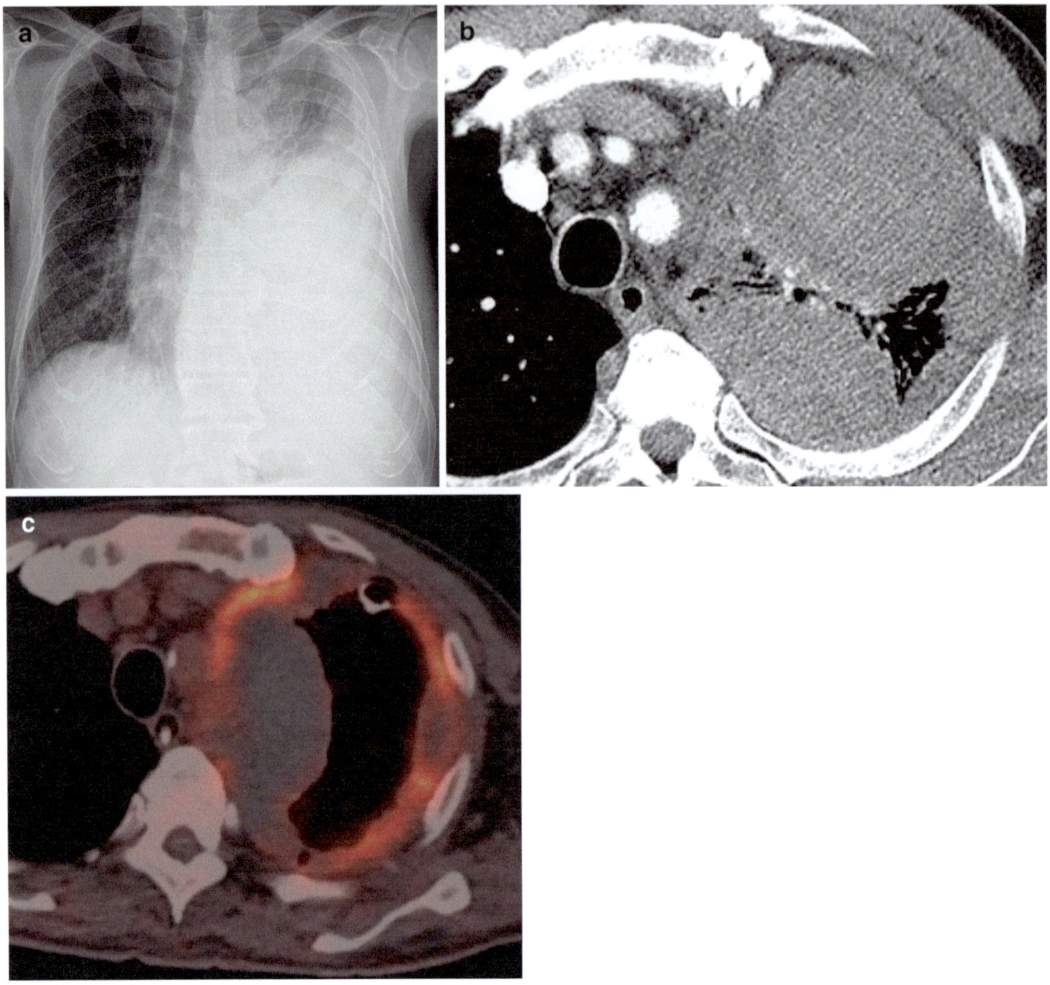

Fig. 13.10 Hemothorax as the initial presentation of malignancy. (**a**) There is a large amount of left pleural fluid on the chest radiograph of a 68-year-old man. (**b**) Chest CT shows that the pleural fluid has high attenuation suggestive of hemothorax. On medical thoracoscopy, a large amount of hemothorax was present; a pleural biopsy confirmed the presence of mesothelioma. (**c**) PET/CT shows diffuse fluorodeoxyglucose uptake along the left pleura

diately, since undrained hemothorax leads to the development of late-onset complications, including empyema or fibrothorax (trapped lung) [24]. In cases of occult hemothorax, the decision to drain or simply observe should be made considering the amount of blood present and the morbidity of chest tube insertion.

Evacuation of a hemothorax is incomplete in up to 20% of cases [25–27]. A retained hemothorax of less than 300 mL may be observed on chest CT [28] (Fig. 13.11). For a larger retained hemothorax, early video-assisted thoracic surgery should be considered within 3–7 days of hospitalization because this reduces the risk of infection and the requirement for thoracotomy [14]. Additional chest tube placement is usually ineffective for clot evacuation.

Over the past decade, there has been a trend toward using smaller chest tubes to evacuate hemothorax [18]. Advanced Trauma Life Support previously recommended placement of a large-bore thoracostomy tube. Recent studies have demonstrated that the diameter (size) of the tube does not affect the effectiveness of hematoma evacuation [29]. Therefore, Advanced Trauma Life Support-10th now recommends placement

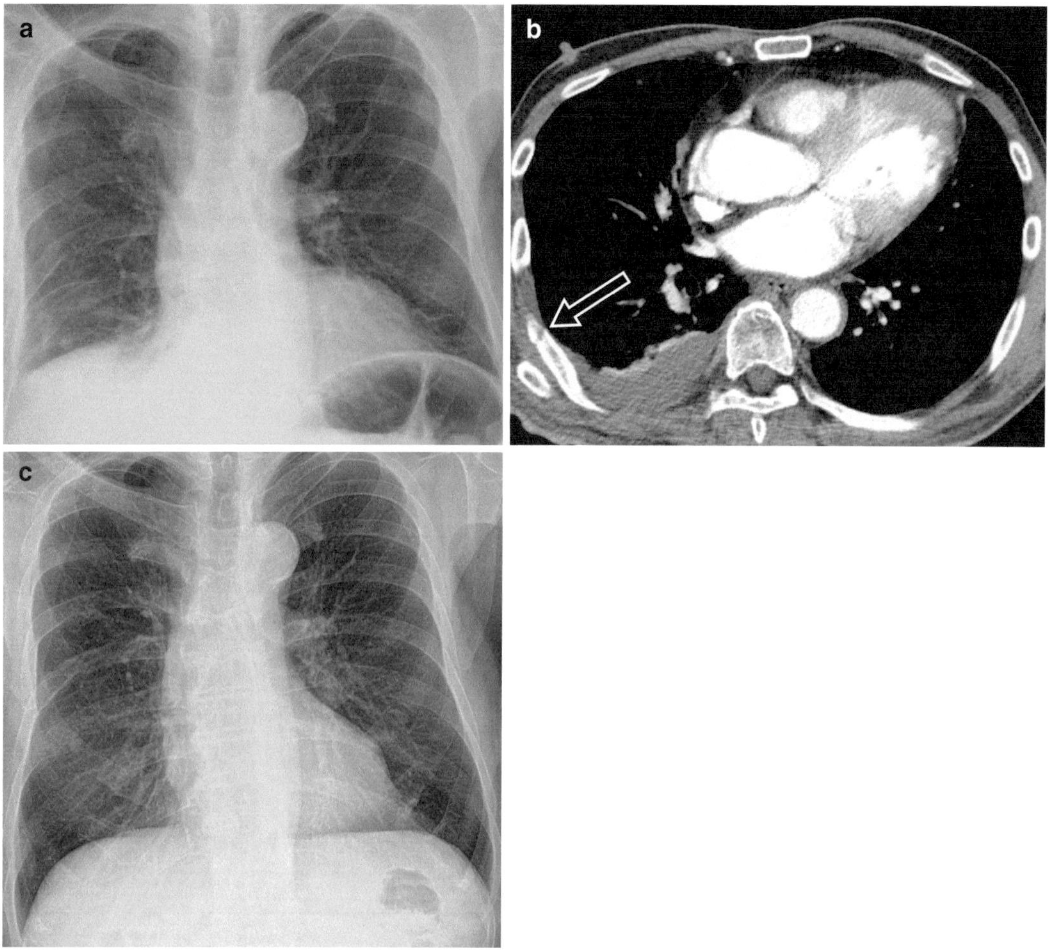

Fig. 13.11 Hemothorax that spontaneously resolved without tube drainage. (**a**) Chest radiograph shows a small amount of right pleural effusion or hemothorax. (**b**) Chest CT demonstrates a right rib fracture (arrow) associated with a small right hemothorax. (**c**) On follow-up chest radiograph, the hemothorax spontaneously resolved without tube drainage

of a smaller 28F to 32F chest tube for acute hemothorax that is visible on chest radiograph [30]. Niinami et al. reported that a 19-French fluted silicone drain is capable of draining fluid at a rate of 11 L/h [31]. Similarly, Kulvatunyou et al. reported that a 14-French pigtail catheter drained blood as effectively as larger-bore traditional chest tubes, with a similar incidence of complications [32].

13.4 Parapneumonic Effusion and Empyema

Pleural infection affects patients of all ages but has a bimodal distribution, with peak incidences in children and the elderly. Men are affected twice as often as women [33, 34]. Although parapneumonic effusion frequently results from community-acquired pneumonia, a sizable proportion of cases manifest without evidence of pneumonia on chest CT and are thought to have been acquired through hematologic spread or direct translocation from the oropharynx [35].

When pleural effusion is identified on chest radiograph in patients with possible pleural infection, it is important to differentiate a complicated parapneumonic effusion requiring chest tube drainage from a simple effusion that may resolve with antibiotics alone [36]. Pleural fluid analysis remains the most reliable diagnostic test to guide management [36–38]. Thus, if parapneumonic effusion is suspected and the thickness of the pleural fluid is more than 10 mm, pleural fluid sampling and analysis should be done to determine patient management and prognosis. Based on the pleural fluid analysis, pleural fluid can be categorized as uncomplicated parapneumonic effusion, complicated parapneumonic effusion, or empyema.

13.4.1 Evolution of Pleural Infection

The evolution of a pleural infection can be divided into three stages. In the first, exudative, stage, there is an outpouring of sterile pleural fluid into the pleural space due to increased permeability. The amount of pleural fluid is generally small. The glucose level and pH of pleural fluid are usually within the normal range, and the white blood cell count and lactate dehydrogenase (LDH) level in pleural fluid are low [39, 40]. At this stage, chest tube drainage is generally not required, and antibiotics alone suffice.

The second, fibropurulent, stage evolves if bacteria invade the sterile exudative effusion. During this stage, leukocytes, bacteria, and cell debris accumulate together with pleural fluid. Fibrin is then deposited over the visceral and parietal pleura, and loculations form within the pleural fluid. The pleural fluid pH and glucose level decrease, and the LDH level rises [35].

The final, organization, stage is characterized by aggressive fibroblast growth over the pleural surfaces to form a pleural peel [35]. This may progress to fibrothorax with decreased lung volume.

13.4.2 Imaging Findings

Chest radiograph plays the primary role for screening of patients with pneumonia for the presence of an effusion to determine the need for thoracentesis [41]. The radiographic appearance of infected pleural fluid collections depends on the volume and viscosity of pleural fluid, the patient's position, and the presence of pleural loculations. It is often difficult to detect and diagnose nondependent loculations that simulate masses or airspace densities on frontal projections (Fig. 13.12), loculated collections along the mediastinal pleura, subpulmonic effusions (Fig. 13.13), or effusions on portable radiographs.

Ultrasonography and chest CT have greater sensitivity for fluid detection and provide additional information that can be used to determine the extent and nature of pleural infection [41]. On ultrasonography, simple pleural effusions typically appear as triangular anechoic collections immediately above the diaphragm. However, infected pleural effusion may show different echogenicity, such as complex septated (Fig. 13.14) or homogeneously echogenic patterns (Fig. 13.15) [42]. Uniformly echogenic collections typically contain blood or debris and almost invariably indicate the presence of an empyema in patients who appear clinically infected [43]. Uniformly echogenic fluid collections may mimic the normal liver or spleen on ultrasonography. By identifying the locational relationship with the diaphragm and visualizing the abdominal organ vascular structures, complicated pleural effusions can easily be differentiated from abdominal organs.

On chest CT, most infected pleural fluid collections have attenuation levels similar to water (0–20 HU). The presence of air in the pleural space without a history of recent procedures (thoracentesis, chest tube placement, or surgical intervention) suggests the possibility of pleural infection. The air bubbles may have formed due to a gas-forming bacterial infection or rupture of necrotizing pneumonia/abscess into the pleural space. Parietal pleural thickening also indicates the presence of a pleural exudate, although this finding is not specific for infection [44]. Pleural

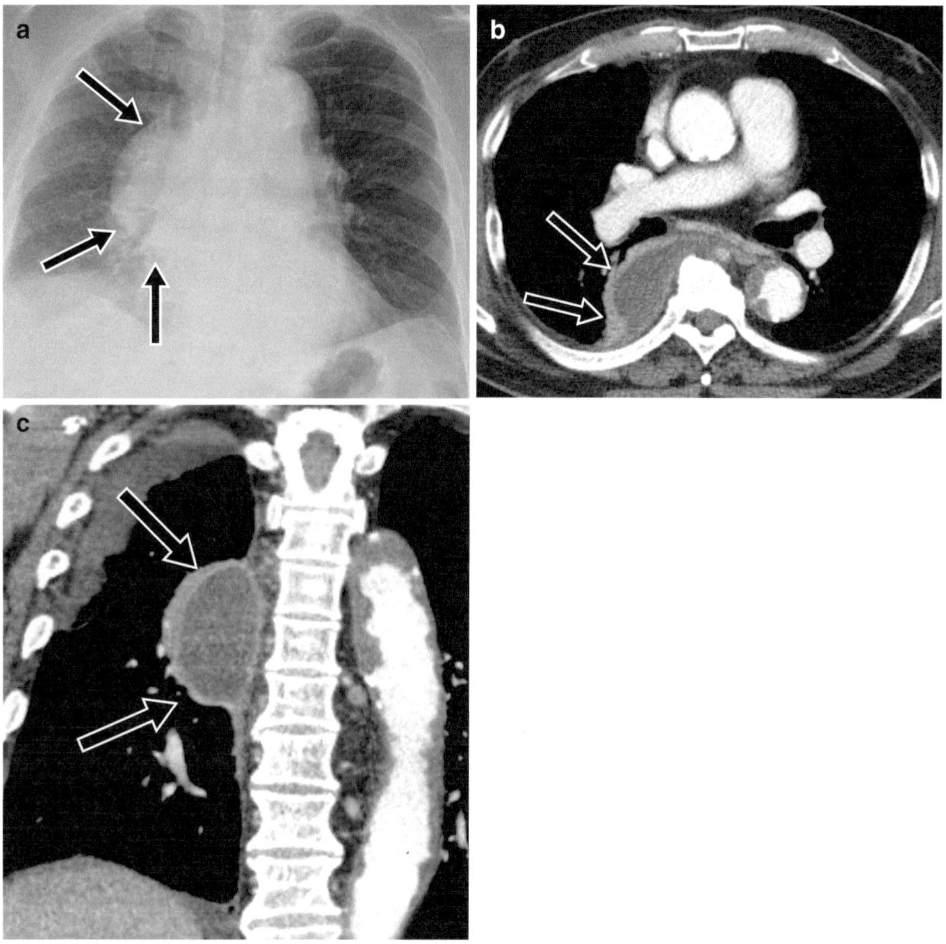

Fig. 13.12 Loculated empyema. (**a**) Chest radiograph shows loculated fluid collections (arrows) that simulate a mass. (**b**, **c**) Chest CT shows loculated pleural effusion (arrows) at the right posterior pleural space. Note that the pleural effusion is lenticular in shape, has a thick, smooth wall, and is surrounded by adjacent atelectatic lung

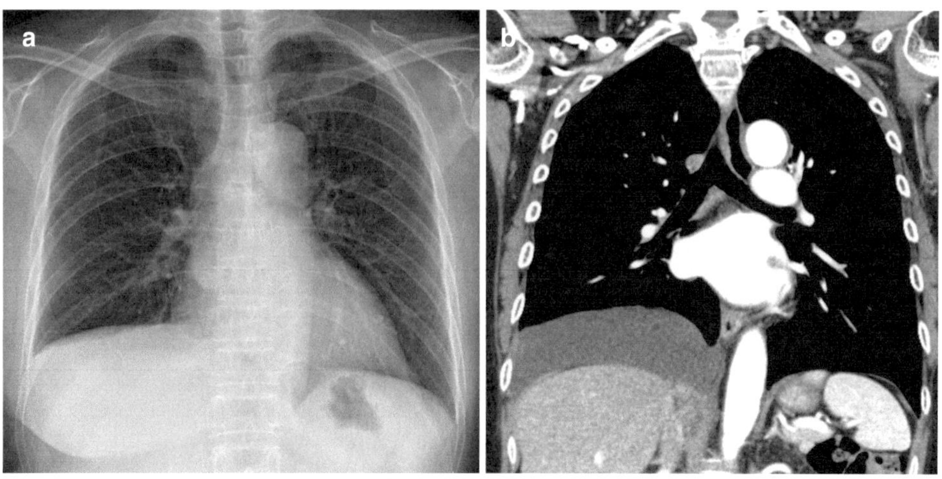

Fig. 13.13 Subpulmonic effusion. (**a**) On chest radiograph, elevation and flattening of the right diaphragm are visible. (**b**) Chest CT demonstrates the presence of subpulmonic pleural effusion

infection typically produces smooth, uniform pleural thickening that is limited to the costal and diaphragmatic pleural surfaces [41]. The detection of mediastinal pleural thickening or nodules along thickened parietal pleural surfaces on CT scan suggests pleural malignancy [41].

It is important to differentiate between pleural empyema and lung abscesses based on chest CT findings, as management differs. Empyema contacts the chest wall at obtuse angles, is usually lenticular in shape, has a smooth wall, and is surrounded by adjacent atelectatic lung. Adjacent bronchi and pulmonary vessels are compressed or distorted by the empyema. On the other hand, a lung abscess contacts the chest wall at acute angles, is usually rounded in shape, has a thick irregular wall, and often has an indistinct boundary with the lung parenchyma (Figs. 13.14 and 13.16). The bronchi and pulmonary vessels terminate abruptly or are connected to the abscess wall and are not compressed or distorted [36, 45, 46].

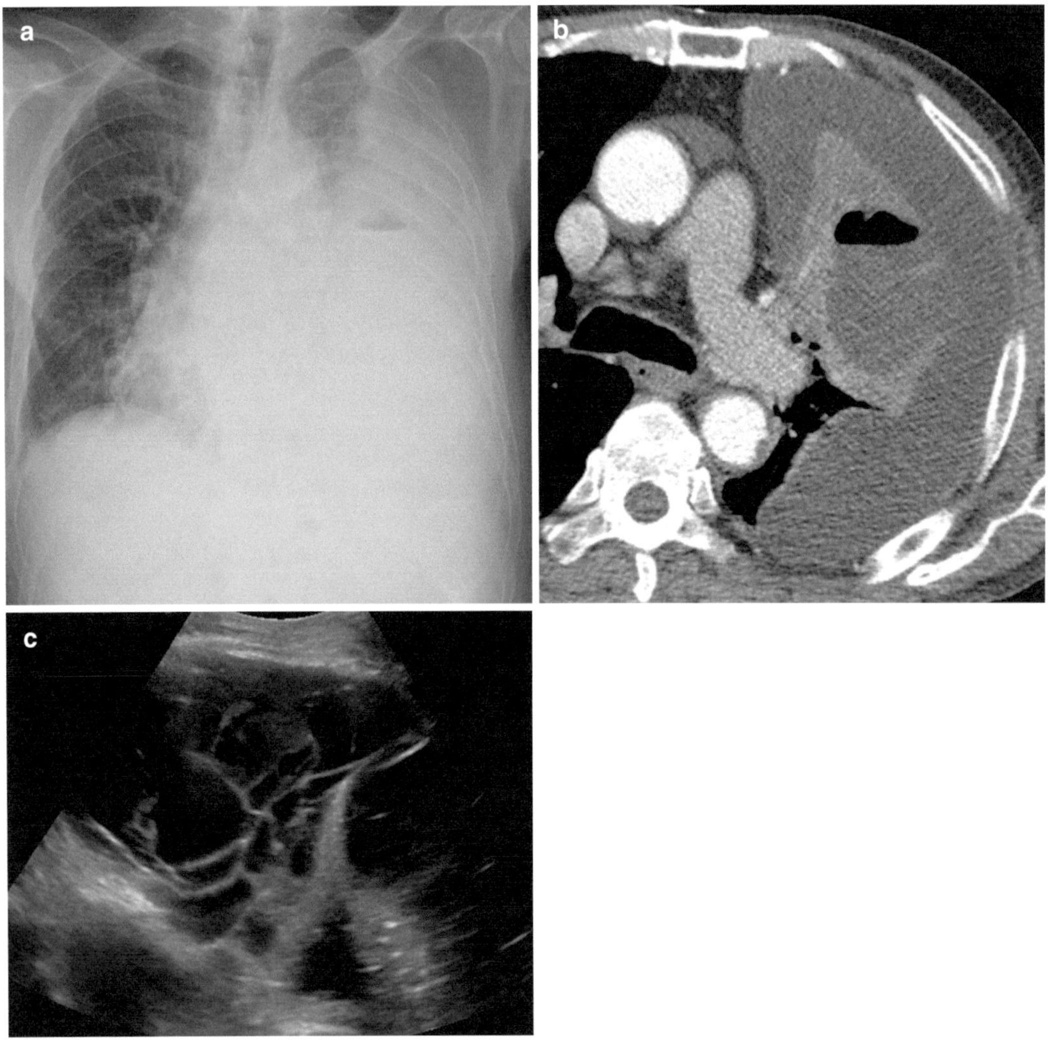

Fig. 13.14 Empyema with lung abscess. (**a**) On chest radiograph, there is a large amount of left pleural fluid. In the middle, a small amount of air with air–fluid level is also seen. (**b**) Chest CT shows a large amount of left pleural effusion with mild pleural thickening. In the left upper lobe, there is a low-attenuating lesion with air–fluid level, suggestive of a lung abscess. (**c**) Ultrasonography demonstrates that the pleural effusion is multi-septated. A percutaneous chest drainage pigtail catheter was inserted and the empyema was drained

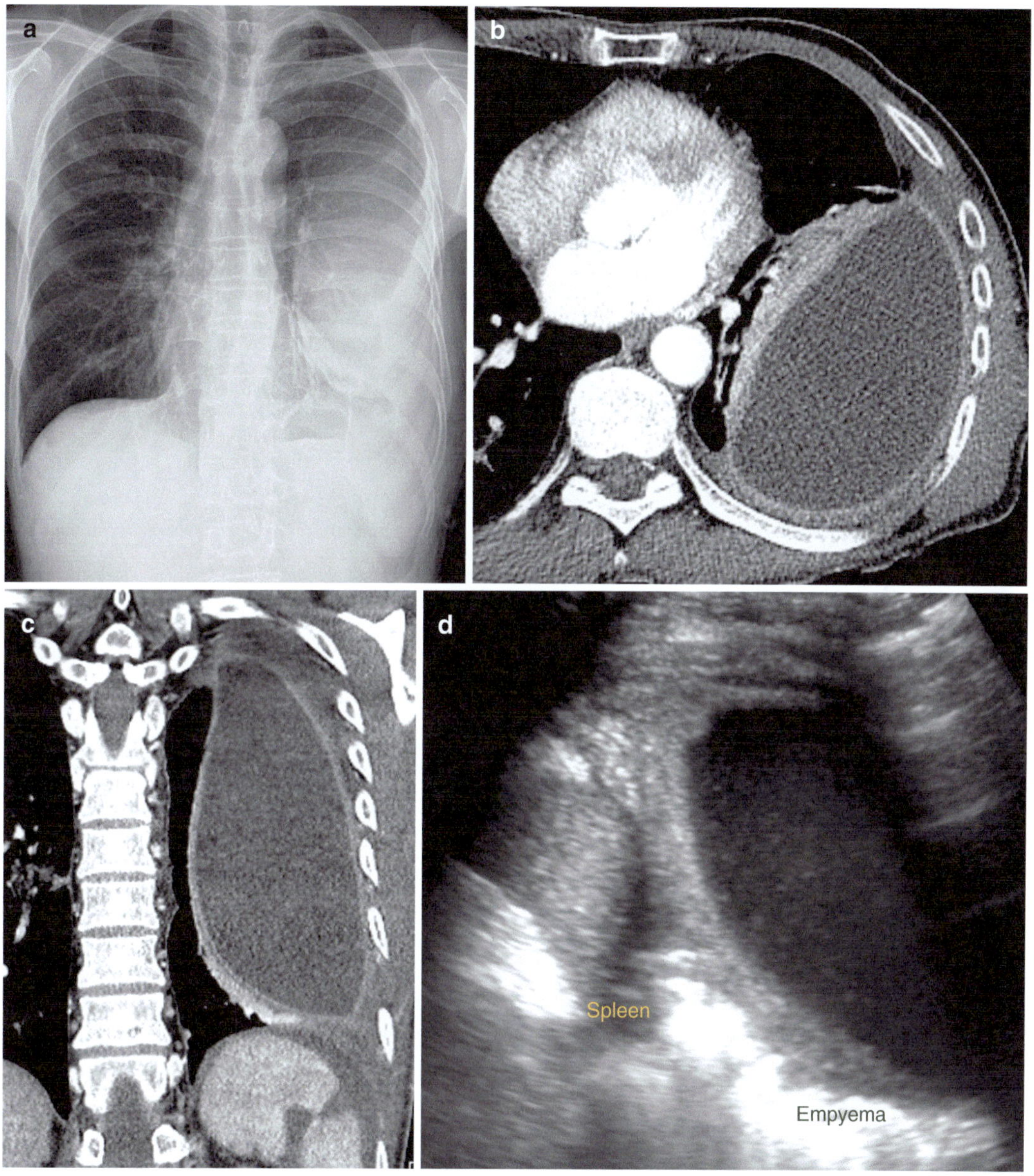

Fig. 13.15 Empyema. (**a**) Chest radiograph shows a large amount of loculated pleural effusion. (**b**, **c**) On chest CT, there is a large amount of left pleural effusion associated with diffuse, smooth pleural thickening. (**d**) On ultrasonography, the left pleural effusion is homogenously echogenic

13.4.3 Treatment

Uncomplicated/simple parapneumonic effusions usually resolve with antibiotics alone. For patients with empyema or complicated parapneumonic effusion, chest tube placement and drainage is required. Empyema is, by definition, pus in the pleural space. The American College of Chest Physicians defines complicated parapneumonic effusion as one of the following: (a) large, free-flowing effusion; loculated effusion; effusion with thickened pleura, (b) positive culture or Gram stain, or (c) pH <7.2 or glucose <60 mg/dL [47]. The British Thoracic Society recommends

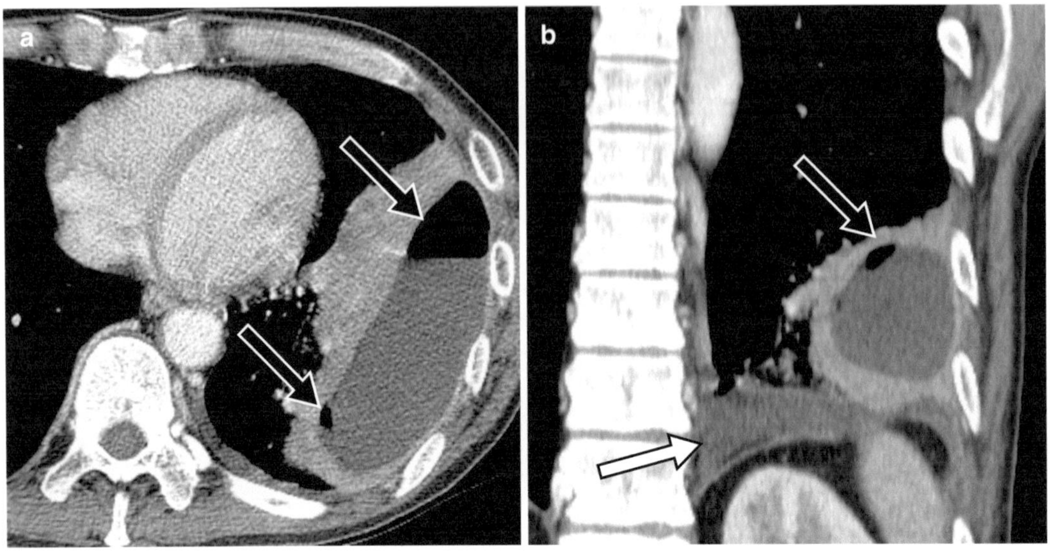

Fig. 13.16 Lung abscess mimicking empyema. (**a**, **b**) On chest CT, there is a large fluid collection with air–fluid level. Note that this fluid collection is surrounded by consolidative lung parenchyma. In the operating room, this fluid collection with air–fluid level was confirmed as a lung abscess (black arrows). There is also pleural effusion (empyema, white arrow) present inferior to the left lower lung

chest tube drainage for (a) patients with frankly purulent or turbid/cloudy pleural fluid, (b) pleural fluid pH < 7.2, or (c) the presence of organisms identified by Gram stain and/or culture from a non-purulent pleural fluid sample. A small-bore catheter (10–14 F) is adequate for most cases of pleural infection [36]. However, there is no consensus on the optimal size of chest tube for drainage.

13.5 Tuberculous Pleurisy

Tuberculous pleurisy is a not uncommon disease encountered at the emergency department in tuberculosis-endemic countries. Indeed, tuberculous pleurisy is one of the most common forms of extrapulmonary tuberculosis. Patients with tuberculous pleurisy should be treated with antituberculous medications using the same treatment regimens as given to patients with pulmonary tuberculosis.

The points of differential diagnosis from parapneumonic effusion are as follows: [1] tuberculous pleurisy shows high adenosine deaminase levels on pleural fluid analysis, [2] nodular lung lesions are common in tuberculosis pleurisy (consolidations are common in parapneumonic effusion), [3] tuberculosis pleurisy may show nodular pleural thickening, and [4] loculation is less common in tuberculosis pleurisy. Lung parenchymal lesions are observed in 39–86% of patients with tuberculous pleursiy (Fig. 13.17) [48, 49]. It should be noted that pleural loculation is more common in parapneumonic effusion than in tuberculous pleurisy. In one study, the percentage of loculation was higher in patients with parapneumonic effusion (79%, 22 of 28) than in those with tuberculous pleurisy (29%, 7 of 24) [50].

As tuberculous pleurisy may show nodular pleural thickening on chest CT, it is sometimes difficult to differentiate between tuberculous pleurisy and malignant pleural effusion. However, nodular pleural thickening with nodules >10 mm is a more common CT finding in malignant pleural effusion. In a previous study, nodular pleural thickening and pleural thickening >10 mm were observed in 9% (12 of 135) and 2% (3 of 135), respectively, of patients with tuberculous pleurisy, whereas they were observed in 57% (39 of 69) and 7% (5 of 69) of patients with malignant pleural effusion [51] (Fig. 13.18).

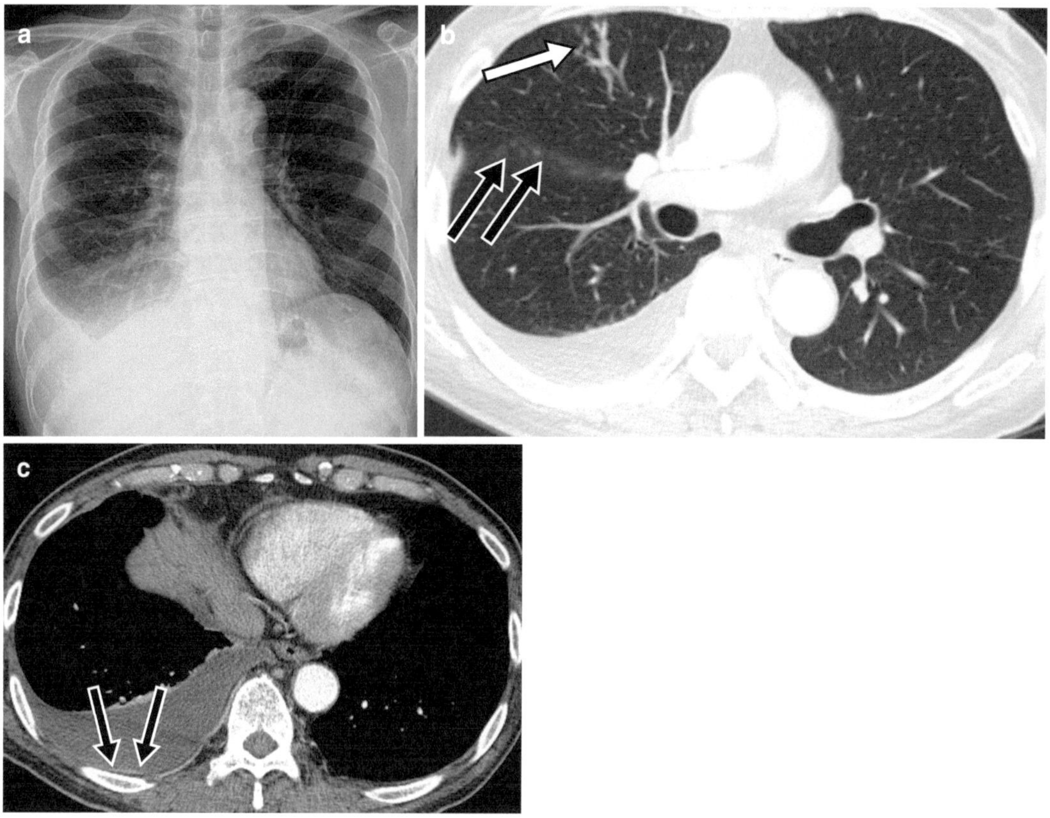

Fig. 13.17 Tuberculosis pleurisy with parenchymal tuberculosis. (**a**) Chest radiograph shows right pleural effusion. (**b**) Chest CT shows several tiny right fissural nodules (black arrows). Tiny nodular and branching opacities (white arrow) are present in the right upper lobe. (**c**) Chest CT shows pleural thickening with contrast enhancement (black arrows). This patient was confirmed to have tuberculosis pleurisy with parenchymal tuberculosis

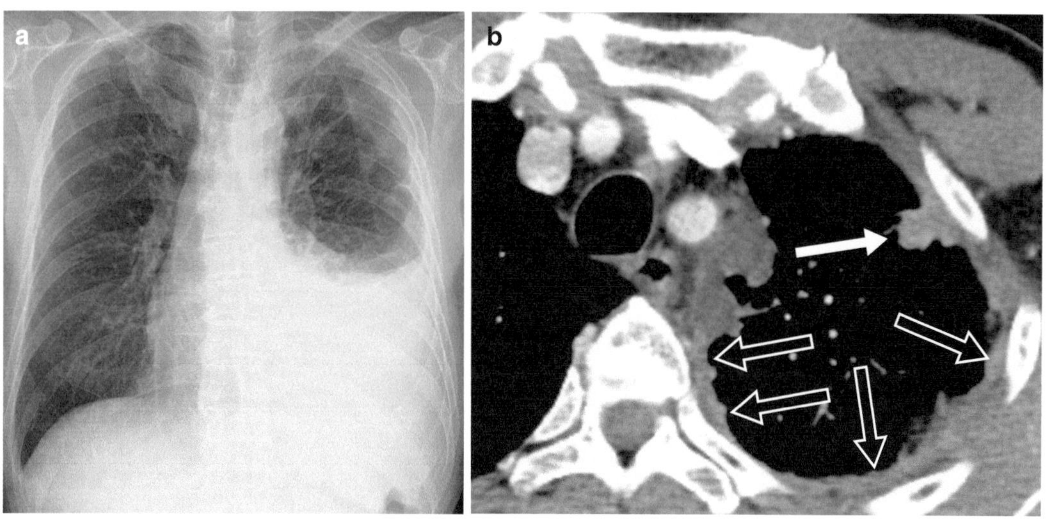

Fig. 13.18 Malignant pleural effusion. (**a**) Chest radiograph shows left pleural effusion. There are also faint nodules in the left upper lung. (**b–d**) Chest CT demonstrates multiple, irregular, uneven nodular thickenings (black arrows) along the left pleura. There is also an enhancing nodule (>10 mm) in the left upper lobe (white arrow), which was later confirmed as left upper lobe lung cancer

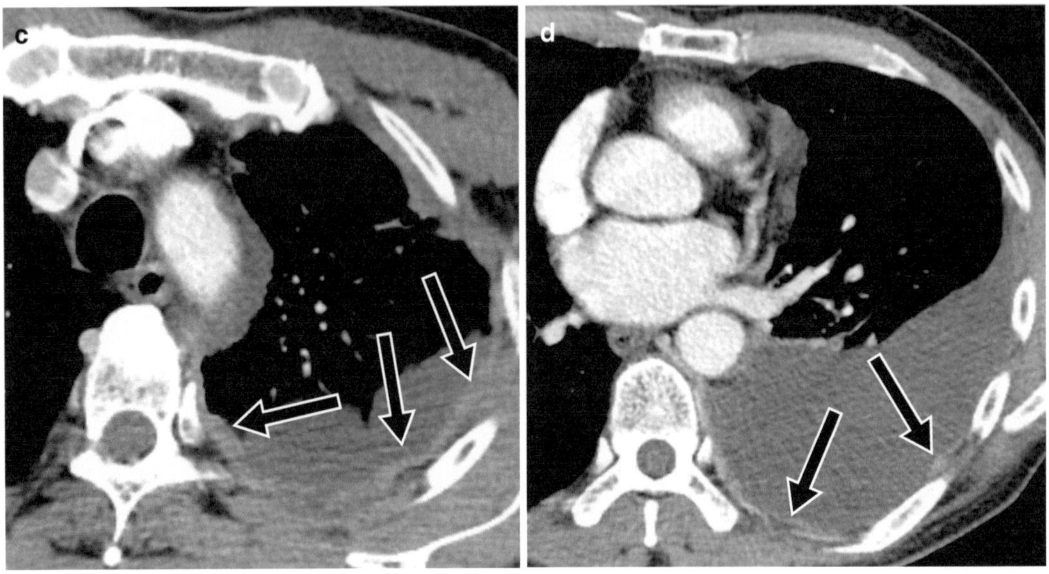

Fig. 13.18 (continued)

13.6 Summary

Pneumothorax can be classified as spontaneous or traumatic. It is important to remember the imaging findings of pneumothorax in supine patients and those of tension pneumothorax. Pneumothorax should be differentiated from skin folds, giant bullous emphysema, and pneumothorax ex vacuo.

Hemothorax can be classified as traumatic, iatrogenic, or non-traumatic. Blood in the pleural space typically has an attenuation of 35–70 HU. It can show a layered appearance on CT, called the "hematocrit sign."

Complicated parapneumonic effusion and empyema should be drained with a chest tube or pigtail catheters. The indications for drainage include (a) purulent, turbid, loculated pleural fluid or pus, (b) positive culture or Gram stain, or (c) pH < 7.2 or glucose <60 mg/dL.

The differential diagnosis of tuberculous pleurisy includes parapneumonic effusion and malignant pleural effusion. Chest CT imaging findings may help make this differential diagnosis.

Key Points

- The presence of pneumothorax should be suspected when the following imaging findings are seen on a supine radiograph: (a) increased lucency at the affected lung base, (b) the "deep sulcus" sign, and (c) sharp delineation of the mediastinal border.
- Undrained hemothorax leads to the development of late-onset complications, including empyema or fibrothorax.
- *Empyema* versus *lung abscess*
  Empyema: Contacts the chest wall at obtuse angles, lenticular in shape, smooth wall, surrounded by adjacent atelectatic lung.
  Lung abscess: Contacts the chest wall at acute angles, rounded in shape, thick irregular wall, indistinct boundary with the lung parenchyma.
- *Tuberculous pleurisy* versus *parapneumonic effusion*
  1. Tuberculous pleurisy shows high adenosine deaminase levels on pleural fluid analysis
  2. Nodular lung lesions are common in tuberculosis pleurisy

3. Tuberculosis pleurisy may show nodular pleural thickening
4. Loculation is less common in tuberculosis pleurisy

- *Tuberculous pleurisy* versus *malignant effusion*

  Nodular pleural thickening with nodules >10 mm is more common in malignant pleural effusion

References

1. Light RW, Lee YCG. Pneumothorax, chylothorax, hemothorax, and fibrothorax. In: Broaddus VC, editor. Murray & Nadel's textbook of respiratory medicine, chapter 81, vol. 2. 6th ed. Philadelphia: Elsevier; 2016. p. 1439.
2. Groskin SA. Selected topics in chest trauma. Semin Ultrasound CT MR. 1996;17(2):119–41. https://doi.org/10.1016/s0887-2171(96)90012-8.
3. Mirvis SE. Imaging of acute thoracic injury: the advent of MDCT screening. Semin Ultrasound CT MR. 2005;26(5):305–31. https://doi.org/10.1053/j.sult.2005.08.001.
4. Miller LA. Chest wall, lung, and pleural space trauma. Radiol Clin N Am. 2006;44(2):213–24. https://doi.org/10.1016/j.rcl.2005.10.006.
5. de Moya MA, Seaver C, Spaniolas K, et al. Occult pneumothorax in trauma patients: development of an objective scoring system. J Trauma. 2007;63(1):13–7. https://doi.org/10.1097/TA.0b013e31806864fc.
6. Rodriguez RM, Canseco K, Baumann BM, et al. Pneumothorax and hemothorax in the era of frequent chest computed tomography for the evaluation of adult patients with blunt trauma. Ann Emerg Med. 2019;73(1):58–65. https://doi.org/10.1016/j.annemergmed.2018.08.423.
7. McPherson JJ, Feigin DS, Bellamy RF. Prevalence of tension pneumothorax in fatally wounded combat casualties. J Trauma. 2006;60(3):573–8. https://doi.org/10.1097/01.ta.0000209179.79946.92.
8. Leigh-Smith S, Harris T. Tension pneumothorax--time for a re-think? Emerg Med J. 2005;22(1):8–16. https://doi.org/10.1136/emj.2003.010421.
9. Light RW. Pleural diseases. 6th ed. Baltimore: Lippincott Williams & Wilkins; 2013.
10. Light RW, Lee YCG. Pneumothorax, chylothorax, hemothorax, and fibrothorax. In: Broaddus VC, editor. Murray & Nadel's textbook of respiratory medicine, chapter 81, vol. 2. 6th ed. Philadelphia: Elsevier; 2016. p. 1449–50.
11. Kaewlai R, Avery LL, Asrani AV, Novelline RA. Multidetector CT of blunt thoracic trauma. Radiographics. 2008;28(6):1555–70. https://doi.org/10.1148/rg.286085510.
12. Talbot BS, Gange CP Jr, Chaturvedi A, Klionsky N, Hobbs SK, Chaturvedi A. Traumatic rib injury: patterns, imaging pitfalls, complications, and treatment. Radiographics. 2017;37(2):628–51. https://doi.org/10.1148/rg.2017160100.
13. Yeh DD, Lee J. Trauma and blast injuries. In: Broaddus VC, editor. Murray & Nadel's textbook of respiratory medicine, chapter 76, vol. 2. 6th ed. Philadelphia: Elsevier; 2016. p. 1359–61.
14. Mowery NT, Gunter OL, Collier BR, et al. Practice management guidelines for management of hemothorax and occult pneumothorax. J Trauma. 2011;70(2):510–8. https://doi.org/10.1097/TA.0b013e31820b5c31.
15. Moore FO, Goslar PW, Coimbra R, et al. Blunt traumatic occult pneumothorax: is observation safe? Results of a prospective, AAST multicenter study. J Trauma. 2011;70(5):1019–23. https://doi.org/10.1097/TA.0b013e318213f727.
16. Kircher LT Jr, Swartzel RL. Spontaneous pneumothorax and its treatment. J Am Med Assoc. 1954;155(1):24–9. https://doi.org/10.1001/jama.1954.03690190030009.
17. Kulvatunyou N, Vijayasekaran A, Hansen A, et al. Two-year experience of using pigtail catheters to treat traumatic pneumothorax: a changing trend. J Trauma. 2011;71(5):1104–7. https://doi.org/10.1097/TA.0b013e31822dd130.
18. Rivera L, O'Reilly EB, Sise MJ, et al. Small catheter tube thoracostomy: effective in managing chest trauma in stable patients. J Trauma. 2009;66(2):393–9. https://doi.org/10.1097/TA.0b013e318173f81e.
19. Sivrikoz MC, Tunçözgür B, Cekmen M, et al. The role of tissue reperfusion in the reexpansion injury of the lungs. Eur J Cardiothorac Surg. 2002;22(5):721–7. https://doi.org/10.1016/s1010-7940(02)00447-5.
20. Light RW, Lee YCG. Pneumothorax, chylothorax, hemothorax, and fibrothorax. In: Broaddus VC, editor. Murray & Nadel's textbook of respiratory medicine, chapter 81, vol. 2. 6th ed. Philadelphia: Elsevier; 2016. p. 1458.
21. Gallardo X, Castañer E, Mata JM. Benign pleural diseases. Eur J Radiol. 2000;34(2):87–97. https://doi.org/10.1016/s0720-048x(00)00167-4.
22. Thoongsuwan N, Kanne JP, Stern EJ. Imaging of blunt chest trauma. RSNA. Syllabus. 2004;2004:71–9.
23. Sangster GP, González-Beicos A, Carbo AI, et al. Blunt traumatic injuries of the lung parenchyma, pleura, thoracic wall, and intrathoracic airways: multidetector computer tomography imaging findings. Emerg Radiol. 2007;14(5):297–310. https://doi.org/10.1007/s10140-007-0651-8.
24. DuBose J, Inaba K, Okoye O, et al. Development of posttraumatic empyema in patients with retained hemothorax: results of a prospective, observational AAST study. J Trauma Acute Care Surg. 2012;73(3):752–7. https://doi.org/10.1097/TA.0b013e31825c1616.
25. Helling TS, Gyles NR 3rd, Eisenstein CL, Soracco CA. Complications following blunt and penetrat-

ing injuries in 216 victims of chest trauma requiring tube thoracostomy. J Trauma. 1989;29(10):1367–70. https://doi.org/10.1097/00005373-198910000-00013.
26. Villegas MI, Hennessey RA, Morales CH, Londoño E. Risk factors associated with the development of post-traumatic retained hemothorax. Eur J Trauma Emerg Surg. 2011;37(6):583–9. https://doi.org/10.1007/s00068-010-0064-3.
27. MacLeod JB, Ustin JS, Kim JT, Lewis F, Rozycki GS, Feliciano DV. The epidemiology of traumatic hemothorax in a level I trauma center: case for early video-assisted thoracoscopic surgery. Eur J Trauma Emerg Surg. 2010;36(3):240–6. https://doi.org/10.1007/s00068-009-9119-8.
28. DuBose J, Inaba K, Demetriades D, et al. Management of post-traumatic retained hemothorax: a prospective, observational, multicenter AAST study. J Trauma Acute Care Surg. 2012;72(1):11–22. https://doi.org/10.1097/TA.0b013e318242e368.
29. Inaba K, Lustenberger T, Recinos G, et al. Does size matter? A prospective analysis of 28-32 versus 36-40 French chest tube size in trauma. J Trauma Acute Care Surg. 2012;72(2):422–7. https://doi.org/10.1097/TA.0b013e3182452444.
30. Galvagno SM Jr, Nahmias JT, Young DA. Advanced trauma life support® update 2019: management and applications for adults and special populations. Anesthesiol Clin. 2019;37(1):13–32. https://doi.org/10.1016/j.anclin.2018.09.009.
31. Niinami H, Tabata M, Takeuchi Y, Umezu M. Experimental assessment of the drainage capacity of small silastic chest drains. Asian Cardiovasc Thorac Ann. 2006;14(3):223–6. https://doi.org/10.1177/021849230601400311.
32. Inaba K. Editorial critique. J Trauma Acute Care Surg. 2012;73(6):1421–2. https://doi.org/10.1097/TA.0b013e318270bb58.
33. Strange C, Sahn SA. The definitions and epidemiology of pleural space infection. Semin Respir Infect. 1999;14(1):3–8.
34. Maskell NA, Davies CW, Nunn AJ, et al. U.K. controlled trial of intrapleural streptokinase for pleural infection. N Engl J Med. 2005;352(9):865–74. https://doi.org/10.1056/NEJMoa042473.
35. Maskell NA, Light RW. Pleural infection. In: Broaddus VC, editor. Murray & Nadel's textbook of respiratory medicine, chapter 80, vol. 2. 6th ed. Philadelphia: Elsevier; 2016. p. 1426.
36. Davies HE, Davies RJ, Davies CW. Management of pleural infection in adults: British Thoracic Society Pleural Disease Guideline 2010. Thorax. 2010;65(Suppl 2):41–53. https://doi.org/10.1136/thx.2010.137000.
37. Light RW. Parapneumonic effusions and empyema. Proc Am Thorac Soc. 2006;3(1):75–80. https://doi.org/10.1513/pats.200510-113JH.
38. Heffner JE, Klein JS, Hampson C. Interventional management of pleural infections. Chest. 2009;136(4):1148–59. https://doi.org/10.1378/chest.08-2956.
39. Porcel JM. Pleural fluid tests to identify complicated parapneumonic effusions. Curr Opin Pulm Med. 2010;16(4):357–61. https://doi.org/10.1097/MCP.0b013e328338a108.
40. Light RW. Management of parapneumonic effusions. Arch Intern Med. 1981;141(10):1339–41.
41. Heffner JE, Klein JS, Hampson C. Diagnostic utility and clinical application of imaging for pleural space infections. Chest. 2010;137(2):467–79. https://doi.org/10.1378/chest.08-3002.
42. Yang PC, Luh KT, Chang DB, Wu HD, Yu CJ, Kuo SH. Value of sonography in determining the nature of pleural effusion: analysis of 320 cases. AJR Am J Roentgenol. 1992;159(1):29–33. https://doi.org/10.2214/ajr.159.1.1609716.
43. Tu CY, Hsu WH, Hsia TC, et al. Pleural effusions in febrile medical ICU patients: chest ultrasound study. Chest. 2004;126(4):1274–80. https://doi.org/10.1378/chest.126.4.1274.
44. Aquino SL, Webb WR, Gushiken BJ. Pleural exudates and transudates: diagnosis with contrast-enhanced CT. Radiology. 1994;192(3):803–8. https://doi.org/10.1148/radiology.192.3.8058951.
45. Müller NL. Imaging of the pleura. Radiology. 1993;186(2):297–309. https://doi.org/10.1148/radiology.186.2.8421723.
46. Stark DD, Federle MP, Goodman PC, Podrasky AE, Webb WR. Differentiating lung abscess and empyema: radiography and computed tomography. AJR Am J Roentgenol. 1983;141(1):163–7. https://doi.org/10.2214/ajr.141.1.163.
47. Colice GL, Curtis A, Deslauriers J, et al. Medical and surgical treatment of parapneumonic effusions: an evidence-based guideline. Chest. 2000;118(4):1158–71. https://doi.org/10.1378/chest.118.4.1158.
48. Ariyürek OM, Cil BE. Atypical presentation of pleural tuberculosis: CT findings. Br J Radiol. 2000;73(866):209–10. https://doi.org/10.1259/bjr.73.866.10884737.
49. Kim HJ, Lee HJ, Kwon SY, et al. The prevalence of pulmonary parenchymal tuberculosis in patients with tuberculous pleuritis. Chest. 2006;129(5):1253–8. https://doi.org/10.1378/chest.129.5.1253.
50. Lee J, Lee SY, Lim JK, et al. Radiologic and laboratory differences in patients with tuberculous and parapneumonic pleural effusions showing non-lymphocytic predominance and high adenosine deaminase levels. Infection. 2015;43(1):65–71. https://doi.org/10.1007/s15010-014-0697-y.
51. Kim JS, Shim SS, Kim Y, Ryu YJ, Lee JH. Chest CT findings of pleural tuberculosis: differential diagnosis of pleural tuberculosis and malignant pleural dissemination. Acta Radiol. 2014;55(9):1063–8. https://doi.org/10.1177/0284185113513894.

Foreign Bodies in the Thorax

14

14.1 Introduction

In the thorax, the airways and esophagus are the two most frequent locations of foreign bodies. Although radiopaque foreign bodies are easily detectable on plain radiographs, they can be overlooked since radiologists or clinicians may regard them as radiopaque materials present outside the body or medical devices. In addition, many foreign bodies (e.g., food boluses) are radiolucent. Thus, imaging diagnosis is often difficult. It is necessary that radiologists and clinicians be familiar with the imaging findings of commonly encountered foreign bodies, secondary signs such as post-obstructive changes, and associated complications.

14.2 Foreign Bodies in Airways

About 75% of cases of foreign body aspiration in the airways occur in children younger than 3 years of age [1, 2], and the most frequent cause is accidental swallowing [3]. Foreign body aspiration in adults usually has an iatrogenic or traumatic cause or occurs in patients who have underlying diseases, such as mental retardation, seizures, alcoholism, brain tumors, and Parkinson's disease, which impair the swallowing reflex [4–7]. In elderly patients, the clinical presentation may be obscure due to uncharacteristic symptoms and an unclear history of foreign body aspiration [8]. In the trauma setting, teeth, dentures, and other dental devices are commonly avulsed by a traumatic event and are then at risk for aspiration [9].

The most commonly aspirated foreign bodies are food and broken fragments of teeth. The clinical and radiologic manifestations depend on the size of the aspirated material, degree (partial or complete), level, and chronicity (acute or chronic) of obstruction [3]. The most common symptom is sudden onset choking and intractable cough, with or without vomiting. Other symptoms include cough, fever, breathlessness, and wheezing [6, 10].

Identification and removal of a foreign body are important to avoid complications such as obstructive pneumonitis, atelectasis, lung abscess, pneumomediastinum, and pneumothorax [10, 11]. Teeth are generally well-visualized on radiographs, but some fish or chicken bones, plastic, wood, glass, and thin metal objects cannot be seen on radiographs. The most reliable imaging finding is that of a foreign body in the lumen of the tracheobronchial tree on CT (Figs. 14.1 and 14.2).

T. J. Kim et al., *Emergency Chest Radiology*, https://doi.org/10.1007/978-981-33-4396-2_14

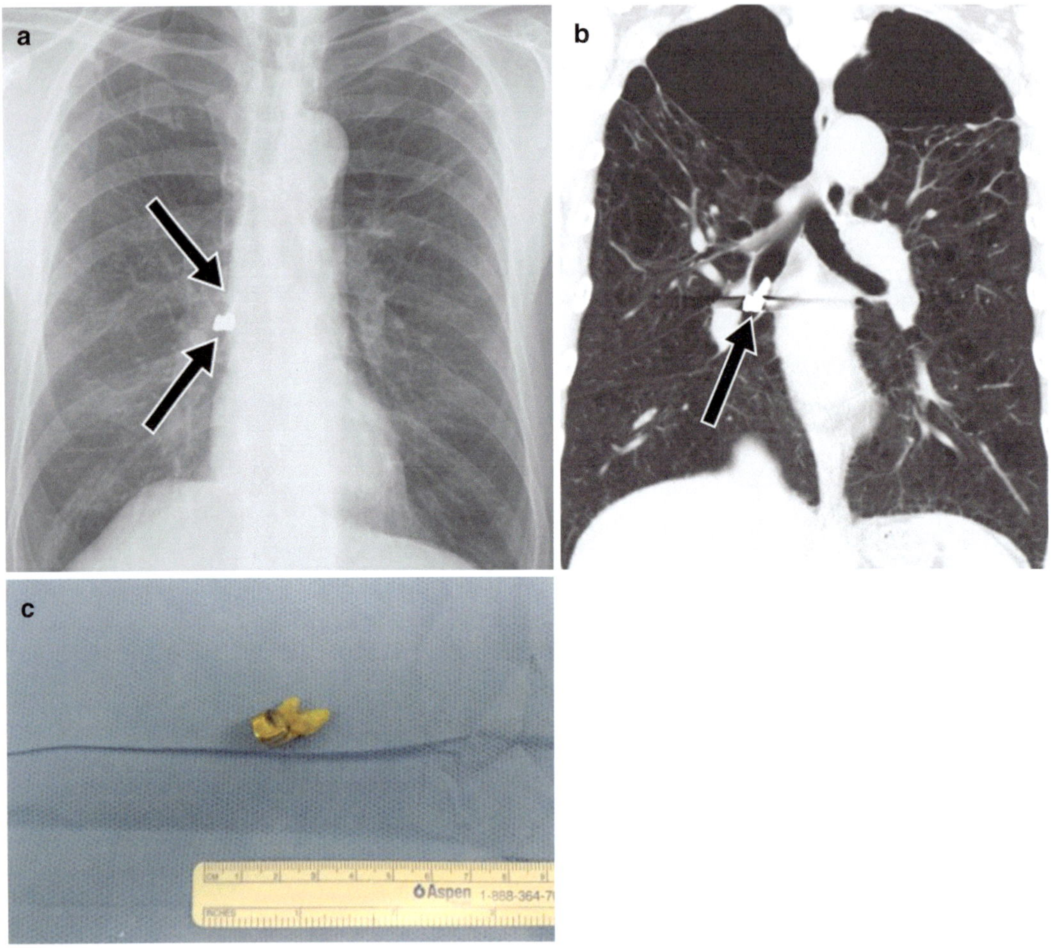

Fig. 14.1 A foreign body (tooth) aspirated into the airway of a 65-year-old man during a dental procedure. (**a**) Chest radiograph demonstrates a radiopaque foreign body (arrows). (**b**) Chest CT shows a radiopaque foreign body (arrow) in the right bronchus intermedius. (**c**) Ventilation bronchoscopic foreign body removal was done, and a tooth was removed

On CT, bones, stones, metal fragments, and denture and teeth fragments usually show high attenuation. Radiopaque foreign bodies should not be mistaken for calcified lymph nodes or bronchial mural calcifications [7]. Of special note, many aspirated foreign bodies such as food boluses are radiolucent [12], and the clinical symptoms are sometimes nonspecific. Thus, radiologists should pay attention to secondary signs such as post-obstructive changes, atelectasis, and pneumonia when making a diagnosis.

The potential secondary changes resulting from foreign body aspiration are as follows. When the aspirate lodges in the main bronchus, patients may present with atelectasis (complete obstruction), air trapping (partial check valve obstruction), or no abnormality (incomplete obstruction). Aspiration into the right main bronchus is more common than that into the left bronchial tree. Aspiration of a large foreign body to the lobar bronchi may cause lobar atelectasis (complete obstruction), air trapping (partial check valve obstruction) (Fig. 14.3), or post-obstructive pneumonia (Fig. 14.2). Aspiration of a small foreign body that obstructs the segmental or subsegmental bronchi may present as an endobronchial lesion, focal recurrent pneumonia, or focal atelectasis at a segmental or subsegmental level [3].

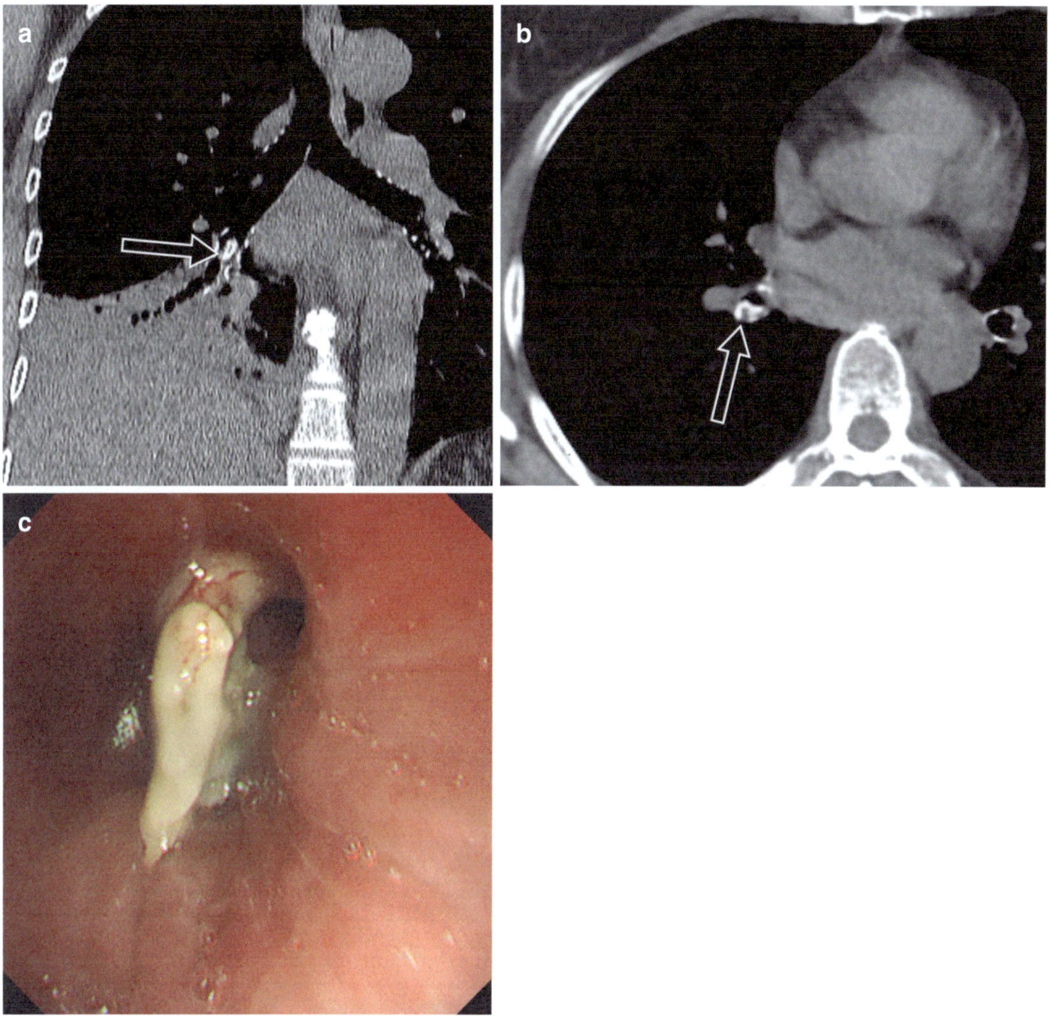

Fig. 14.2 A foreign body (fish bone) in a 68-year-old man who complained of persistent cough and pneumonia after aspiration of the fish bone. (**a**, **b**) Chest CT shows a radiopaque foreign body (arrow) in the right truncus basalis. There is distal obstructive pneumonia in the right lower lobe. (**c**) The foreign body (fish bone) was identified with bronchoscopy and bronchoscopic foreign body removal was performed

14.3 Foreign Bodies in the Esophagus

Esophageal foreign bodies are common medical emergencies [13]. Most ingested objects pass spontaneously without intervention [14, 15]. However, the esophagus is vulnerable to perforation and pressure necrosis from lodged foreign bodies owing to the thinness of the esophageal wall, the lack of supporting adventitia, and the relatively weak blood supply. Between 10% and 20% of ingested foreign bodies require endoscopic removal (Fig. 14.4), and surgery is needed in about 1% of cases (Fig. 14.5) [14, 16, 17]. Sharp or pointed foreign bodies, button batteries, and objects that cause obstruction require emergent removal.

When there is a history of foreign body ingestion, radiographic evaluation of the neck, chest, and/or abdomen is performed [14]. However, many ingested foreign bodies (35% or more, such as objects made of plastic, wood, etc.) are

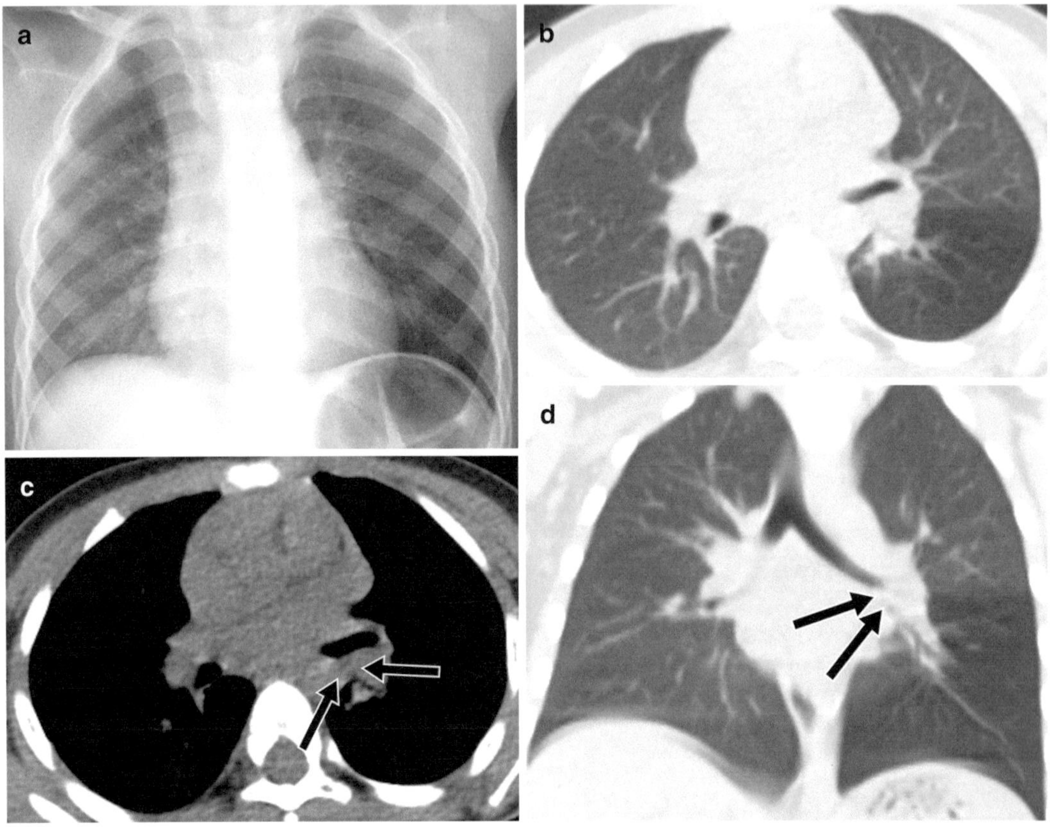

Fig. 14.3 A foreign body (nut) aspirated into the airway of a 21-month-old child. (**a**, **b**) Chest radiography and CT shows hyperlucency and air-trapping in the left lower lobe. There is no visible radiopaque foreign body. (**c**, **d**) An intra-luminal filling defect is present in the left lower lobar bronchus (arrows). The nut was identified with bronchoscopy and foreign body removal was performed

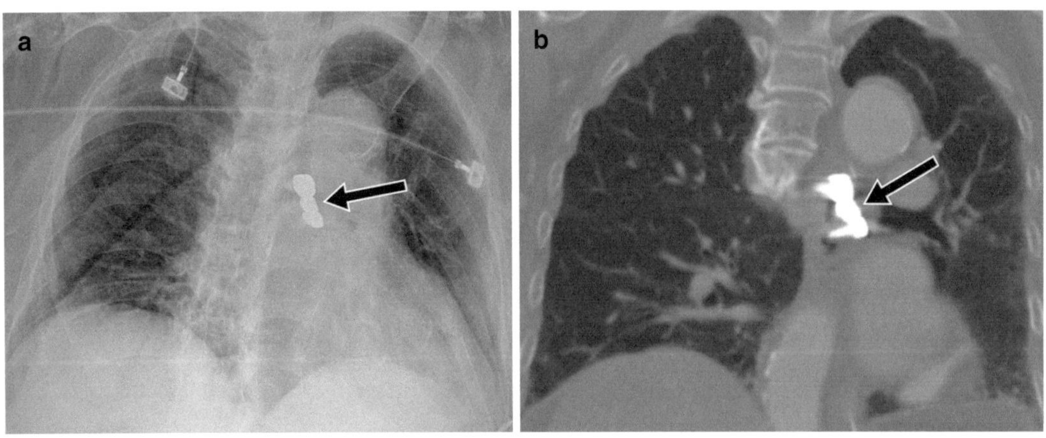

Fig. 14.4 Foreign bodies (teeth) ingested into the esophagus of an 82-year-old bed-ridden woman who complained of hematochezia. (**a**) Chest radiograph demonstrates a radiopaque foreign body (arrow). (**b**) Chest CT shows a radiopaque foreign body in the mid-thoracic esophagus (arrow). (**c**) Foreign bodies (teeth) with multiple accompanying ulcers in the esophagus were identified with esophagogastroduodenoscopy. Endoscopic removal was successful

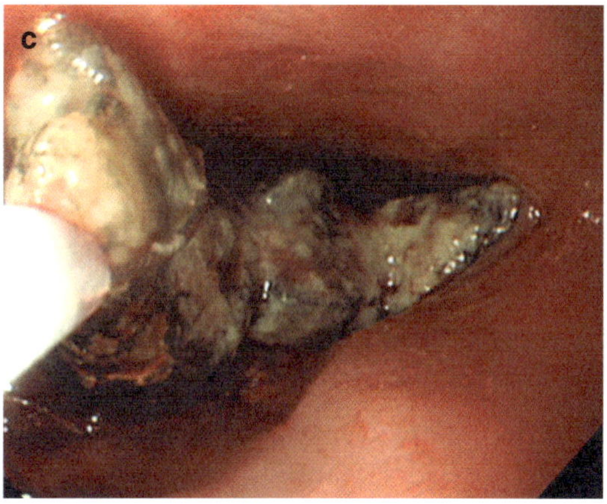

Fig. 14.4 (continued)

not radiopaque even though they can cause symptoms or complications [18]. Therefore, a negative radiographic examination does not guarantee the absence of an esophageal foreign body [19]. CT may be useful in select cases when more definitive diagnosis or localization is required before endoscopic intervention, or when perforation or another complication is suspected.

In children, coins are the most commonly ingested foreign bodies [20]. Because they lack sharp edges and are generally nontoxic, ingested coins that reach the stomach can be managed conservatively. On the other hand, ingested batteries require aggressive management. Disk batteries carry a high risk of corrosive injury to the

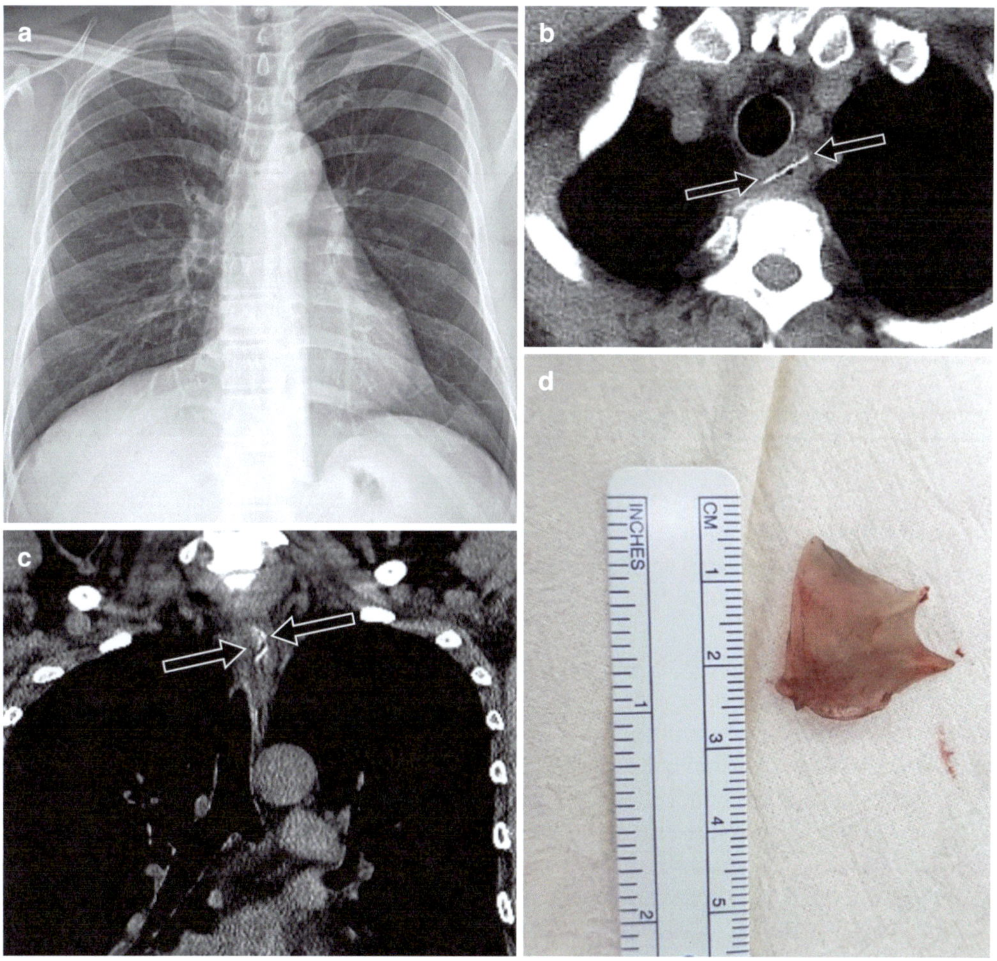

Fig. 14.5 A foreign body (fish bone) ingested into the esophagus which was surgically removed in a 59-year-old man. (**a**) Chest radiograph shows no abnormal findings. (**b**, **c**) Chest CT shows a sharp, linear radiopaque foreign body (arrows). (**d**) Video-assisted thoracoscopic surgery was done to remove the foreign body (fish bone), as endoscopic removal may lead to injuries of the pharynx and teeth

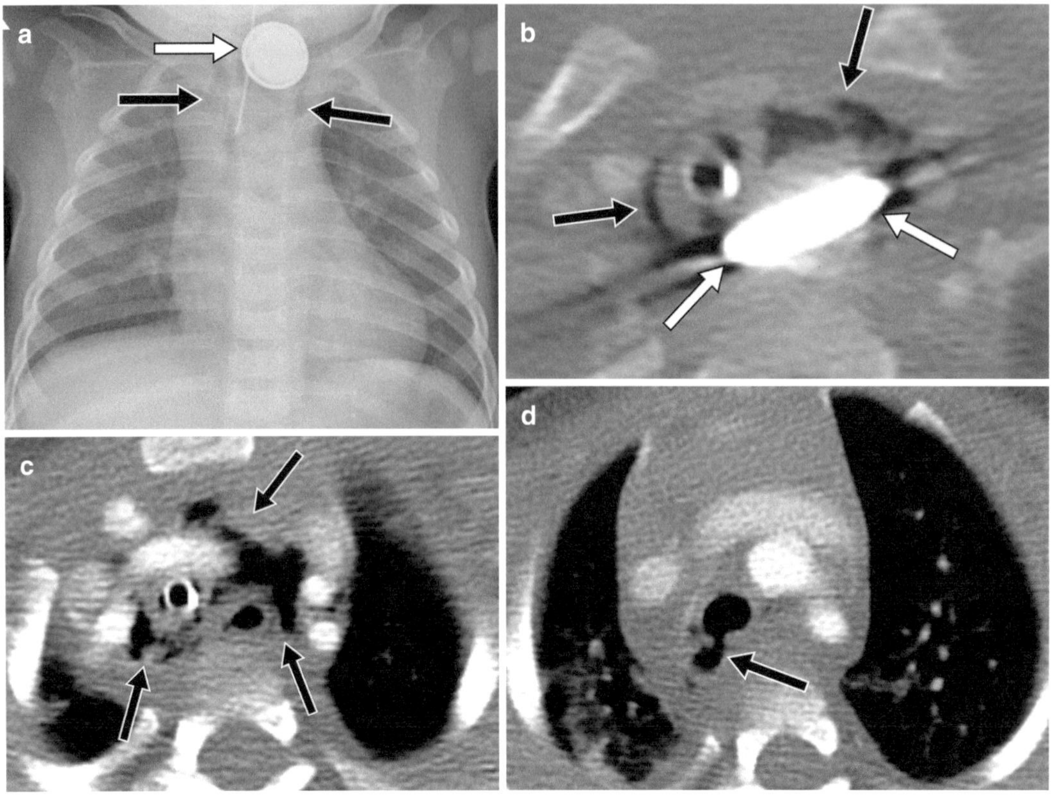

Fig. 14.6 A foreign body (disc battery) ingested into the esophagus which resulted in esophageal perforation in a 10-month-old baby. (**a**) Chest radiograph shows a round, radiopaque foreign body (white arrow) at the upper esophageal level. There are multiple air densities surrounding the foreign body (black arrows). (**b**, **c**) There is a foreign body in the upper esophagus (white arrows). Adjacent air densities suggest the presence of pneumomediastinum (black arrows) and esophageal perforation. (**d**) This patient also had a tracheoesophageal fistula. Note that there is a wall defect in the posterior wall of the trachea (arrow)

gastrointestinal tract, including esophageal burns, fistula formation, and perforation [21] (Fig. 14.6). In this case, esophageal damage can occur within the first 1–2 h; thus, urgent endoscopic removal is indicated [22].

In adults, animal bones, fish bones, and unchewed boluses of meat are major causes of esophageal foreign body impaction [13]. Most ingested foreign bodies pass through the gastrointestinal tract without problem [17, 23]. Less than 1% of ingested foreign bodies cause perforation of the gastrointestinal tract [19]. However, when the esophageal foreign body is a sharp fish bone, the risk of complications is greater because the bone could easily penetrate the esophageal wall, cause deep cervical and mediastinal infection, or damage the great vessels. Esophageal perforation typically appears within 24 h after foreign body ingestion, and it may form a fistula, including aortoesophageal, esophago-tracheal, esophago-bronchial, or esophagopericardial fistulas [24–26]. Thus, when a sharp or pointed esophageal foreign body is suspected, chest CT is the first-line imaging modality in the emergency setting after a negative physical examination [14, 27].

14.4 Other Foreign Bodies

Although the incidence is much rarer, foreign bodies can be found in other parts of the body such as the pleural space/lungs (Figs. 14.7 and 14.8), pulmonary artery (Fig. 14.9), heart (Fig. 14.10), or chest wall (Fig. 14.11). There

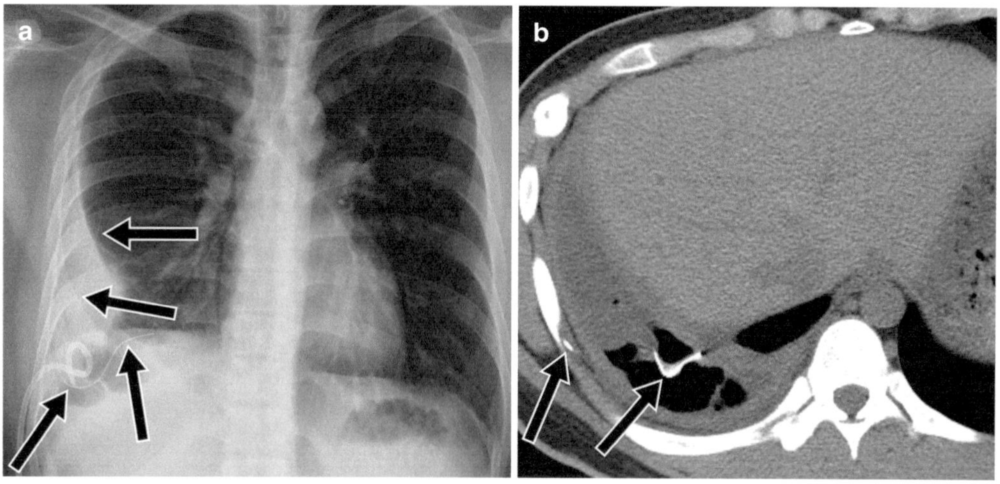

Fig. 14.7 Retained guidewire in the pleural space in a 20-year-old man. (**a**) Chest radiography shows right loculated pleural effusion. Right pigtail catheter insertion was performed for effusion drainage. There is a foreign body (a retained guidewire) in the pleural cavity (black arrows). (**b**) Chest CT shows a retained guidewire in the right pleural space (black arrows). Video-assisted thoracoscopic foreign body removal surgery and decortication was performed

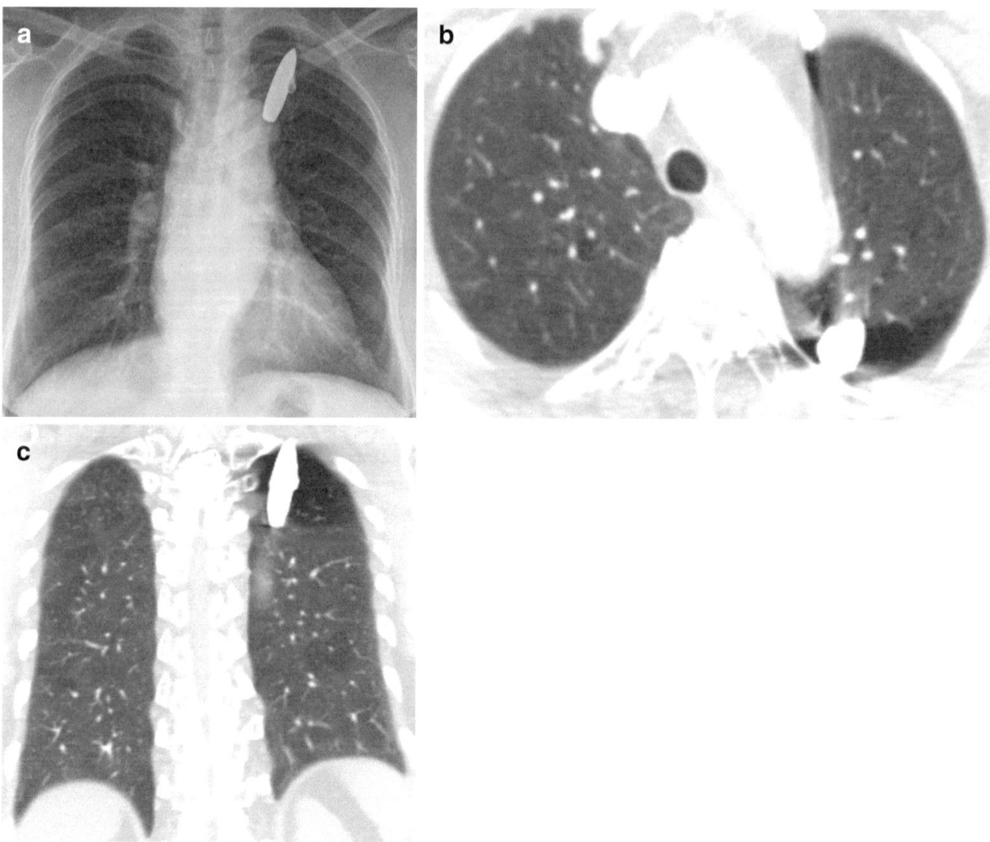

Fig. 14.8 A foreign body (bullet) in the left upper thorax in a 63-year-old woman who was shot during a war that occurred 57 years prior. (**a**) Chest radiograph shows a bullet in the left upper lung. (**b**, **c**) Chest CT shows a bullet in the left upper lung apex. Surgical removal was performed, as this patient had to undergo magnetic resonance imaging

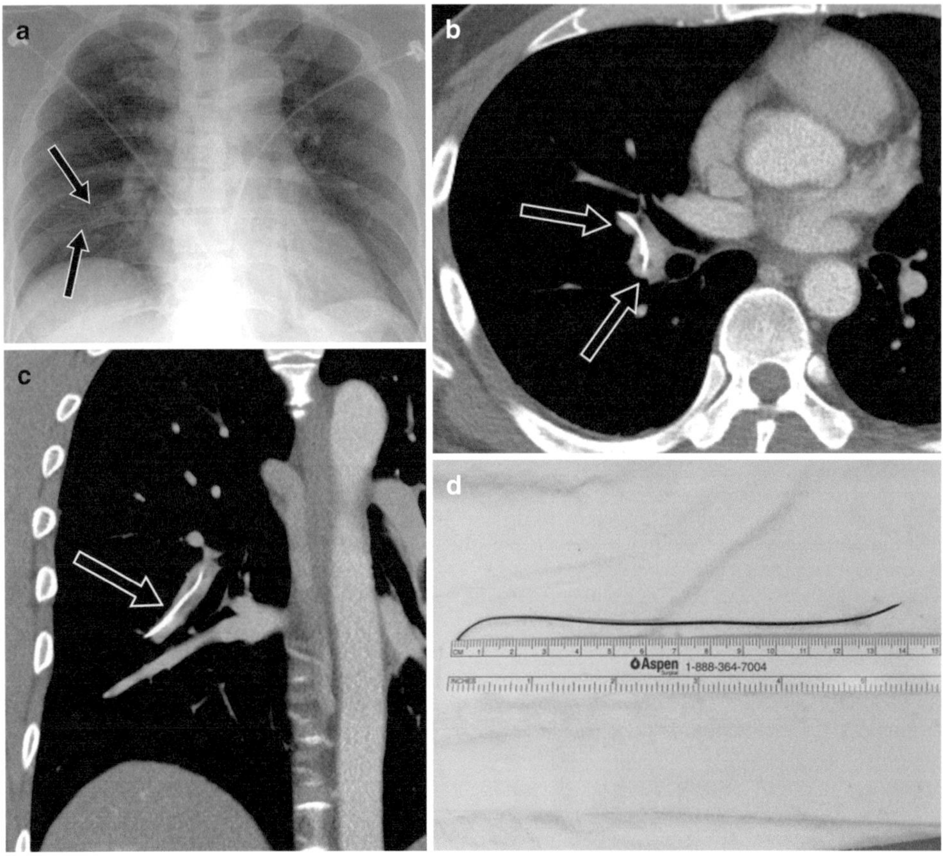

Fig. 14.9 Foreign body (guidewire) embolization in the pulmonary artery in a 48-year-old man. (**a**) Chest radiography shows a foreign body (guidewire) in the right lower lung (arrows). (**b**, **c**) Chest CT shows an embolized foreign body (guidewire) in the pulmonary artery (arrows). (**d**) Surgical removal was successful

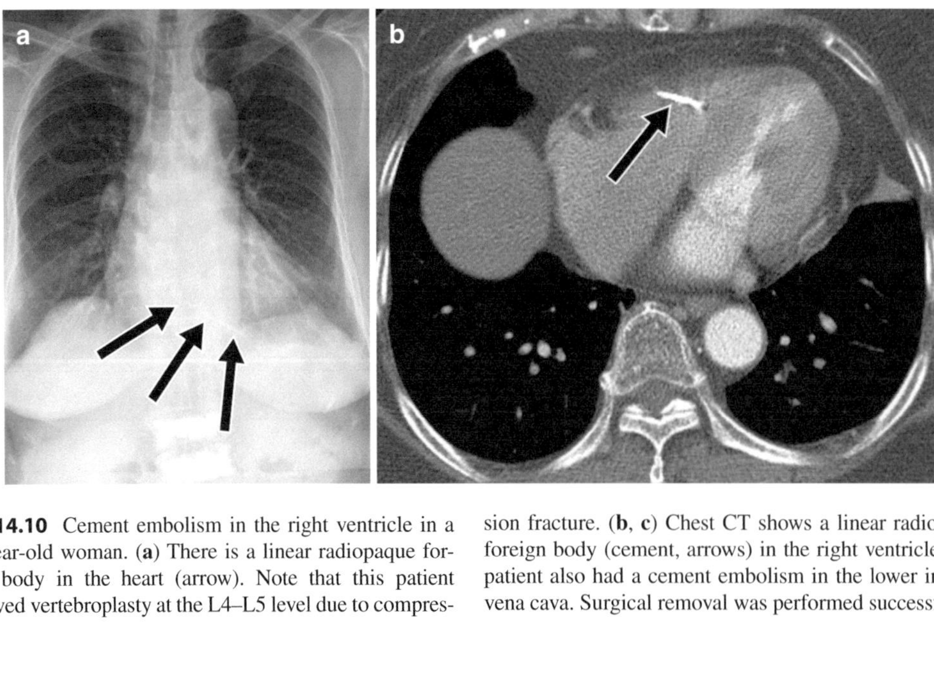

Fig. 14.10 Cement embolism in the right ventricle in a 66-year-old woman. (**a**) There is a linear radiopaque foreign body in the heart (arrow). Note that this patient received vertebroplasty at the L4–L5 level due to compression fracture. (**b**, **c**) Chest CT shows a linear radiopaque foreign body (cement, arrows) in the right ventricle. This patient also had a cement embolism in the lower inferior vena cava. Surgical removal was performed successfully

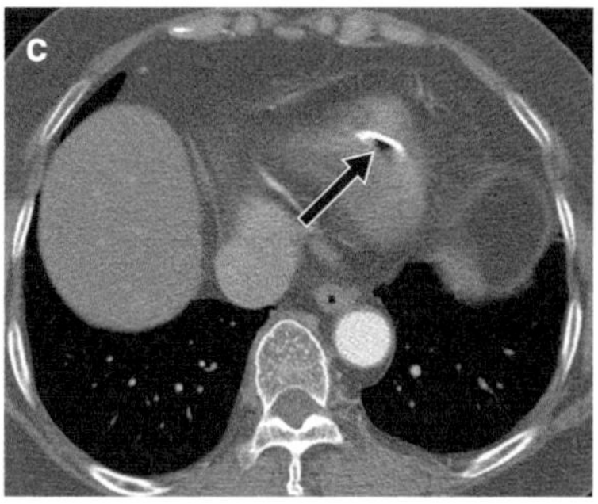

Fig. 14.10 (continued)

are three major causes of such foreign bodies: iatrogenic, traumatic-intentional, and accidental [28]. The incidence of iatrogenic foreign bodies has increased due to the frequent use of interventional techniques in modern medicine [29]. Small, blunt, peripherally located foreign bodies may not require removal. However, other foreign bodies may require removal, as leaving them in the chest may predispose the patient to infection, foreign body migration [28], thrombosis, or sepsis.

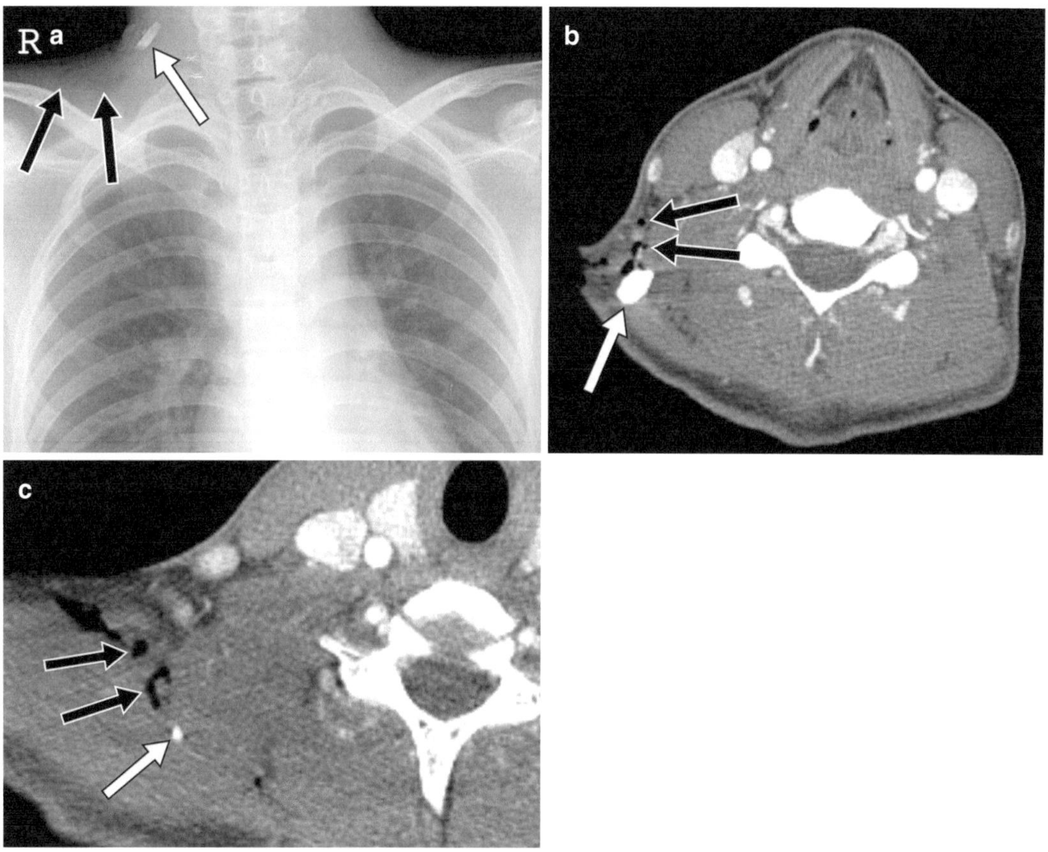

Fig. 14.11 A foreign body in the lower neck in a 14-year-old boy with multiple lacerations in the right lower neck and shoulder after a fall. A glass door was broken during the fall. (**a**–**c**) Chest radiograph and CT show radiopaque foreign bodies (pieces of glass, white arrows) and adjacent air densities (black arrows) in the right lower neck and shoulder

14.5 Summary

Foreign bodies are found in the airways, esophagus, and other body parts. Although teeth, dentures, or other metal objects are radiopaque, many aspirated or ingested foreign bodies are radiolucent (e.g., food boluses). To ensure accurate diagnosis and treatment of radiolucent foreign bodies, radiologists should pay attention to the secondary signs such as post-obstructive changes and potential complications. Leaving a foreign body behind in the chest may cause complications such as infection, migration, thrombosis, or sepsis.

Key Points

- On radiograph, radiopaque foreign bodies should not be mischaracterized as radiopaque materials outside the body or medical devices.
- When a radiolucent foreign body is present, it is important to identify secondary signs such as post-obstructive changes and potential complications such as esophageal perforation.
- Ingestion of disk batteries and sharp or pointed esophageal foreign bodies raises a particular concern of esophageal injury.

References

1. Hsu W, Sheen T, Lin C, Tan C, Yeh T, Lee S. Clinical experiences of removing foreign bodies in the airway and esophagus with a rigid endoscope: a series of 3217 cases from 1970 to 1996. Otolaryngol Head Neck Surg. 2000;122(3):450–4. https://doi.org/10.1067/mhn.2000.98321.
2. Baharloo F, Veyckemans F, Francis C, Biettlot MP, Rodenstein DO. Tracheobronchial foreign bodies: presentation and management in children and adults. Chest. 1999;115(5):1357–62. https://doi.org/10.1378/chest.115.5.1357.
3. Kim M, Lee KY, Lee KW, Bae KT. MDCT evaluation of foreign bodies and liquid aspiration pneumonia in adults. AJR Am J Roentgenol. 2008;190(4):907–15. https://doi.org/10.2214/ajr.07.2766.
4. Schloss MD, Pham-Dang H, Rosales JK. Foreign bodies in the tracheobronchial tree: a retrospective study of 217 cases. J Otolaryngol. 1983;12(4):212–6.
5. Weissberg D, Schwartz I. Foreign bodies in the tracheobronchial tree. Chest. 1987;91(5):730–3. https://doi.org/10.1378/chest.91.5.730.
6. Limper AH, Prakash UB. Tracheobronchial foreign bodies in adults. Ann Intern Med. 1990;112(8):604–9. https://doi.org/10.7326/0003-4819-112-8-604.
7. Zissin R, Shapiro-Feinberg M, Rozenman J, Apter S, Smorjik J, Hertz M. CT findings of the chest in adults with aspirated foreign bodies. Eur Radiol. 2001;11(4):606–11. https://doi.org/10.1007/s003300000619.
8. Lin L, Lv L, Wang Y, Zha X, Tang F, Liu X. The clinical features of foreign body aspiration into the lower airway in geriatric patients. Clin Interv Aging. 2014;9:1613–8. https://doi.org/10.2147/cia.s70924.
9. Wilcox SR, Arbelaez C, Nadel ES, Brown DF. Foreign body aspiration after high-velocity trauma. J Emerg Med. 2009;37(4):411–4. https://doi.org/10.1016/j.jemermed.2009.09.005.
10. Chen CH, Lai CL, Tsai TT, Lee YC, Perng RP. Foreign body aspiration into the lower airway in Chinese adults. Chest. 1997;112(1):129–33. https://doi.org/10.1378/chest.112.1.129.
11. Williams GS, Modi C, Singh T, Bhabra M. A case of black magic. South Med J. 2008;101(5):552–3. https://doi.org/10.1097/SMJ.0b013e31815d2420.
12. Pugmire BS, Lim R, Avery LL. Review of ingested and aspirated foreign bodies in children and their clinical significance for radiologists. Radiographics. 2015;35(5):1528–38. https://doi.org/10.1148/rg.2015140287.
13. Kim EY, Min YG, Bista AB, Park KJ, Kang DK, Sun JS. Usefulness of ultralow-dose (submillisievert) chest CT using iterative reconstruction for initial evaluation of sharp fish bone esophageal foreign body. AJR Am J Roentgenol. 2015;205(5):985–90. https://doi.org/10.2214/ajr.15.14353.
14. Mosca S, Manes G, Martino R, et al. Endoscopic management of foreign bodies in the upper gastrointestinal tract: report on a series of 414 adult patients. Endoscopy. 2001;33(8):692–6. https://doi.org/10.1055/s-2001-16212.
15. Li ZS, Sun ZX, Zou DW, Xu GM, Wu RP, Liao Z. Endoscopic management of foreign bodies in the upper-GI tract: experience with 1088 cases in China. Gastrointest Endosc. 2006;64(4):485–92. https://doi.org/10.1016/j.gie.2006.01.059.
16. Eisen GM, Baron TH, Dominitz JA, et al. Guideline for the management of ingested foreign bodies. Gastrointest Endosc. 2002;55(7):802–6. https://doi.org/10.1016/s0016-5107(02)70407-0.
17. Webb WA. Management of foreign bodies of the upper gastrointestinal tract: update. Gastrointest Endosc. 1995;41(1):39–51. https://doi.org/10.1016/s0016-5107(95)70274-1.
18. Arana A, Hauser B, Hachimi-Idrissi S, Vandenplas Y. Management of ingested foreign bodies in childhood and review of the literature. Eur J Pediatr. 2001;160(8):468–72. https://doi.org/10.1007/s004310100788.

19. Hunter TB, Taljanovic MS. Foreign bodies. Radiographics. 2003;23(3):731–57. https://doi.org/10.1148/rg.233025137.
20. Wyllie R. Foreign bodies in the gastrointestinal tract. Curr Opin Pediatr. 2006;18(5):563–4. https://doi.org/10.1097/01.mop.0000245359.13949.1c.
21. Sinclair K, Hill ID. Button and cylindrical battery ingestion. In: Burns MM, editor. UpToDate. Waltham, MA: UpToDate; 2020.
22. Votteler TP, Nash JC, Rutledge JC. The hazard of ingested alkaline disk batteries in children. JAMA. 1983;249(18):2504–6.
23. Singh B, Kantu M, Har-El G, Lucente FE. Complications associated with 327 foreign bodies of the pharynx, larynx, and esophagus. Ann Otol Rhinol Laryngol. 1997;106(4):301–4. https://doi.org/10.1177/000348949710600407.
24. Lam HC, Woo JK, van Hasselt CA. Esophageal perforation and neck abscess from ingested foreign bodies: treatment and outcomes. Ear Nose Throat J. 2003;82(10):786–94.
25. Cheng LC, Chiu CS. Foreign body-induced aorto-oesophageal fistula: a review of five cases and their management. Hong Kong Med J. 2006;12(3):219–21.
26. Nandi P, Ong GB. Foreign body in the oesophagus: review of 2394 cases. Br J Surg. 1978;65(1):5–9. https://doi.org/10.1002/bjs.1800650103.
27. Ma J, Kang DK, Bae JI, Park KJ, Sun JS. Value of MDCT in diagnosis and management of esophageal sharp or pointed foreign bodies according to level of esophagus. AJR Am J Roentgenol. 2013;201(5):W707–11. https://doi.org/10.2214/ajr.12.8517.
28. Weissberg D, Weissberg-Kasav D. Foreign bodies in pleura and chest wall. Ann Thorac Surg. 2008;86(3):958–61. https://doi.org/10.1016/j.athoracsur.2008.05.036.
29. Wolf F, Schernthaner RE, Dirisamer A, et al. Endovascular management of lost or misplaced intravascular objects: experiences of 12 years. Cardiovasc Intervent Radiol. 2008;31(3):563–8. https://doi.org/10.1007/s00270-007-9201-8.

15 Contrast Extravasation on Chest CT

15.1 Introduction

The most common cause of hemoptysis is systemic hypervascularization of the lungs by bronchial and non-bronchial systemic arteries in contact with the pleura [1, 2]. The actual hemorrhage usually occurs from fragile thin-walled anastomoses between distant bronchial arterial branches and pulmonary arteries that are under high systemic arterial pressure. This type of bleeding is too small to be directly visualized [3] and usually does not manifest as contrast media extravasation on CT.

Contrast extravasation is a relatively uncommon imaging finding on chest CT. Although the incidence is rare, detection of contrast extravasation on chest CT is essential. Localizing the culprit lesion from which bleeding occurs provides clinically useful information that can guide angiographic or surgical intervention [4]. Overlooking the signs of contrast extravasation may result in persistent bleeding and even death. Thus, radiologists must be familiar with the clinical manifestations and imaging findings of contrast extravasation.

15.2 Contrast Extravasation on Chest CT

Contrast extravasation can be divided into two categories: uncontained or contained (pseudoaneurysm) [4, 5]. If the size increases and the affected areas remain hyper-attenuating on delayed-phase CT, extravasation is uncontained and represents active hemorrhage [5]. If the areas are well-circumscribed and the size of the extravasation is stable on delayed-phase CT, contained contrast extravasation (pseudoaneurysm) is present. Unlike true aneurysm, pseudoaneurysm does not involve all layers of the arterial wall; therefore, it is at higher risk of rupture. Although uncontained extravasation requires more emergent intervention or surgery [5] than contained extravasation, both require further work-up, interventional procedures, or surgeries [6]. Some cases of venous bleeding or bleeding from a pulmonary artery may resolve spontaneously as the pulmonary arteries are under low arterial pressure; however, many such cases require embolization or surgery.

The origin of contrast extravasation may be either an artery or a vein. Differentiation may be accomplished using multiphasic imaging including arterial and portal venous phases [7]. In patients with arterial bleeding, extravasation foci can be identified on arterial phase images; these areas are often persistent and enlarged on portal venous phase images. In patients with isolated venous bleeding, no abnormality is identified on arterial phase images but extravasation foci are identified on the subsequent portal venous phase images [7]. However, multiphase chest CT angiography is not routinely performed, and it is often difficult to differentiate between arterial and venous bleeding.

Contrast extravasation on chest CT can be observed in various settings: secondary to pulmonary tuberculosis (Rasmussen aneurysm), following trauma, as a complication of surgery, as a

T. J. Kim et al., *Emergency Chest Radiology*, https://doi.org/10.1007/978-981-33-4396-2_15

complication of interventional procedures such as thoracentesis, as a result of a tumor or pneumonia, etc. Pulmonary artery pseudoaneurysms secondary to pulmonary tuberculosis are known as Rasmussen aneurysms and usually involve the upper lobes in patients with chronic pulmonary tuberculosis or reactivated tuberculosis [8]. Granulation tissue destroys the elastic fibers of the artery and results in aneurysm formation. Tumors (pulmonary metastasis and primary lung cancer) and pneumonia (bacterial and fungal) can also cause erosion of the pulmonary arteries and result in pseudoaneurysm formation [8]. In this chapter, we present several representative cases involving contrast extravasation on chest CT (Figs. 15.1, 15.2, 15.3, 15.4, 15.5, 15.6, 15.7, 15.8, 15.9, and 15.10).

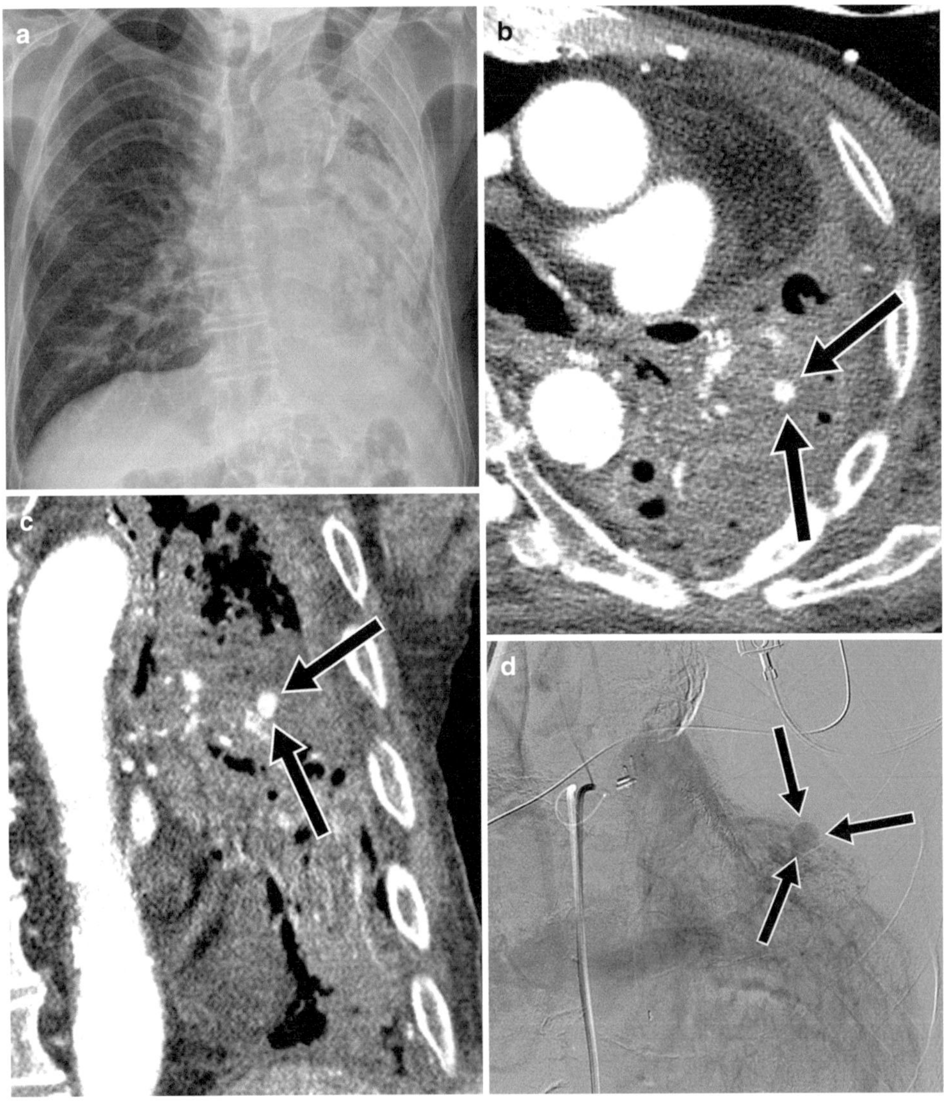

Fig. 15.1 Rasmussen aneurysm in an 85-year-old man. (**a**) Chest radiograph demonstrates destruction of the left lung by previous tuberculosis. (**b**, **c**) Chest CT was performed because this patient complained of hemoptysis. There is a pseudoaneurysm (arrows) within the destroyed left lung. (**d**) On angiography, a pulmonary artery aneurysm (arrows) is noted adjacent to the left bronchial–pulmonary shunt. Embolization was performed for this aneurysm

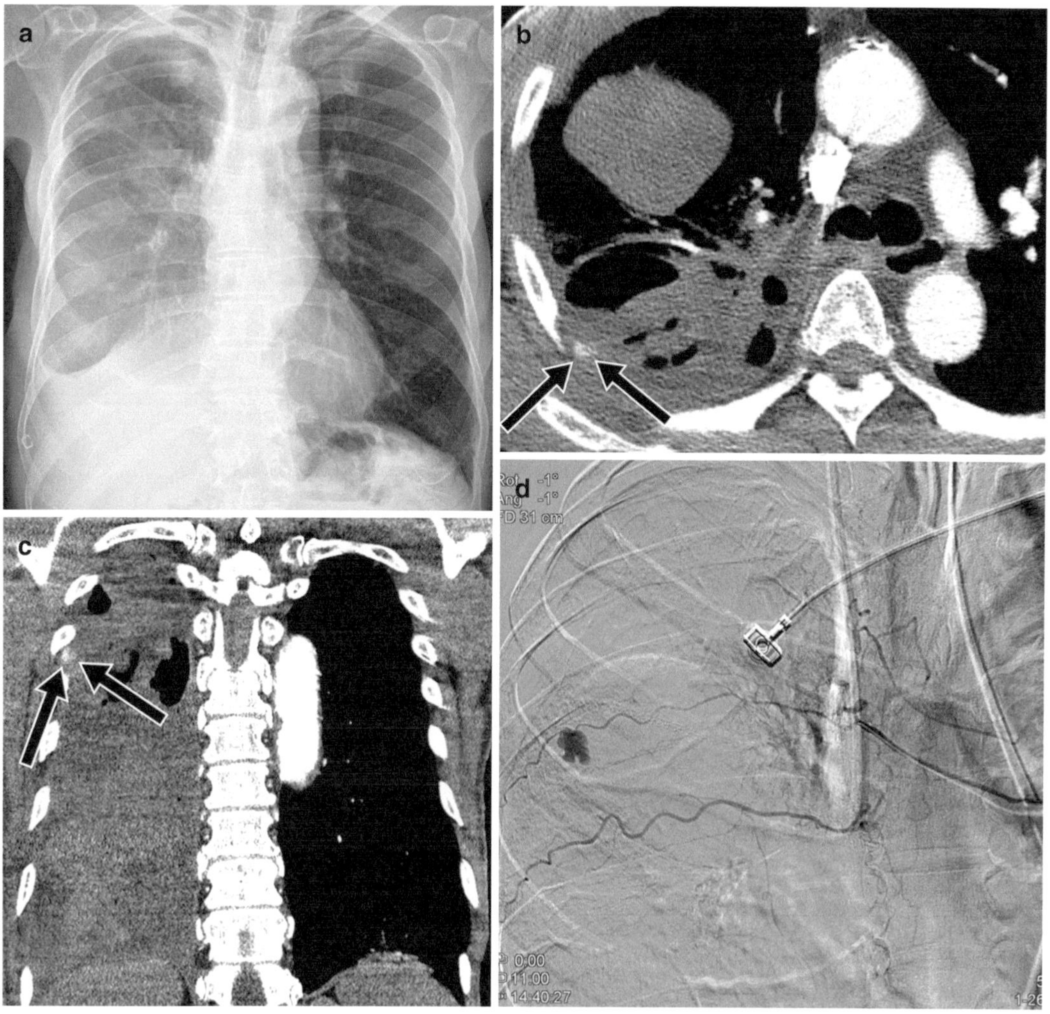

Fig. 15.2 Active bleeding from the intercostal artery after lobectomy in a 79-year-old man. (**a**) Chest radiograph obtained 1 month after surgery shows a large amount of right pleural effusion or hemothorax. (**b**, **c**) Chest CT demonstrates a large amount of right hemothorax with air bubbles in the right pleural space. There is contrast extravasation from the right fifth intercostal artery (arrows). (**d**) On angiography, contrast extravasation was seen at the fifth intercostal artery. Embolization was performed

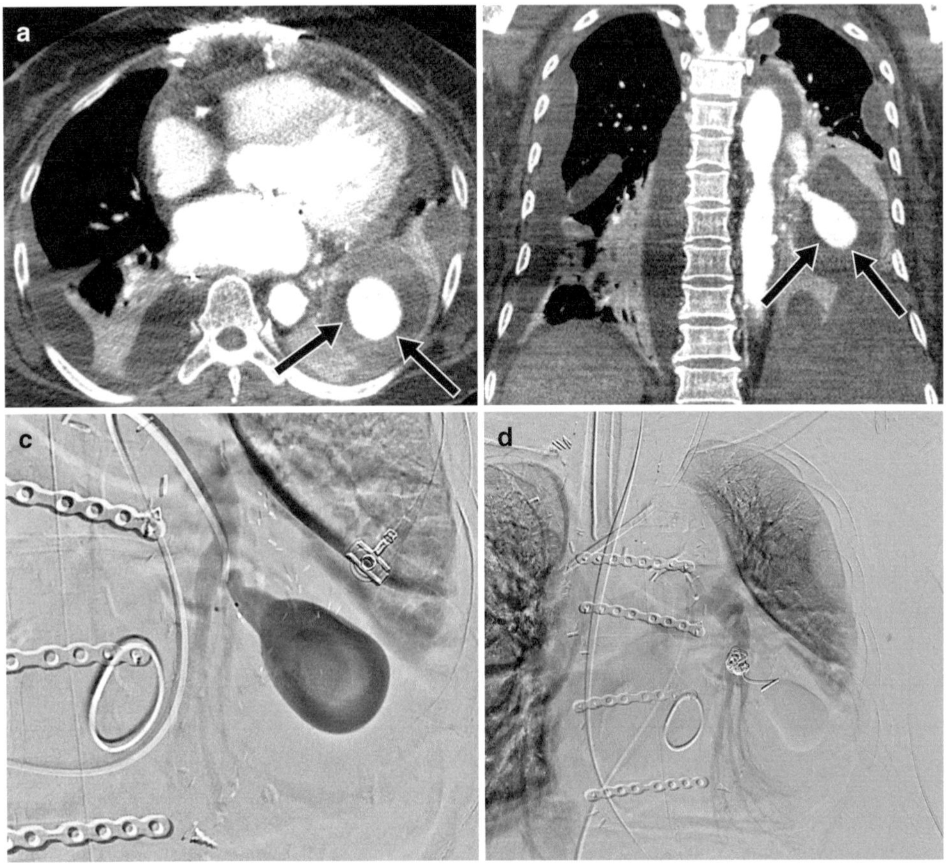

Fig. 15.3 A huge pulmonary artery pseudoaneurysm that occurred after coronary artery bypass grafting surgery and postoperative mediastinitis in a 76-year-old woman. (**a**, **b**) Chest CT shows a 3.0-cm pseudoaneurysm (arrows) in the left lower segmental pulmonary artery with an arterio–pleural fistula. There is a large left hemothorax. (**c**) Angiography shows a huge pseudoaneurysm in the territory of the left inferior pulmonary artery. (**d**) After embolization, contrast extravasation disappeared

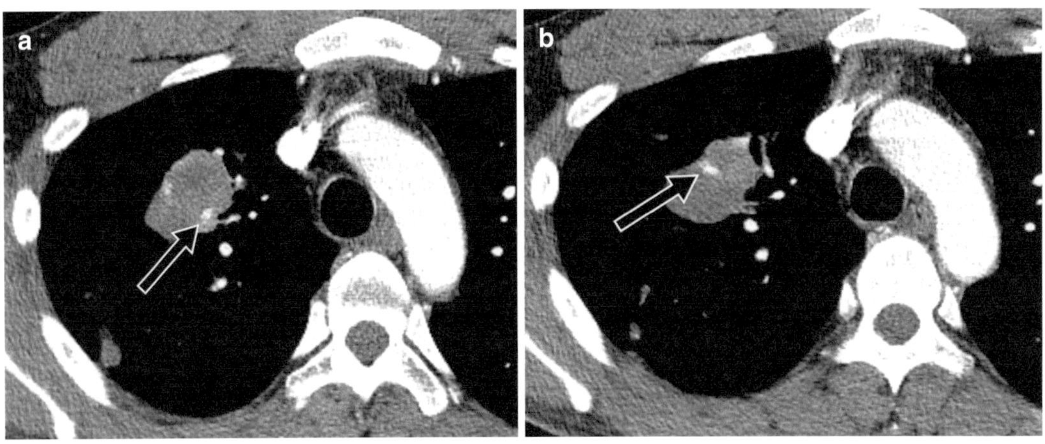

Fig. 15.4 Pseudoaneurysm related to pulmonary metastasis from choriocarcinoma in a 34-year-old man. (**a–c**) Chest CT shows hypervascularity at the lung metastasis in the right upper lobe, with suspicious pseudoaneurysm (arrow). (**d**) On angiography, the right bronchial arteries were connected to the pseudoaneurysm (arrows). Embolization was performed

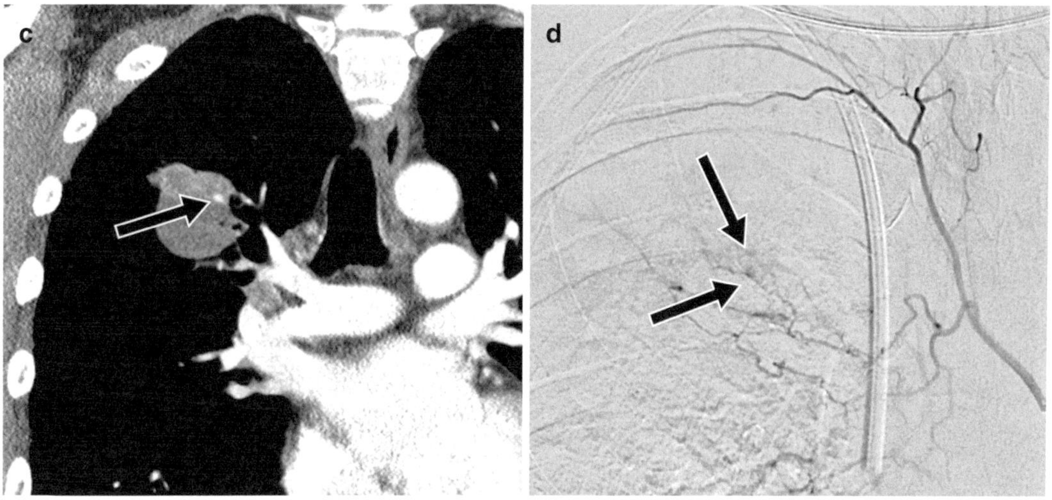

Fig. 15.4 (continued)

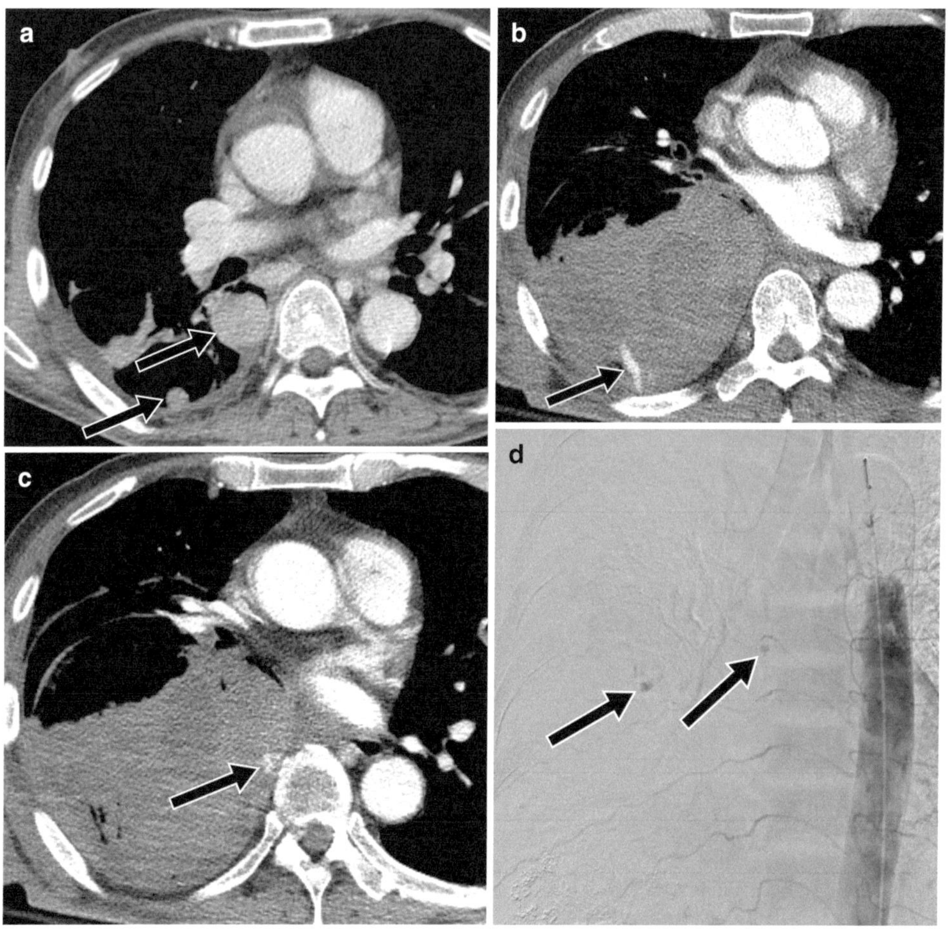

Fig. 15.5 Intercostal arterial bleeding associated with lung metastases from hepatocellular carcinoma in a 61-year-old man. (**a**) Chest CT shows metastases in the right lower lobe (arrows). (**b**, **c**) Chest CT performed 1 month later shows a large right hemothorax and contrast extravasation foci (arrow). (**d**) On angiography, multiple active bleeding foci (arrows) were noted from the right seventh to ninth intercostal arteries. Embolization was performed

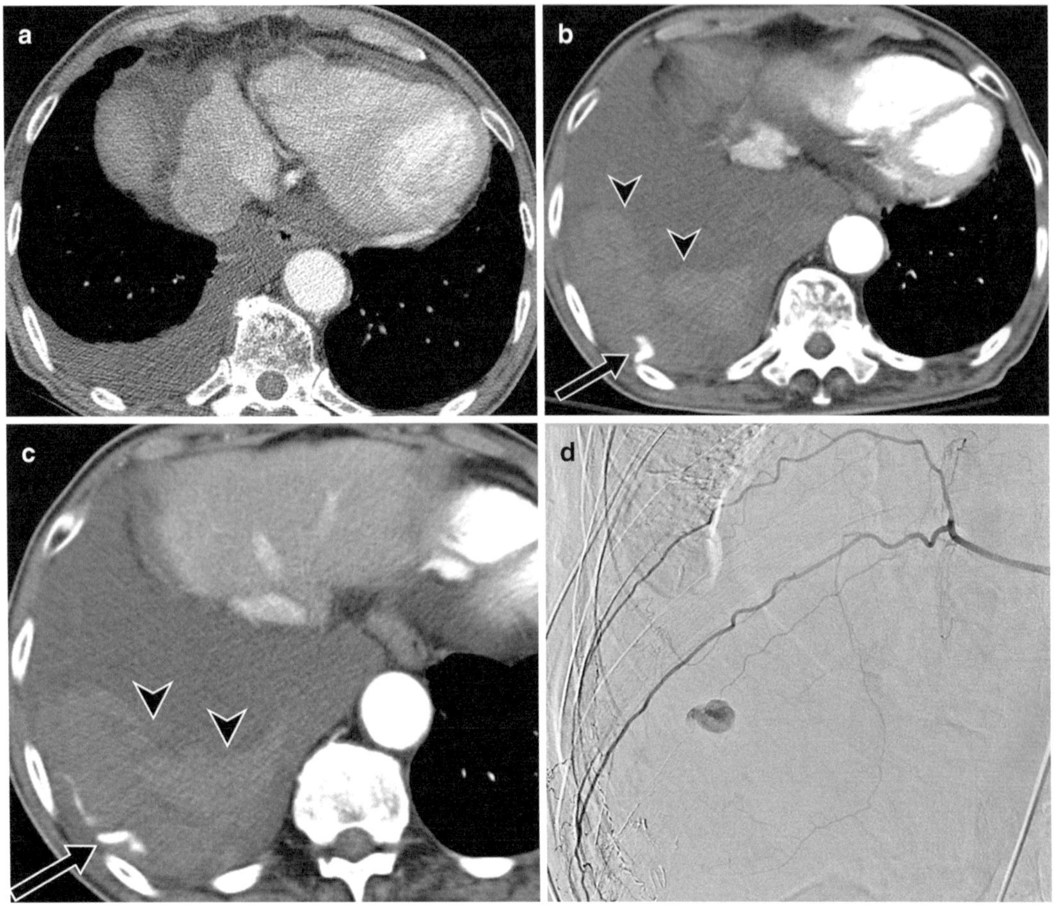

Fig. 15.6 Intercostal artery laceration after thoracentesis in a 78-year-old man. (**a**) Chest CT shows right pleural effusion. (**b**, **c**) Chest CT performed after thoracentesis shows contrast extravasation from the right tenth intercostal artery (arrow). There is a large hematoma in the right hemothorax (arrowheads), leading to mediastinal shifting. (**d**) Angiography shows contrast extravasation from the right tenth intercostal artery. Embolization was performed

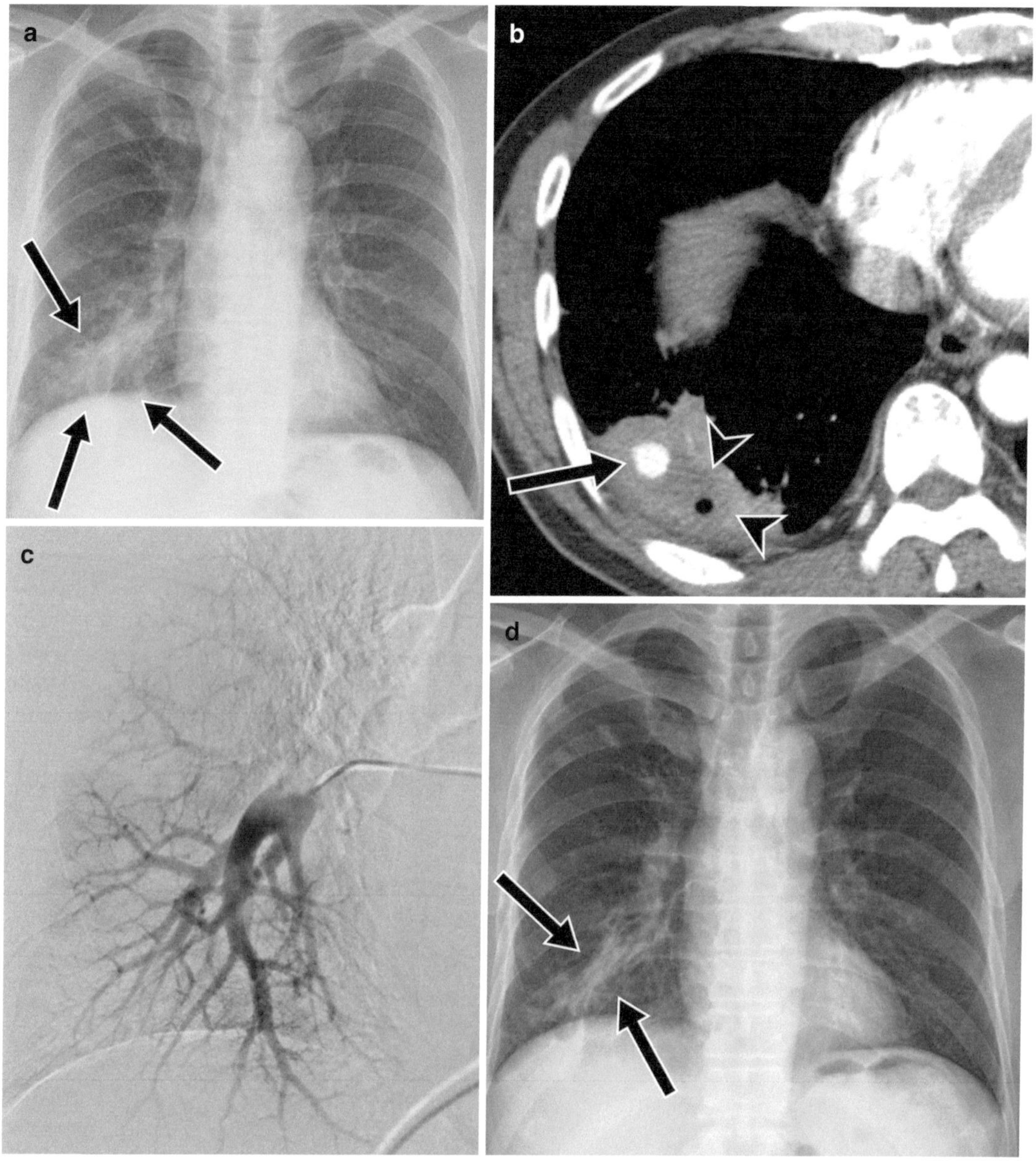

Fig. 15.7 Pulmonary artery pseudoaneurysm associated with a lung abscess in a 65-year-old man. (**a**) Chest radiograph shows patchy increased opacity in the right lower lung (arrows). (**b**) Chest CT shows consolidation in the right lower lobe with a lung abscess (arrowheads). There is a pseudoaneurysm (arrow) from the branch pulmonary artery in the right lower lobe. (**c**) On pulmonary artery angiography, there was no contrast extravasation. The pulmonary artery pseudoaneurysm spontaneously occluded. (**d**) Follow-up chest radiography performed 2 weeks later shows a decrease of right lower lobe consolidation (arrows)

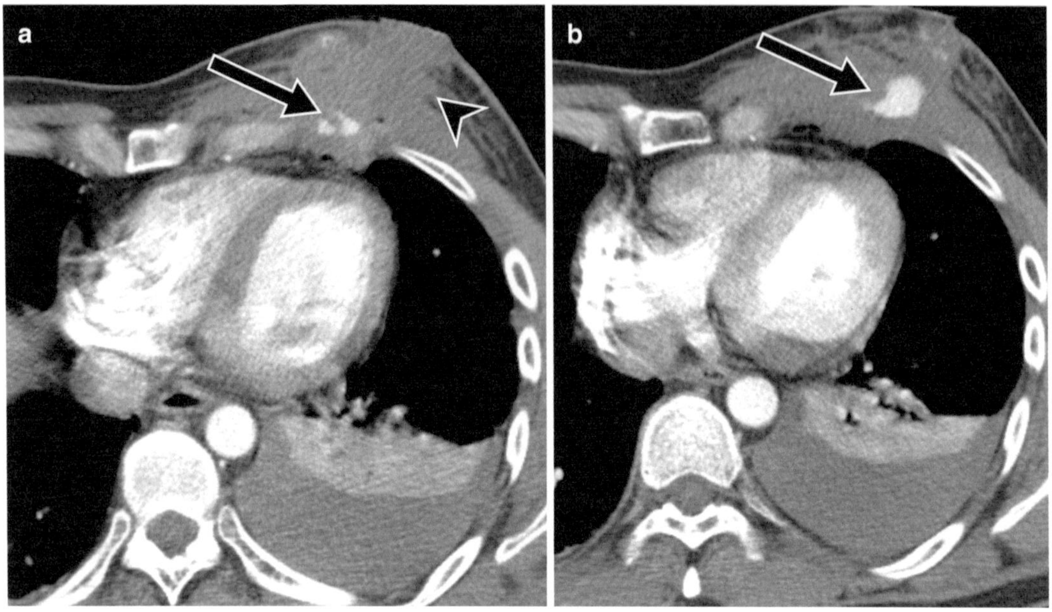

Fig. 15.8 Contrast extravasation at the chest wall due to a stab wound in a 34-year-old woman. (**a**, **b**) Chest CT shows a hematoma (arrowhead) in the left chest wall with multiple contrast extravasation foci (arrow). Left hemothorax is also noted

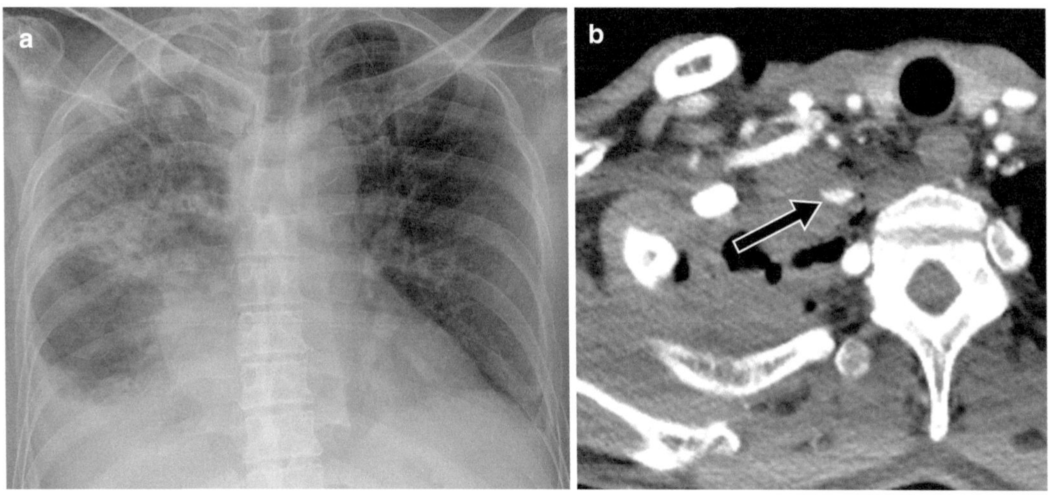

Fig. 15.9 Trauma-related active bleeding in a 58-year-old man. (**a**) Chest radiograph shows right pleural effusion or hemothorax. Patchy consolidations are also noted in the right lung. (**b**, **c**) Chest CT shows right hemothorax. There is contrast extravasation at the right lung apex (arrows). (**d**) Angiography shows contrast extravasation (arrows) from the right thyrocervical branch. Embolization was performed

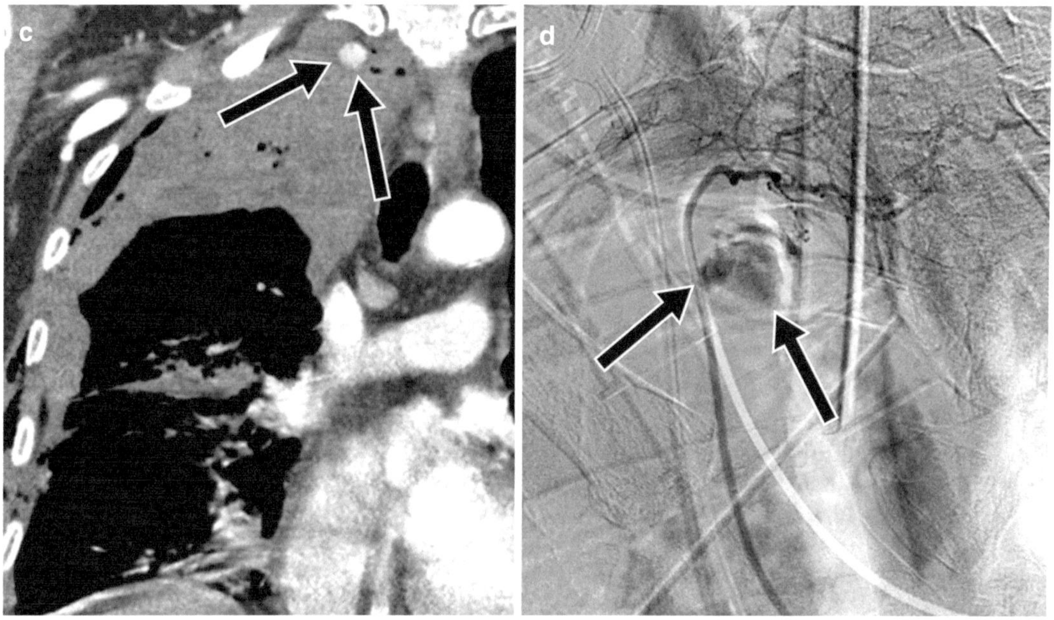

Fig. 15.9 (continued)

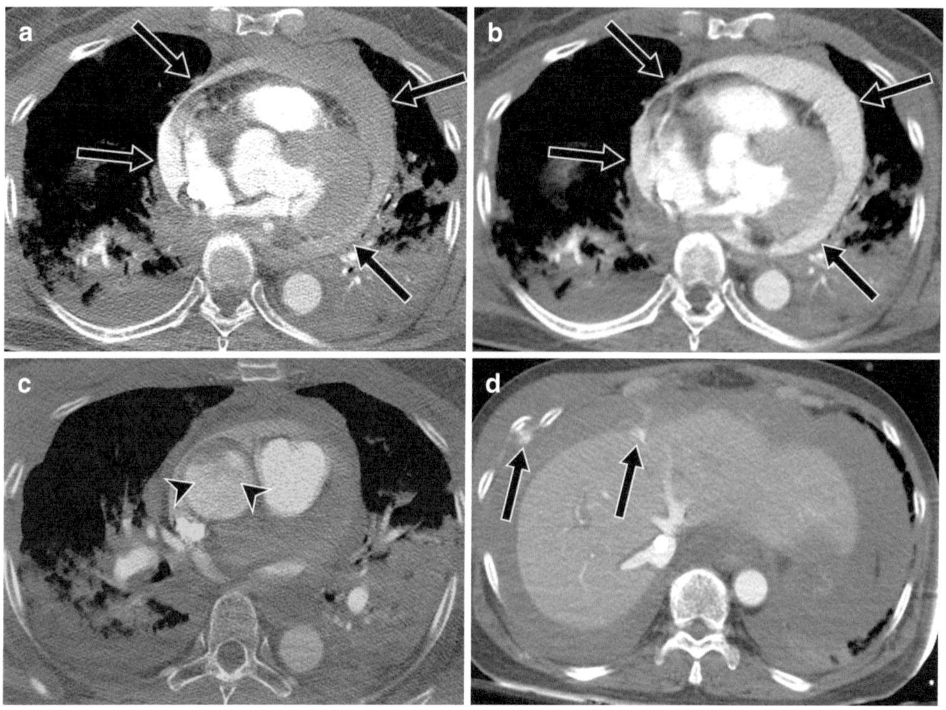

Fig. 15.10 Contrast extravasation into the pericardial sac in a 66-year-old woman with a trauma history who received thrombolysis for a pulmonary embolism. (**a**, **b**) Chest CT shows contrast extravasation (arrows) into the pericardial space, suggesting hemopericardium. There may be a rupture in a cardiac chamber or in the aorta. (**c**) There is an intimal flap (arrowheads) in the ascending aorta, suggesting traumatic aortic dissection. (**d**) There is also contrast extravasation from an intercostal artery and the liver surface (arrows)

15.3 Summary

Although the incidence is rare, contrast extravasation on chest CT is observed in various clinical settings. Detection of contrast extravasation on chest CT is essential as it can provide clinically useful information that can guide angiographic or surgical intervention.

Key Points

- Overlooking the signs of contrast extravasation may result in persistent bleeding and even death.
- Contrast extravasation is observed on chest CT in many clinical scenarios, such as secondary to pulmonary tuberculosis (Rasmussen aneurysm), trauma, surgery, interventional procedures, tumor, and pneumonia.

References

1. Yoon W, Kim JK, Kim YH, Chung TW, Kang HK. Bronchial and nonbronchial systemic artery embolization for life-threatening hemoptysis: a comprehensive review. Radiographics. 2002;22(6):1395–409. https://doi.org/10.1148/rg.226015180.
2. Khalil A, Fartoukh M, Tassart M, Parrot A, Marsault C, Carette MF. Role of MDCT in identification of the bleeding site and the vessels causing hemoptysis. AJR Am J Roentgenol. 2007;188(2):W117–25. https://doi.org/10.2214/ajr.05.1578.
3. Bruzzi JF, Rémy-Jardin M, Delhaye D, Teisseire A, Khalil C, Rémy J. Multi-detector row CT of hemoptysis. Radiographics. 2006;26(1):3–22. https://doi.org/10.1148/rg.261045726.
4. Yao DC, Jeffrey RB Jr, Mirvis SE, et al. Using contrast-enhanced helical CT to visualize arterial extravasation after blunt abdominal trauma: incidence and organ distribution. AJR Am J Roentgenol. 2002;178(1):17–20. https://doi.org/10.2214/ajr.178.1.1780017.
5. Anderson SW, Varghese JC, Lucey BC, Burke PA, Hirsch EF, Soto JA. Blunt splenic trauma: delayed-phase CT for differentiation of active hemorrhage from contained vascular injury in patients. Radiology. 2007;243(1):88–95. https://doi.org/10.1148/radiol.2431060376.
6. Catalano O, Cusati B, Nunziata A, Siani A. Active abdominal bleeding: contrast-enhanced sonography. Abdom Imaging. 2006;31(1):9–16. https://doi.org/10.1007/s00261-005-0369-6.
7. Anderson SW, Lucey BC, Rhea JT, Soto JA. 64 MDCT in multiple trauma patients: imaging manifestations and clinical implications of active extravasation. Emerg Radiol. 2007;14(3):151–9. https://doi.org/10.1007/s10140-007-0600-6.
8. Nguyen ET, Silva CI, Seely JM, Chong S, Lee KS, Müller NL. Pulmonary artery aneurysms and pseudoaneurysms in adults: findings at CT and radiography. AJR Am J Roentgenol. 2007;188(2):W126–34. https://doi.org/10.2214/ajr.05.1652.

MIX
Papier aus verantwortungsvollen Quellen
Paper from responsible sources
FSC® C105338

If you have any concerns about our products,
you can contact us on
ProductSafety@springernature.com

In case Publisher is established outside the EU,
the EU authorized representative is:
Springer Nature Customer Service Center GmbH
Europaplatz 3, 69115 Heidelberg, Germany

Printed by Libri Plureos GmbH
in Hamburg, Germany